CW01367214

W. Hach V. Hach-Wunderle

Phlebography and Sonography of the Veins

Springer
Berlin
Heidelberg
New York
Barcelona
Budapest
Hong Kong
London
Milan
Paris
Santa Clara
Singapore
Tokyo

W. Hach V. Hach-Wunderle

Phlebography and Sonography of the Veins

With 394 Figures, Some in Color

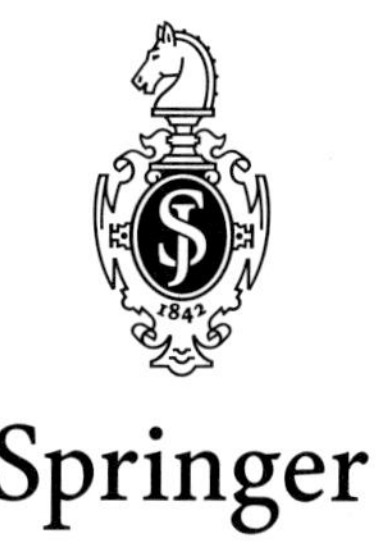

Springer

Professor Dr. med. Wolfgang Hach
Facharzt für Chirurgie und Innere Medizin (Röntgendiagnostik)
Wissenschaftliches Institut für Angiologie
Zeil 51, 60313 Frankfurt

Priv.-Doz. Dr. med. Viola Hach-Wunderle
Abteilung für Innere Medizin, William Harvey-Klinik
Am Kaiserberg 6, 61231 Bad Nauheim

Title of the German Edition:
Hach/Hach-Wunderle, Phlebographie der Bein- und Beckenvenen
4., vollständig überarbeitete Auflage
© 1996 Schnetztor-Verlag GmbH Konstanz

ISBN 3-540-53772-4 Springer-Verlag Berlin Heidelberg New York

Library of Congress Cataloging-in-Publication Data
Hach, Wolfgang. [Phlebographie der Bein- und Beckenvenen. English] Phlebography and sonography of the veins/W. Hach, V. Hach-Wunderle. p.cm. Includes bibliographical references and index.
ISBN 3-540-53772-4 [alk. paper]
1. Veins-Radiography. 2. Veins-Ultrasonic imaging. I. Hach-Wunderle, V. (Viola) II. Title.
[DNLM: 1. Thrombophlebitis-radiography. 2. Phlebography. 3. Ultrasonography.
WG 610 H117p 1996a] RC695.H2713 1997 616.1'40754-dc20 DNLM/DLC 96-13128

English Translation: Terry C. Telger, 6112 Waco Way, Fort Worth, TX 76133, USA
Cover design: Erich Kirchner, Heidelberg
Data version, printing and binding: G. Appl, Wemding

SPIN: 1001 9459 21/3135 – 5 4 3 2 1 0 – Printed on acid-free paper

Dedicated
to our wife and mother Helga
to Alois and Marius

Preface

Since the first German edition of this book was published in 1967 to the publication of the fourth this year, our knowledge of venous disease has greatly increased. During this time the role of phlebography as a diagnostic method has changed. In the past it was considered the "gold standard" for scientific research and differential diagnosis. Today, phlebography in combination with color-coded duplex sonography can provide diagnostic information with a high sensitivity and specificity. However, the physical features of these two methods are so different that they will never be congruous or replace each other. Certain problems are still solved better by one or the other. Therefore, we coined the term "golden partnership." Together, phlebography and duplex sonography provide optimal and reliable results in the diagnostic imaging of venous disease. One requirement is, however, that the phlebogram meets the highest demands in technical quality and interpretation.

X-ray study of the veins has provided us with a good deal of new information, which first was substantiated scientifically and published in the German language. These results have been translated into English for the first time, and we would like to take this opportunity to thank T. Telger for his excellent translation.

The new edition of this book required extensive reworking and additions to the existing chapters. Outdated methods were left out and new ones included. Comparisons with sonography, which are so important from a practical point of view, and the physical methods of measurement have been extensively presented. All the figures have been redone and a number of X-rays replaced by digital images. For this we are thank Dr. H. Meents, Bad Nauheim, Germany.

The English edition of this book produced by Springer-Verlag is of the usual high quality, we greatly appreciate Springer's willingness to take all our special wishes into consideration. We are especially grateful to I. Haas and Dr. U. Heilmann for their excellent cooperation. The excellent graphics were produced by Christiane von Solodkoff, Neckargemünd. The secretarial work of P. Wieboris and G. Kristel, Bad Nauheim, Germany, is also greatly appreciated.

A good phlebogram will always play the leading role in the "golden partnerships" of diagnostic phlebology. It is our hope that the present book will offer a contribution to this.

Frankfurt, November 1996

Viola Hach-Wunderle
Wolfgang Hach

Contents

Historical Review of Phlebography

The first roentgenographic examination of the veins in a living person was performed by Berberich and Hirsch in 1923, who injected a small dose of strontium bromide into the brachial vein. In the same year McPheeters and Rice performed similar tests with Lipiodol. In 1929, introduction of the relatively well tolerated water-soluble contrast agent Uroselectan made it safe to begin systematic research. Ratschow (1930), Barber and Orley (1931), Pomeranz and Tunick (1933), and Schwarz (1934) studied the conditions of venous drainage in varices. In 1935 Frimann-Dahl made the first successful phlebographic diagnosis of acute femoral vein thrombosis. In the same year Hutter first demonstrated the pelvic veins and inferior vena cava by the transfemoral injection of contrast medium. Luke introduced retrograde pressure phlebography in 1941 for assessing valvular function in the deep veins of the thigh. In 1956 Gullmo improved the method, establishing what has now become the standard technique.

In the 1960s and 1970s, May and Nissl did extensive research on the lower extremity venous system and established guidelines for the coordination of clinical and radiographic findings. The introduction of ascending pressure phlebography into routine clinical use by Hach (1973) made possible a comprehensive evaluation of all the lower extremity venous systems and pelvic vessels. This technique has also provided a sound, reproducible scientific basis for approaching the most common and most important venous disorder, primary varicose veins. Ascending pressure phlebography has led to the discovery of a number of new disease states and to the development of corresponding surgical treatments.

The development of nonionic contrast media was a milestone on the road towards establishing an open indication. In addition, the technical requirements for an optimal protection against radiation were fulfilled.

The routine use of the digital subtraction technique, which begain in the 1970s, represented a major advance in phlebography and in angiographic diagnosis as a whole. It has added a new dimension to evaluations of the retroperitoneal vessels and visceral veins, and it has superseded conventional pelvic phlebography in almost all applications. The investigation of organ diseases via the vein system has now been completely taken over by computed tomography and magnetic resonance imaging.

In recent years real-time sonography and duplex scanning have added whole new aspects to vascular diagnostic imaging. Modern instruments can provide detailed images of the vascular contents, vessel wall, and perivascular structures, as well as a detailed assessment of the factors affecting flow. Ultrasound not only can resolve some questions in phlebology noninvasively, without the use of bulky radiographic equipment, but frequently provides an adjunct to contrast radiography that can expand the scope of diagnostic information. The search for new avenues in diagnostic imaging has never been as intensive as it is today.

References

Barber RHT, Orley A (1932) Some x-ray observations in varicose disease of the leg. Lancet II: 72

Berberich J, Hirsch S (1923) Die röntgenologische Darstellung der Arterien und Venen am lebenden Menschen. Klin Wschr 2: 2226

Frimann-Dahl J (1935) Postoperative Röntgenuntersuchungen. Acta Chir Scand 76: Suppl 36, 1

Gullmo AL (1956) On the technique of phlebography of the lower limb. Acta Radiol 46: 603

Hach W (1974) Die aszendierende Preßphlebographie, eine Routinemethode zur Beurteilung der oberflächlichen Stammvenen. In: Friedrich HC, Hamelmann H (Hrsg) Ergebnisse der Angiologie, Bd 8. Schattauer, Stuttgart New York

Hutter K (1935) Zur Röntgendarstellung von Beckengefäßen bei urologischen Fällen. Acta Radiol 16: 94

Luke, JC (1941) The diagnosis of chronic enlargement of the leg. Surg Gynec Obstet 73: 472

May R, Nissl R (1973) Die Phlebographie der unteren Extremität. Thieme, Stuttgart
Pomeranz MM, Tunick IS (1933) Varicography. Surg Gynec Obstet 57: 689
Ratschow M (1930) Uroselektan in der Vasographie unter spezieller Berücksichtigung der Varikographie. Fortschr Röntgenstr 42: 37
Schwarz E (1934) Die Krampfadern der unteren Extremität mit besonderer Berücksichtigung ihrer Entstehung und Behandlung. Ergebn Chir Orthop 27: 256
Sicard JA, Forestier G (1923) Injections intravasculaires d'huile iodée sous contrôle radiologique. C R Soc Biol (Paris) 88: 1200

Normal Roentgen Anatomy of the Lower Extremity and Pelvic Veins

All the veins of an extremity function as an *integrated system*. The vessels chiefly responsible for venous drainage of the lower limb are the deep intrafascial veins, for which the foot veins, muscle veins, superficial veins, and communicating veins serve merely as tributaries. A knowledge of the specific flow conditions in the lower extremity is essential in order to select an appropriate method for the differentiated roentgen diagnosis of venous disorders and to interpret abnormal circulatory patterns correctly.

The venous system of the body is subject to endless variations, so it is most difficult to describe a roentgen "norm." There may be *anomalies*, defined as a significant congenital abnormality that does not adversely affect function, or *malformations*, which have pathologic significance. The topographic development of the venous system is complete by the end of the eighth week of intrauterine life.

A knowledge of *embryology*, then, is necessary in order to understand the anatomic variants, anomalies, and malformations that may be encountered in the venous system. This information will be presented within its appropriate context.

Veins of the Foot

The foot contains both a superficial and a deep venous system, separated by the pedal fascia. The systems communicate with each other through numerous perforating veins. The largest blood volume is contained in the dense, venous network of the sole, the *plantar venous rete*, and in the muscle veins of the metatarsal region. In contrast to the leg veins, drainage occurs not just through the intrafascial vessels but also through the venous plexuses at the medial and lateral margins of the foot, which drain to the large superficial veins on the dorsum of the foot and thence to the great and small saphenous trunks (Dos Santos 1938).

The anatomic arrangement of the foot veins is such that a marked acceleration of blood flow occurs during walking ("venous hurry"; Ascar and Shanel 1975). Weight bearing on the sole of the foot expels blood from the plantar plexus. Also, tightening of the plantar ligament and other ligaments causes a contraction of the pedal vault, with emptying of the sinus-like plantar veins. When the foot is relaxed and non-weight-bearing, the plantar network refills, and expansion of the preformed intrafascial spaces exerts a suction effect on the deep venous plexuses. This imparts a rhythmic, reciprocating action to venous hemodynamics much like that of a *pressure-suction pump*.

From a clinical standpoint, radiographic visualization of the foot veins is rarely indicated except for very special inquiries. The vessels are consistently demonstrated by ascending pressure phlebography when contrast medium is injected into the dorsal vein of the great toe.

Superficial Veins

The vessels from the toes drain into a distally convex arcade called the *dorsal venous arch* of the
foot. The medial limb of this subcutaneous venous 1, 2
arch, called the *medial marginal vein*, merges with the root of the great saphenous vein. It receives
numerous small tributaries from the medial bor- 3
der of the foot, the medial marginal collateral veins (Kubik 1982). The lateral limb of the venous arch, called the *lateral marginal vein*, is continuous proximally with the small saphenous trunk. Through this arrangement, both saphenous trunks receive flow from the vessels that drain the superficial dorsal and plantar venous networks.

Other communicating vessels connect the center of the venous arch with the dorsal foot veins. These veins pass beneath the cruciform ligament, their proximal continuation becoming the anterior tibial veins above the ankle joint.

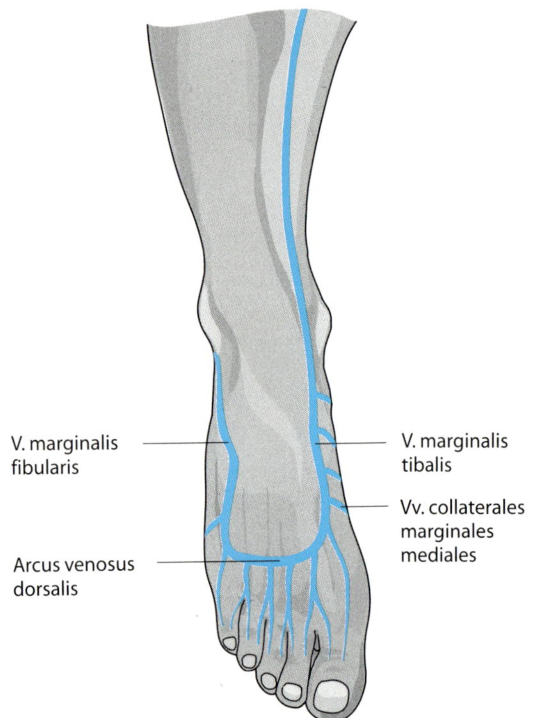

1. Superficial veins of the foot

Demonstration of the foot veins by ascending phlebography
Puncture of the dorsal vein of the great toe
Patient in semiupright or horizontal position
Leg relaxed for contrast injection
Exposures taken with passive plantar flexion and slight internal rotation of the foot, also lateral view

At the level of the ankle joint, there is a relatively
constant connection between the posterior tibial
vein and great saphenous vein, the *medial malleolar vein* (Kubik 1982). This vessel provides a route
by which contrast medium injected into the super- 97
ficial medial foot veins can pass directly into the
deep leg veins, permitting opacification of the intrafascial vascular systems.

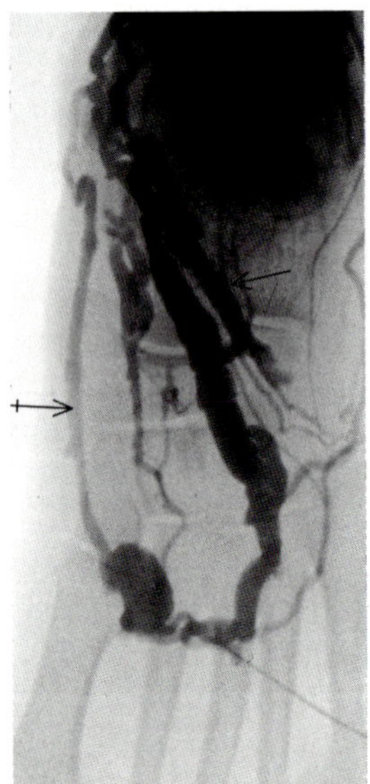

2. Foot veins demonstrated by ascending phlebography in internal rotation. → Duplication of the plantar vein and its junction with the posterior tibial veins, ↔ medial marginal vein

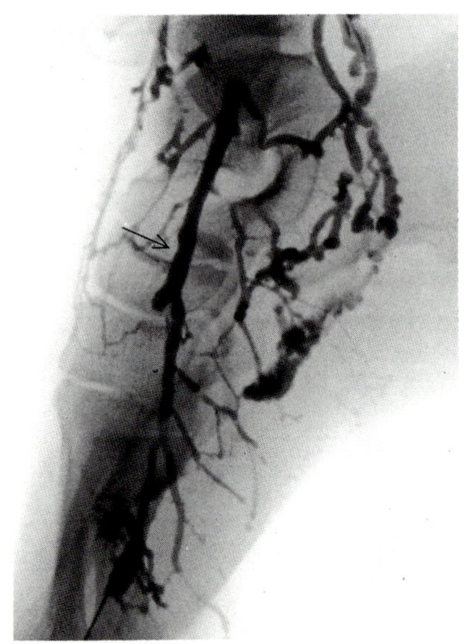

3. Foot veins demonstrated by ascending phlebography. → Medial marginal vein

Deep Veins

4 The *plantar vein* runs parallel to its homonymous
artery. It forms a laterally convex arch that receives many small tributaries from surrounding
2 muscles and bone as well as perforating veins. Fre-
5 quently the plantar vein is paired and fusiform in
shape. It contains few valves, and sometimes it
contains none. Proximal to the ankle joint it merges with the posterior tibial veins, which drain a
substantial portion of the venous blood from the
foot.

Perforating Veins

Most of the perforating veins in the foot are valveless (Kubik 1982) and thus permit flow into either
the deep or superficial venous system, the course
of the vessels favoring the latter route. The perforating vessels include *Kuster's veins*, located about 6
the medial and lateral malleoli (Kuster et al. 1981;
May 1981). They open into superficial venous networks that give rise to the great and small saphenous veins; their radiographic visualization has
no clinical significance.

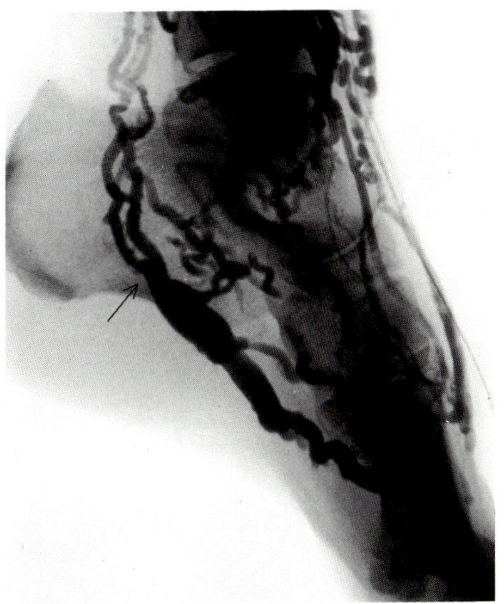

4. Foot veins demonstrated by ascending phlebography, lateral view. → Plantar vein at junction with posterior tibial veins

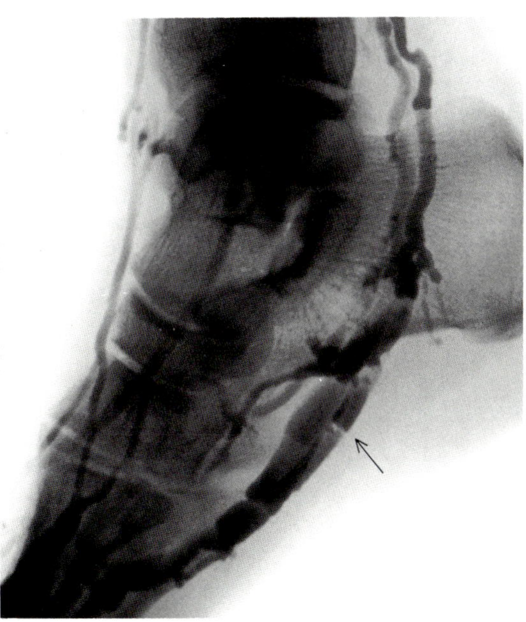

5. Foot veins demonstrated by ascending phlebography, lateral view. Duplication of the plantar vein (→) and posterior tibial veins

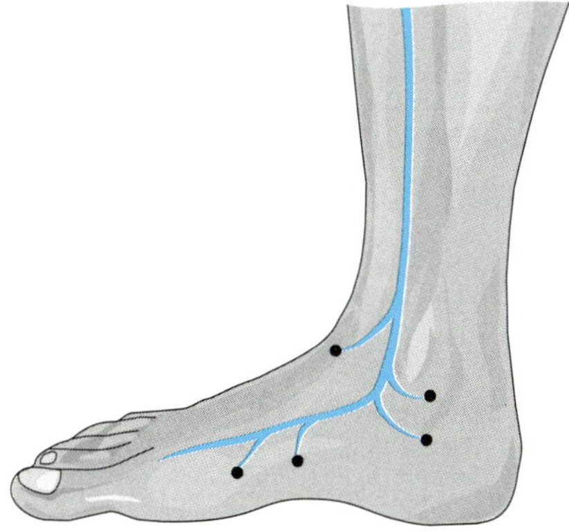

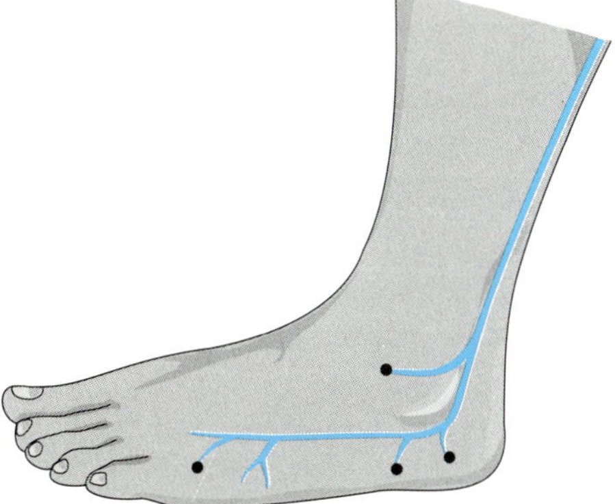

6. Kuster's perforating veins. *Left,* medial aspect of the foot; *right,* lateral aspect of the foot

References

Askar O, Shanel AA (1975) The veins of the foot. J Cardiovasc Surg 16: 53

Dos Santos JC (1938) Direct phlebography, conception, technique, first results. J Internat Chir 3: 625

Kubik S (1982) Die Anatomie des Fußes mit besonderer Berücksichtigung der Faszien, Faszienräume und der Gefäßversorgung. In: Brunner U (Hrsg) Der Fuß. Huber, Bern

Kuster G, Lofgren EF, Hollinshead WH (1981) Anatomy of the veins of the foot. Surg Gynec Obstet 127: 187

May R (1981) Die Nomenklatur der chirurgisch wichtigsten Verbindungsvenen. In: May R, Partsch H, Staubesand J (Hrsg) Venae perforantes. Urban & Schwarzenberg, München

Veins of the Leg

The venous drainage of the leg consists anatomically and physiologically of four systems: the superficial veins, the deep veins, the perforating veins, and the muscle veins.

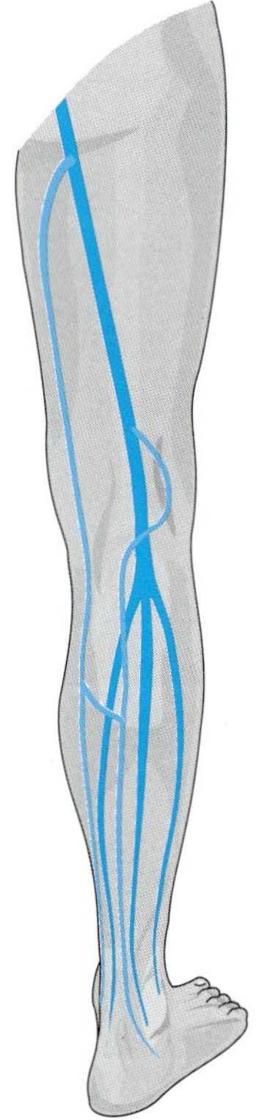

7. Superficial (*light blue*) and deep (*dark blue*) leg veins

Superficial Venous System

The superficial veins lie external to the crural fascia in the subcutaneous fat. They present numerous variations in course and development, and a "norm" can be said to exist only for the larger vessels. It is clinically useful to distinguish *four different groups* of superficial veins based on their topographic relationships. The great and small saphenous trunks carry the largest amount of blood from the venous plexuses of the skin and subcutaneous tissues to the deep leg veins, either directly or via specific perforating veins. The main saphenous tributaries in the leg, often called the "side branches" of the saphenous trunks, align with the longitudinal axis of the limb.

The third group, the reticular veins, are of regional importance and display a seemingly random course. The final group is the short perforating veins that directly interconnect the superficial and deep trunks. Like the saphenous veins, they penetrate the fascia to establish transfascial connections.

Characteristics of the superficial veins		
Vessels	Course relative to the long axis of the lower limb	Relationship to the fascia
Saphenous veins	Aligned	Perforating
Parietal branches	Aligned	Perforating or non-perforating
Reticular veins	Not aligned	Non-perforating
Perforating veins	Not aligned	Perforating

Great Saphenous Vein

The great saphenous vein, the longest vein in the body, arises from the medial limb of the dorsal venous arch of the foot, the medial marginal vein. Passing in front of the medial malleolus and behind the medial condyle of the femur, the vein ascends on the medial side of the leg to the saphenous opening (fossa ovalis) and enters the common femoral vein 2–3 cm below the inguinal ligament. It receives numerous superficial vessels in its course that are not delineated by routine phlebography. The four largest tributaries, the "side

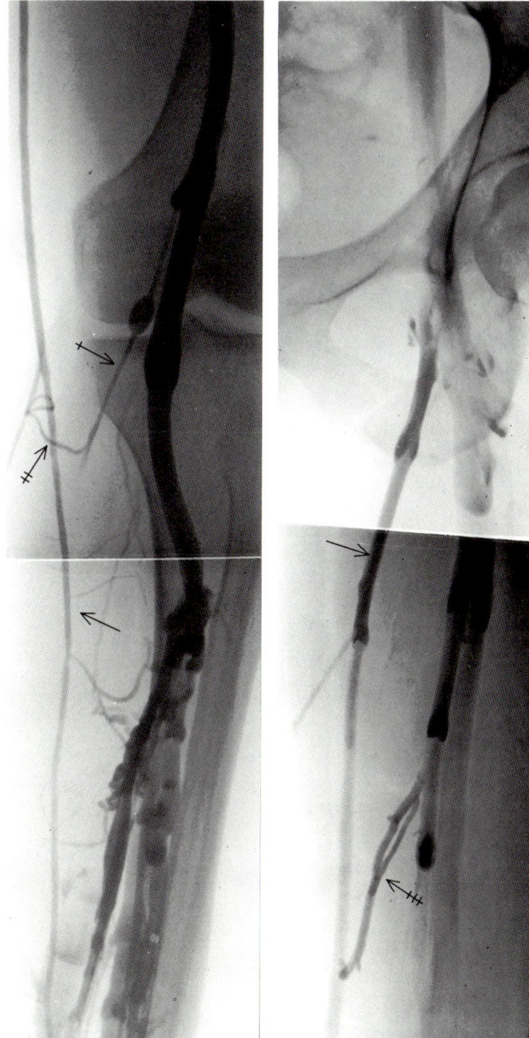

8. Great saphenous vein of the left leg, demonstrated by ascending pressure phlebography. → Great saphenous vein, +→ small saphenous vein with two competent valves, ++→ thin connecting vessel between short and great saphenous trunks, +++→ Dodd's perforating vein. *Left,* lateral view of the lower leg; *right,* view of the thigh in slight external rotation

Demonstration of the competent great saphenous vein by noncompression phlebography
Puncture of the medial marginal vein
No tourniquet
Patient in semiupright position
Leg relaxed and non-weight-bearing for contrast injection
Manual direction of contrast medium
Spot films in slight internal and external rotation
Caution: Risk of thrombophlebitis

branches," are relatively constant and are of greater clinical importance. Additionally there are one or two oblique anastomoses that convey blood
from the small saphenous vein to the great saphe- 8
nous. Before its entrance into the common femoral vein, the great saphenous vein forms a short arch as it traverses the cribriform fascia. This segment is known as the "crosse" in phlebologic nomenclature. The superior epigastric vein, external pudendal vein, and superficial circumflex iliac vein converge upon the saphenous trunk in this area to form the *subinguinal venous confluence.* In
operations for saphenous trunk varicosity, these 9
vessels must be carefully isolated and ligated 10
("crossectomy") as a precaution against recurrent varicose disease.

The etymology of the word "crosse" has been elucidated by Jecht (1983). The French word *crosse* means a bishop's staff or crosier, which is curved at the top like a shepherd's crook. The root of the word can be traced to the Germanic *krutje,* meaning a stick with a curved handle.

▷

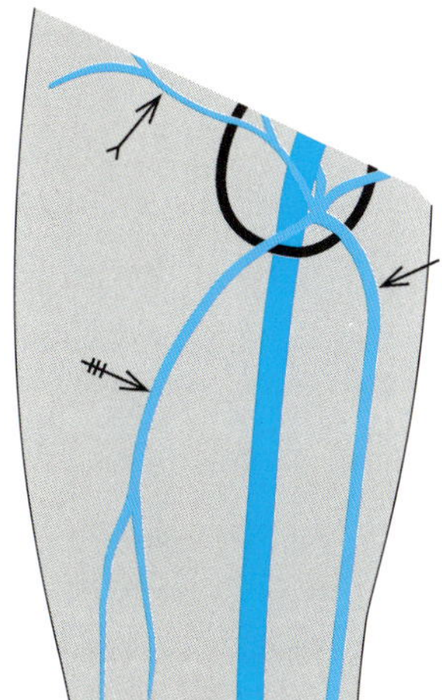

9. Subinguinal venous confluence. → Great saphenous vein, +→ superficial epigastric vein, ++→ external pudendal vein, ≻→ superficial circumflex iliac vein, +++→ lateral accessory saphenous vein

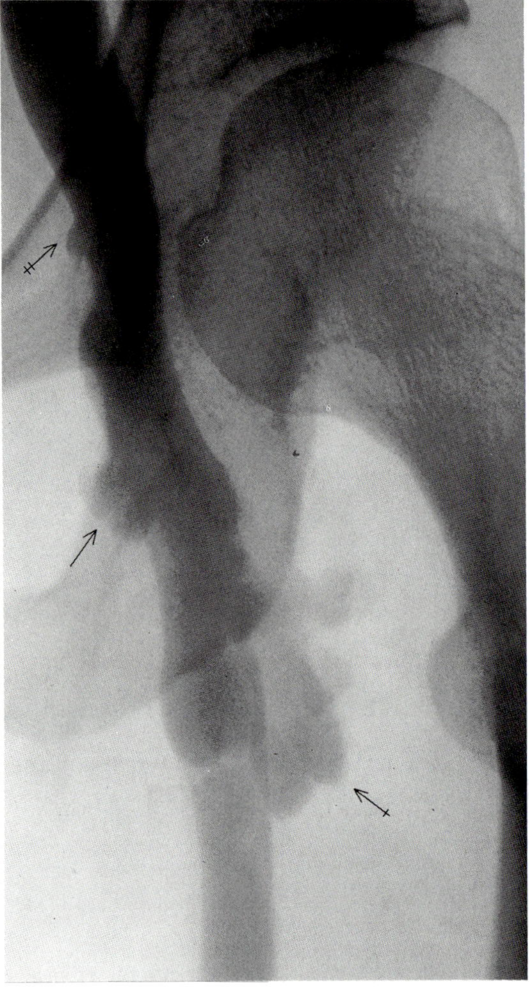

10. Subinguinal venous confluence (*left side*), demonstrated by ascending pressure phlebography. → Great saphenous vein, ↔ profunda femoris vein, ↮ superficial epigastric vein

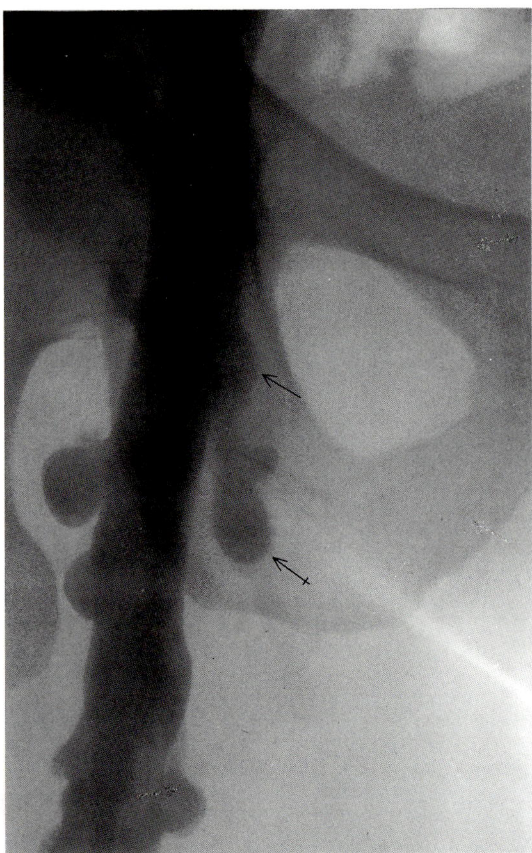

12. Termination of great saphenous vein demonstrated by ascending pressure phlebography. → Terminal valve, ↔ distal sluice valve

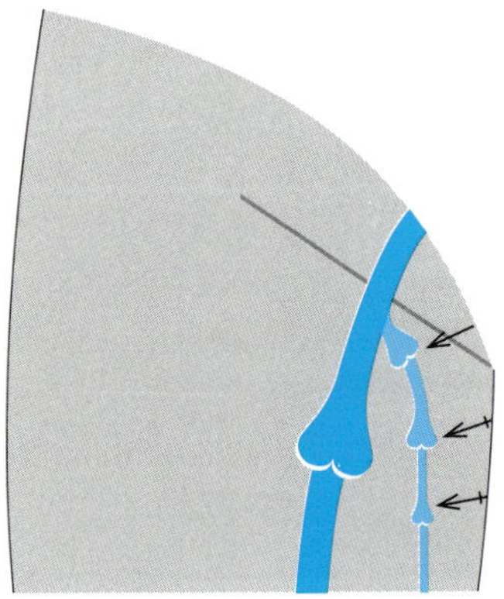

11. Normal saphenofemoral junction. → Saphenous vein sinus with terminal valve, ↔ sluice valves

The *lumen* of the great saphenous vein measures approximately 2 mm at the medial malleolus, 4 mm in the thigh, and 6 mm at the saphenofemoral junction. This progressive caliber increase can be appreciated on phlebograms, the vessel appearing almost threadlike distally and straw-sized near its termination.

The venous valves are spaced 5–10 cm apart and 8
are usually located below the sites of smaller merging veins. The *terminal valve* of the great saphenous vein is of considerable importance in the pathogenesis of saphenous trunk varicosity. It is located 0.5–1.5 cm below the entrance of the great saphenous vein into the common femoral vein

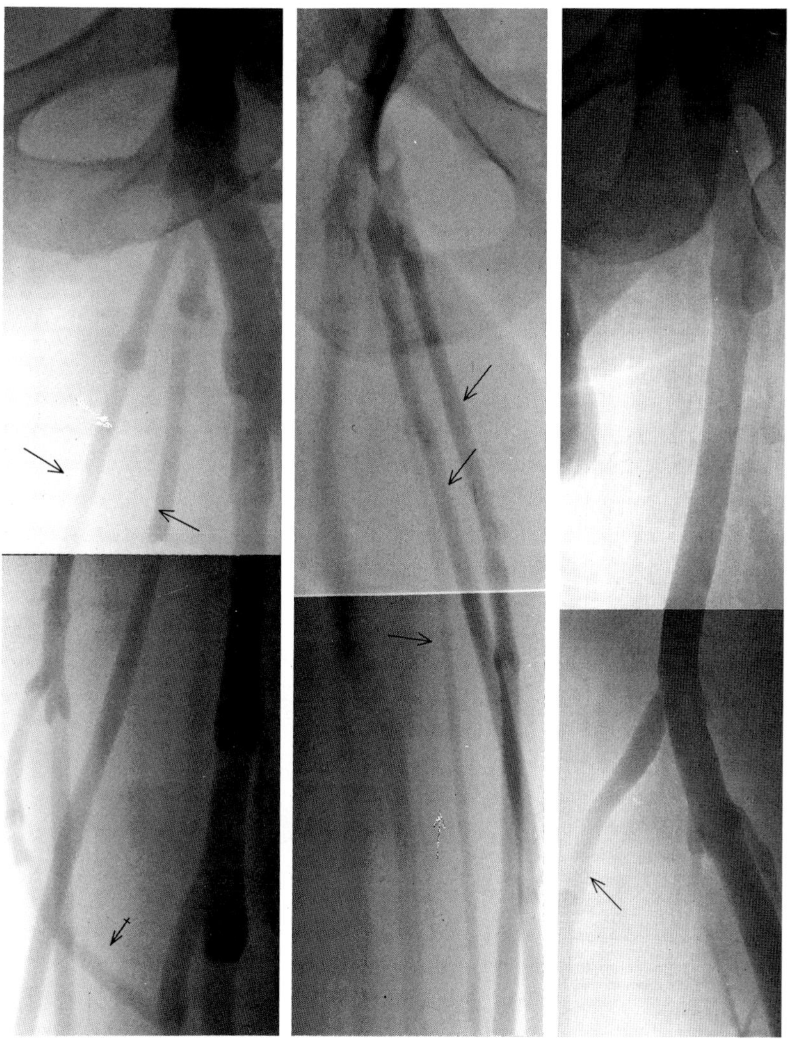

13. Ascending pressure phlebogram demonstrates proximal duplication of the great saphenous vein (→), with both trunks entering a common sinus. ↔ Giacomini anastomosis

14. Tripled great saphenous vein (→) in the thigh, shown by ascending pressure phlebography. Vessels are dilated by collateral function secondary to postthrombotic syndrome of the leg and pelvic veins with extensive recanalization

15. Anomalous distal entry of the incompetent great saphenous vein (→) into the superficial femoral vein in the midthigh, demonstrated by ascending pressure phlebography. Finding was confirmed by operation

11 and separates the broad *ostial sinus* from the
smaller lumen of the competent venous trunk.
Distal to the the terminal valve, spaced at about
12 3 cm intervals, are two parietal valves, below
which the caliber of the venous trunk is again reduced. These subterminal valves function as sluices, so we refer to them as *sluice valves*. When the terminal valve and sluice valves become incompetent due to congenital or acquired pathology of the valve cusps, the regurgitant flow causes a progressive proximal-to-distal dilatation of the great saphenous vein, and varicosity develops. Accordingly, the abrupt change in vascular caliber immediately distal to the sluice valves, called the
telescope sign, provides a useful radiographic 131
criterion for the functional competence of the 44
valves (see p. 89).

The great saphenous vein displays numerous *variations* that can be significant in the surgery of primary varicose disease. A knowledge of possible anomalies is essential for arterial or cardiac operations that involve the use of an autogenous great saphenous vein graft.

The great saphenous vein is *duplicated* in 3.8%–27% of
13 cases (Haeger 1962; May and Nissl 1973), and rarely it is
14 tripled. This is an important consideration in terms of recurrence after varicose vein surgery and dissection of the vein for grafting in cardiovascular operations. *An-*
15 *omalous distal entry* of the great saphenous vein into the superficial femoral vein below the saphenous opening has an incidence less than 0.1% according to our studies. This anomaly is important in operations for saphenous trunk varicosity and in dissecting the saphenous vein for grafting. Variations in the subinguinal venous confluence are very common, the "normal" pattern occurring in only 37% of cases (Lanz and Wachsmuth 1972). *Anomalous proximal entry* of the great saphenous vein into the inferior epigastric vein (May and Nissl 1973) is important in varicose saphenous vein operations.

Demonstration of the great saphenous crosse by sonography
Linear 7-MHz transducer
Patient in supine position
Slight external rotation of the lower limb
Avoidance of transducer pressure
Scans on transverse and longitudinal planes

The numerous variations of the subinguinal venous confluence are not significant in terms of phlebographic imaging. Rarely, crossing of the great saphenous vein by the external pudendal artery may cause islet formation on X-rays; a similar topographic relationship can exist between the common femoral vein and deep femoral artery.

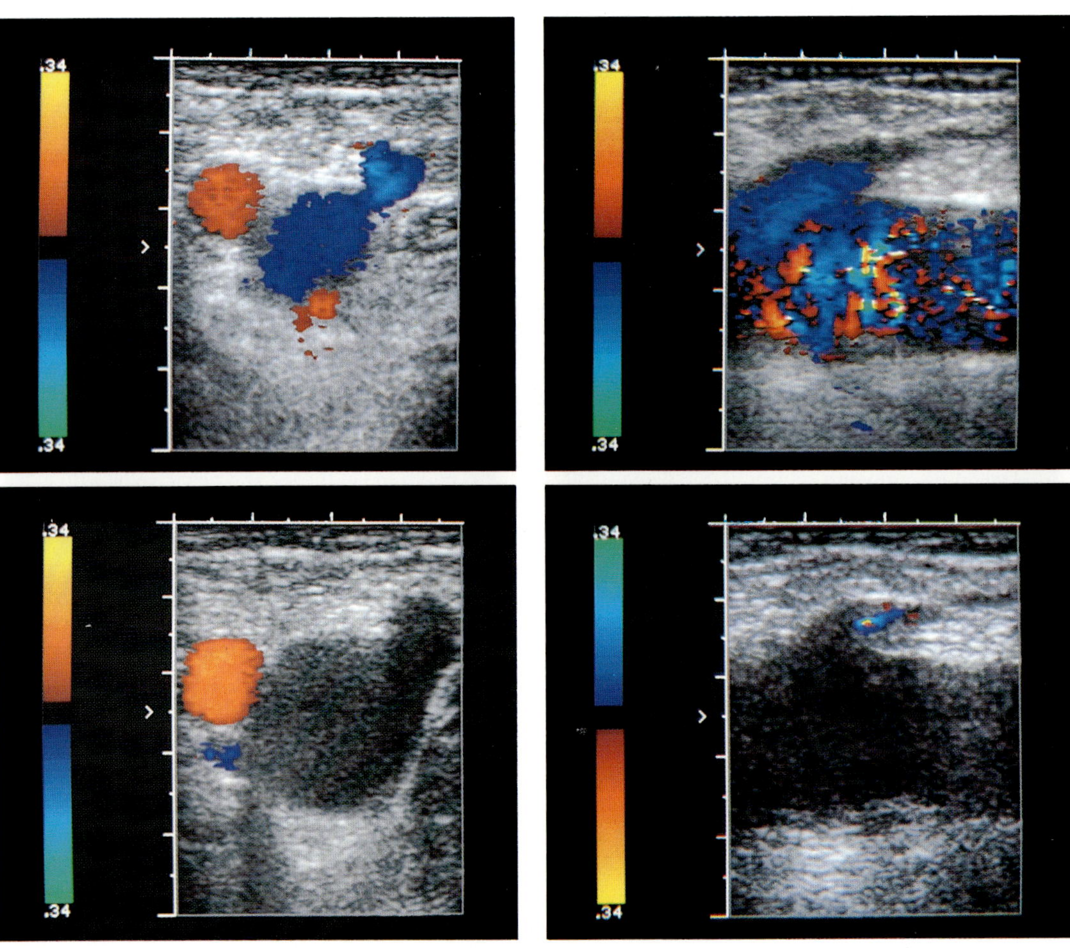

16. Terminal area of the great saphenous vein demonstrated by color-coded duplex sonography. Cross-section at the level of the terminal valve after expiration (*top left*) and during a Valsalva maneuver (*bottom left*). Longitudinal section with discrete turbulence in the common femoral vein after expiration (*top right*) and during the Valsalva maneuver (*bottom right*). (Acuson, 7-MHz transducer)

16 Around the crosse, the great saphenous vein and its increased caliber near the confluence can be easily demonstrated *sonographically*; it follows an arched course. Further distally, a normal vessel can only be identified by detailed examination.

Side Branches of the Great Saphenous Vein

The "side branches" of the great saphenous vein are small-caliber vessels that arise from small reticular veins; hence they are not demonstrated by ascending phlebography under normal circumstances. Varicose deterioration with incompetence of the venous valves must be present before these tributaries will opacify. We use the term "side branches" because it is common in clinical parlance; actually it is a misnomer, since veins receive tributaries and do not give off branches.

17 In the lower leg the ***anterior arch vein*** (vena arcuata cruris anterior; Staubesand 1980) ascends parallel to and about two to three fingerwidths from the anterior tibial margin. It enters the great saphenous vein a hand's width below the joint line of
the knee. It does not communicate with the deep 206
leg veins.

The ***posterior arch vein*** (vena arcuate cruris pos- 207
terior; Staubesand 1980) forms an arcade uniting 17
the three Cockett's perforating veins on the imaginary Linton's line, which runs one fingerwidth behind the posterior tibial border (Dodd and Cockett 1956). This vessel has special clinical importance owing to its transfascial communica- 204
tions with the posterior tibial veins. Distal to the
knee, the posterior arch vein drains into the great 205
saphenous vein, often joined by an oblique ana- 8
stomosis from the small saphenous vein.

The most important tributary in the thigh is the ***lateral accessory saphenous vein,*** formerly called
the lateral femoral subcutaneous vein. It origi- 18
nates from reticular vessels on the lateral side of the knee. It displays varying modes or types of termination. In the femoral type the vein courses laterally to medially in a large arc over the front of the midthigh to its site of termination in the great saphenous vein. It does not communicate directly the deep venous system. Hence, ascending pressure phlebography can demonstrate the vessel only if there is coexisting varicosity of the great saphenous trunk.

In the inguinal type of termination, the vein again 18
arises on the lateral side of the thigh but joins the great saphenous vein at a higher level, entering it in the region of the sluice valves – generally below

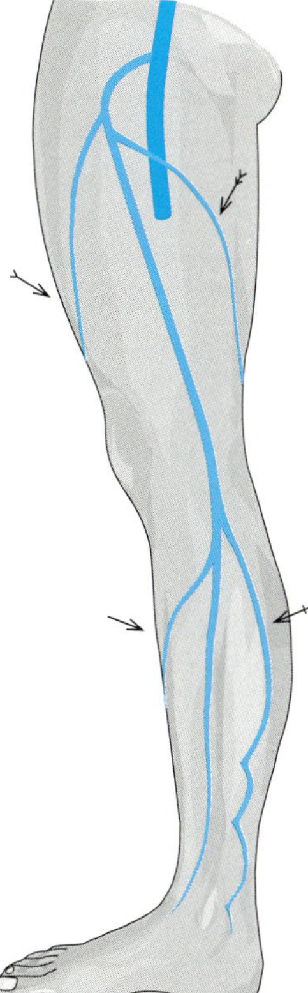

17. Side branches of the great saphenous vein. → Anterior arch vein, ↔ posterior arch vein, ↣ lateral accessory saphenous vein, ⤖ medial accessory saphenous vein

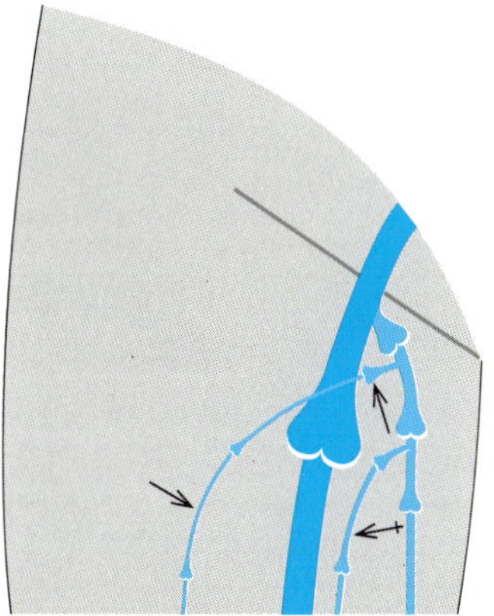

18. Variations in the termination of the lateral accessory saphenous vein. → Inguinal infravalvular type, ↔ femoral type

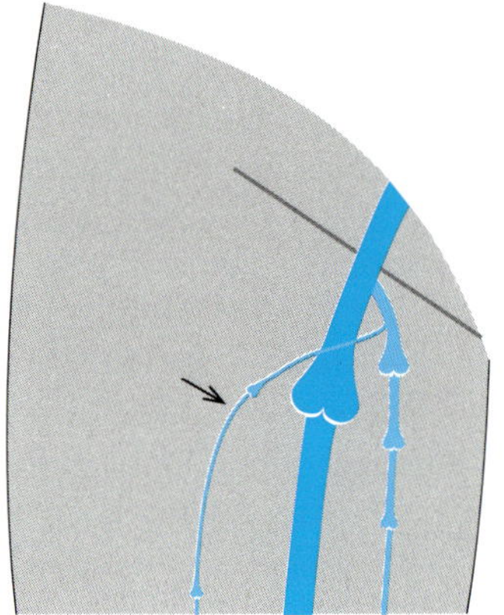

19. Inguinal supravalvular termination of the lateral accessory saphenous vein (→). This pattern, associated with an abnormally enlarged ostial sinus of the great saphenous vein, marks the start of a type I primary varicose circuit

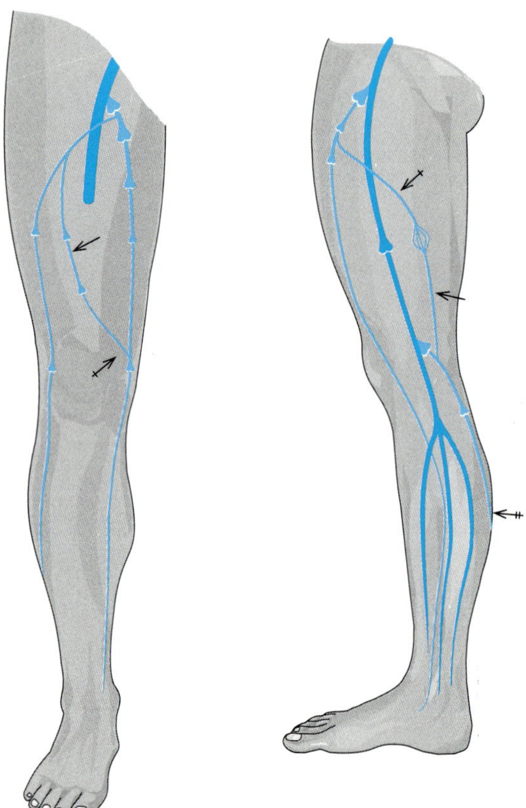

20 *(left)*. Curved, parallel connection of the lateral accessory saphenous vein (→) to the great saphenous vein with a distal accessory anastomosis (↔)

21 *(right)*. Giacomini's anastomosis between the femoropopliteal vein (→) and the medial accessory saphenous vein (↔). ↠ Small saphenous vein

the terminal valve of the great saphenous vein, rarely above it.

An important anomaly of the ostial sinus of the great saphenous vein can profoundly affect the lateral accessory saphenous vein. When the sinus is
congenitally enlarged, the terminal valve is locat- 19
ed farther distally than normal, so the lateral accessory saphenous vein enters the sinus proximal to the terminal valve itself. This establishes a direct (transfascial) connection between the tributary vein and the deep venous system, predis-
posing the vessel to varicose deterioration, which 197
can lead to the pathologic type I recirculation pattern (see p. 124). 140

The femoral and inguinal segments of the great saphenous vein are sometimes linked by a curved,
parallel connection formed by the lateral acces- 20
sory saphenous vein (distal accessory anastomosis). Varicose change in the accessory vein can 170
lead to the "side-branch" type of incomplete sa- 172
phenous trunk varicosity (see Fig. 137 d).

The ***medial accessory saphenous vein*** arises from
reticular vessels on the posterior and medial as- 17
pects of the thigh. It passes around the medial side to enter the great saphenous vein at the inferior
border of the saphenous opening. Generally it is 6
smaller than the lateral accessory vein. Of practical importance is a transfascial communication 21
with the ostial sinus of the small saphenous vein
through the femoropopliteal vein, first described 28
by Giacomini in 1873 (Giacomini's anastomosis). 30
This connection can lead to the development of a 31
"posterior" type of incomplete great saphenous
trunk varicosity. 177

Short Saphenous Vein

The small saphenous vein begins as a continuation of the lateral limb of the dorsal venous arch of
the foot, the lateral marginal vein. Contrast injec- 1
tion through the marginal vein will plainly demonstrate the small saphenous trunk when a noncompression technique is used. The vessel passes behind the lateral malleolus and ascends on the posterior aspect of the lower leg. Generally it merges with the popliteal vein 5–7 cm above the level 7
of the knee joint, forming a slight loop as it enters the vein. The small femoropopliteal vein descends
from the thigh to enter the small saphenous vein 21
just before its termination.

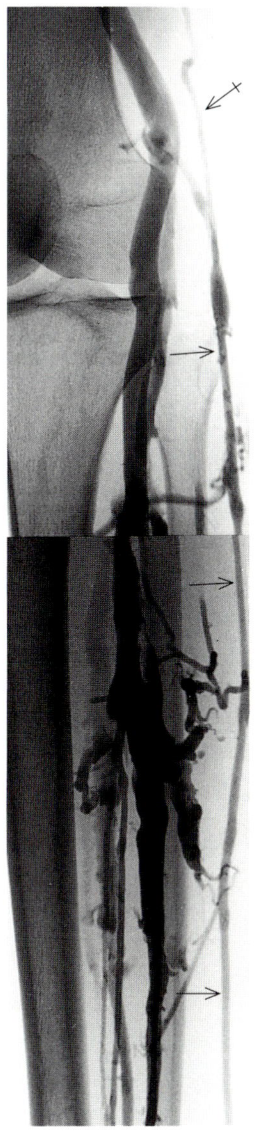

22. Small saphenous vein (→), demonstrated by ascending noncompression phlebography of the internally rotated limb. ↔ Femoropopliteal vein

Demonstration of the competent small saphenous vein by noncompression phlebography
Puncture of the lateral marginal vein
No tourniquet
Patient in semiupright position
Leg relaxed and non-weight-bearing for contrast injection
Internal-rotation and lateral spot films
Caution: risk of thrombophlebitis

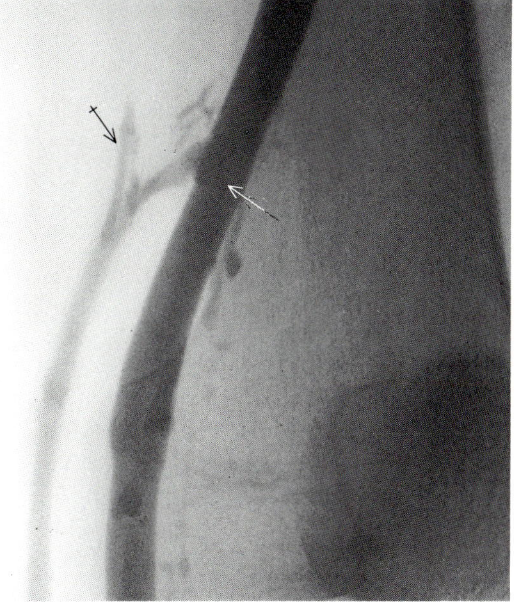

23. Terminal valve and ostial sinus (→) of the small saphenous vein with the telescope sign. Antegrade filling of the femoropopliteal vein (↔) by centripetal flow. Ascending pressure phlebography, lateral view

The normal small saphenous vein appears radiographically as a small-caliber vessel about the 22
thickness of a knitting needle. It contains an average of 8 venous valves spaced about 4 cm apart. Its
terminal valve, located just below its entrance into
the popliteal vein, separates a small ostial sinus 39
from the small lumen of the venous trunk,
performing a sluice function similar to that
described in the great saphenous vein. The phlebographic documentation of different vascular
calibers above and below the valve plane, called 23
the *telescope sign*, is considered proof of the functional competence of the valve. An incompetence 185
terminal valve leads to varicosity of the small
saphenous trunk.

In 32 % of cases the small saphenous vein and the
gastrocnemius veins enter the popliteal vein by a 24
common trunk (May and Nissl 1973). Sometimes 63
these vessels are difficult to distinguish from one 64
another on lateral projections. One distinction is
that the valves of the *gastrocnemius veins* become
more numerous distally, and the veins themselves
have somewhat larger, spindle-shaped lumina. Positive differentiation can be made by taking an exposure with the limb internally rotated. In this view
the muscle veins ascend obliquely in a medical- 25

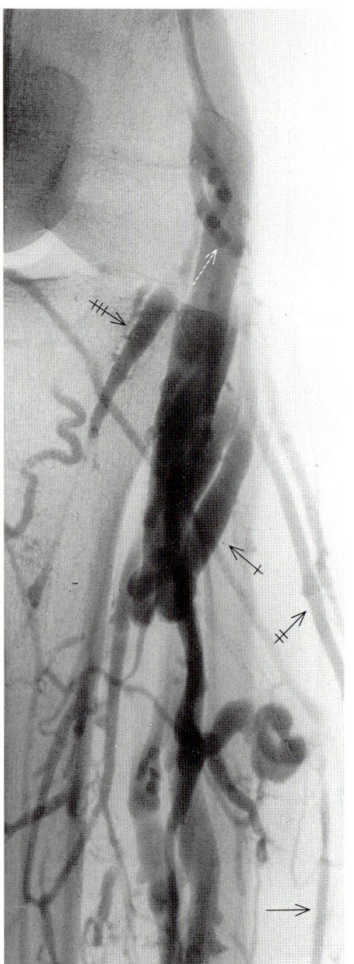
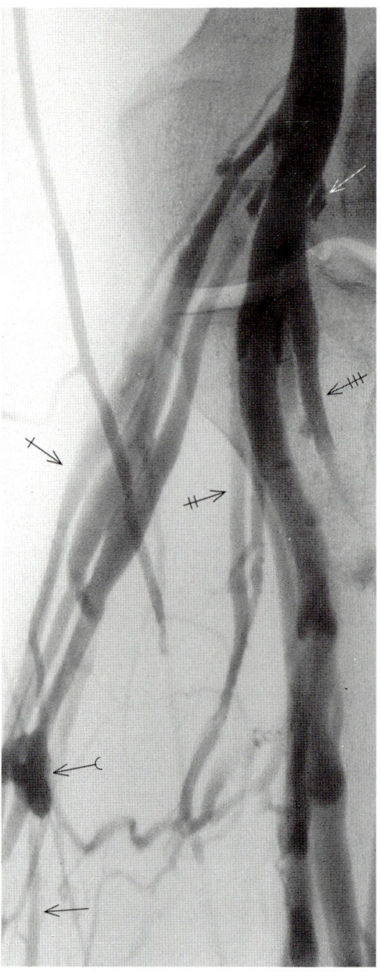

△

24. Termination of the small saphenous vein and gastrocnemius veins in a common trunk. The small saphenous vein (→) is recognized by its gently looping curve. The film shows three vessels of the medial head of the gastrocnemius muscle (⇸), two vessels of the lateral head (⇻), and two veins of the popliteus muscle (⇼). An incompetent May's perforating vein (↣) is shown distally. Ascending pressure phlebography: *left*, internal rotation view; *right*, lateral view

to-lateral direction, crossing over the tibial condyle. Generally two to four vessels are present in each gastrocnemius head. By contrast, the small saphenous vein runs straight up past the fibula and is almost always single in this region.

Unlike the other vessels of the superficial venous system, the small saphenous vein is only partly subcutaneous. Usually it enters the subfascial space through the *crural fascia* in the middle or

Differentiation of the gastrocnemius veins and small saphenous vein on a phlebogram of the internally rotated limb		
Roentgen-criteria	Gastro-cnemius veins	Small saphe-nous vein
Number of trunks	2–4	1
Course of vessel	Medial-to-lateral oblique	Vertical
Shape of vessel	Frequently spindleshaped	Always tubular
Caliber	Increases proximally	Remains constant outside sluice region
Spacing of venous valves	1–3 cm, decreasing proximally	Constant, >4 cm

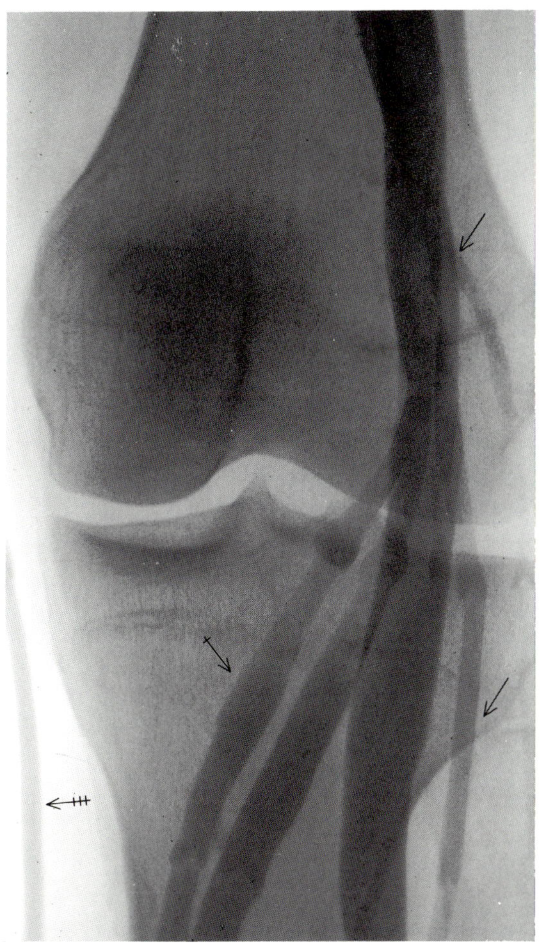

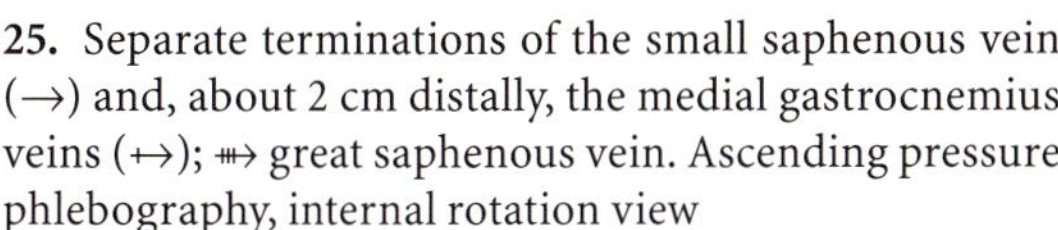

25. Separate terminations of the small saphenous vein (→) and, about 2 cm distally, the medial gastrocnemius veins (↔); ⇸ great saphenous vein. Ascending pressure phlebography, internal rotation view

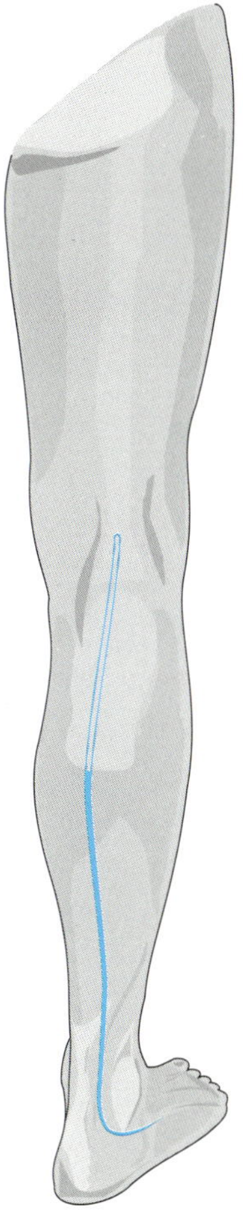

26. A small saphenous vein piercing the fascia at the midcalf level

proximal third of the lower leg, and rarely at the
26 level of the malleolus. A high fascial perforation in the popliteal fossa is uncommon (Moosmann and Hartwell 1964).

Ignorance of this topography often leads to diagnostic
184 errors. A strongly dilated, incompetent small saphenous vein may not be palpable beneath the tough fascia. As a result, only the more distal, extrafascial varices are detected and sclerosed, and the therapy is unsuccessful.

May's perforating vein passes from the small saphenous trunk to the gastrocnemius veins. Located at the level of the muscular attachment of the Achilles tendon, this vessel assumes some clinical
219 significance when incompetent.

Several anastomotic veins carry blood from the 27
small saphenous vein to the great saphenous vein, 8
with a corresponding redirection of the flow. With varicosity of the small saphenous trunk, an "anterior ulcer" can develop through a corresponding distal connection (see p. 121). 193

The small saphenous vein can present numerous 28
variations with which the surgeon should be familiar:

- ***Low termination.*** This denotes entry of the small saphenous vein into one of the three deep veins of the lower leg, usually the peroneal vein. With a prevalence of 9.7% (Kosinski 1926), this anomaly is important in operations for saphenous trunk varicosity.

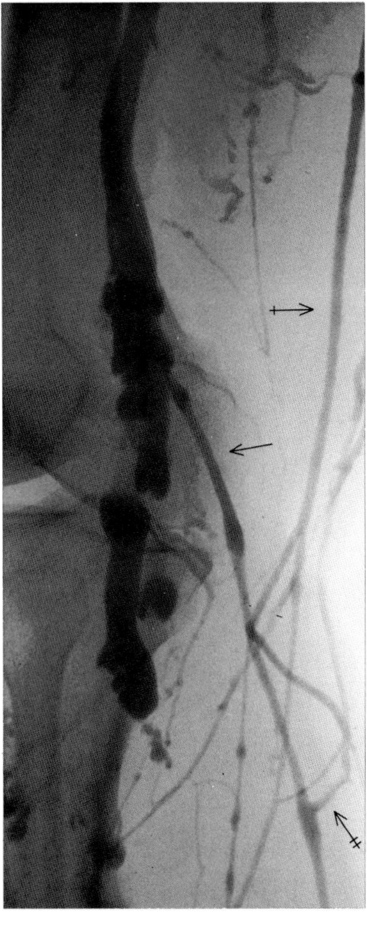
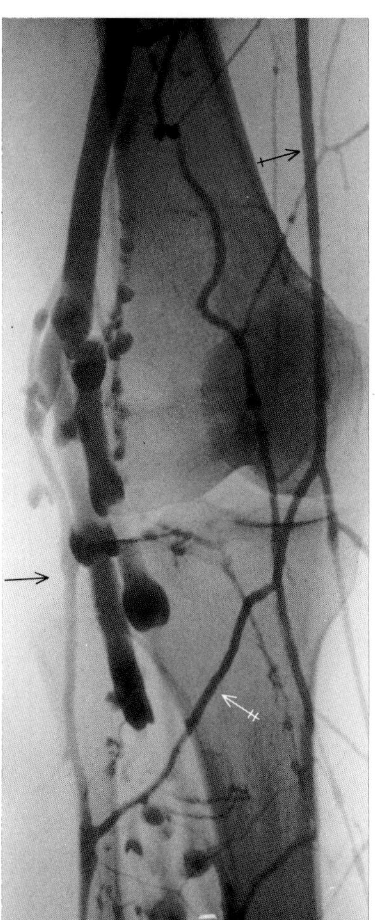

27. Anastomotic vessel (⇻) between the small saphenous vein (→) and great saphenous vein (⇸). Duplication of the popliteal vein. Ascending pressure phlebography: *left*, internal rotation view; *right*, lateral view

- ***Anomalous distal termination.*** The small saphenous vein enters the popliteal vein at or below the level of the knee joint in 14% of cases (Haeger 1962).

192 - ***Anomalous proximal termination.*** The small saphenous vein enters the superficial femoral artery in 7.35% of cases (May and Nissl 1973). This anomaly is important in operations for saphenous varicosity.
- ***Direct connection with the internal iliac vein.*** The mostly intrafascial small saphenous vein opens directly into the femoropopliteal vein, which in turn enters one of the gluteal veins and thus communicates with the internal iliac venous system. This represents the phylogenically oldest communication with the central veins. The reported prevalence of the anomaly is 17.4% (May and Nissl 1973), though we believe it is much lower. The extrafascial form occasionally occurs as part of a congenital anomaly.
- ***Atypical entry into the profunda femoris vein.*** This involves a large opening into the profunda femoris with no communication with the popliteofemoral trunks. It can be demonstrated in 16.6% of patients by systematic intraoperative phlebography (Gillot 1975).
- ***High connection with the great saphenous vein.*** The small saphenous vein unites directly with the femoropopliteal vein, which then communicates with the medial accessory saphenous vein high in the thigh and drains into the great saphenous vein. The epifascial course of the vessel distinguishes it from Giacomini's anastomosis, formed intrafascially by the femoropopliteal vein and medial accessory vein (s. p. 12). Prevalence reports range from 2.3% (May and

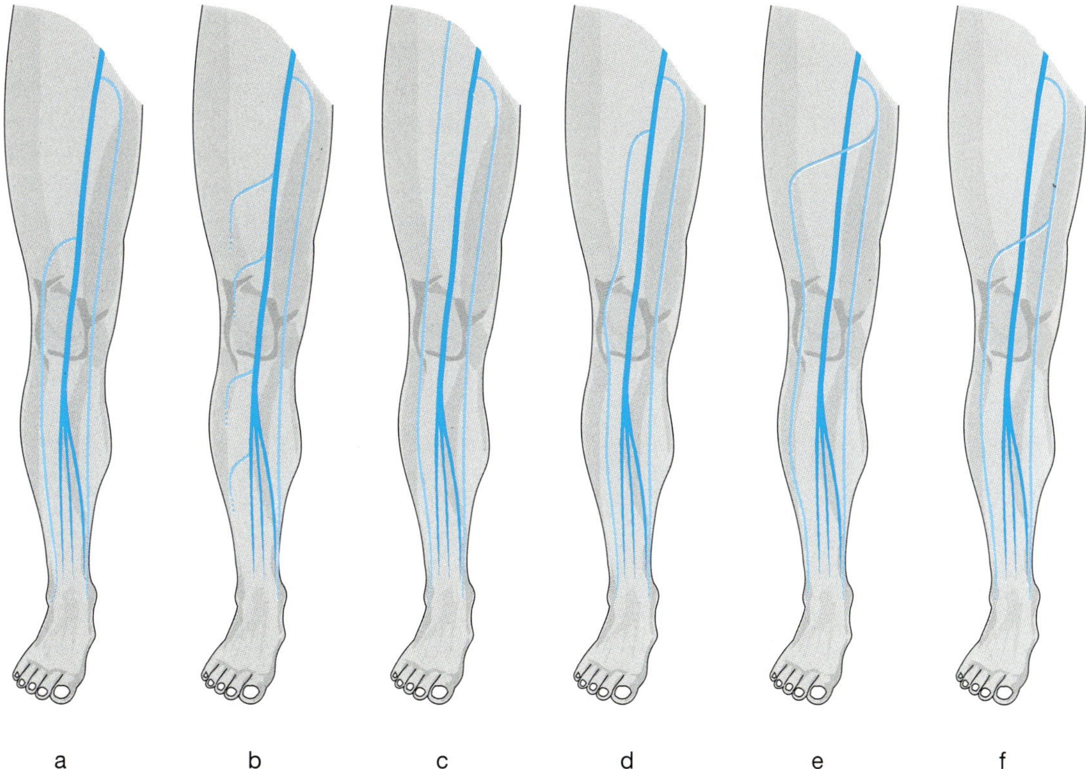

28 a–f. Variations in the termination of the small saphenous vein. **a** Normal course. **b** Anomalous proximal and distal terminations. **c** Gluteal or iliac termination. **d** Termination in the profunda femoris vein. **e** Giacomini's variation. **f** High union with the great saphenous vein. *Dark gray,* intrafascial course; *light gray,* extrafascial course

Demonstration of the small saphenous cross by sonography
Linear 7-MHz transducer
Patient in the prone position
Avoidance of transducer pressure
Scans on transverse and longitudinal planes
Often the vein cannot be identified

Nissl 1973) to 4.2% (Gillot 1975) to as high as 12% (Kosinski 1926), although it is much rarer in our experience. The anomaly is important in operations for saphenous trunk varicosity.

For sonographic examination of the small saphenous vein, the patient is placed in the prone or lateral recumbent position. The vein is often so thin, however, that it is difficult or impossible to identify, and diagnostic uncertainty results. The main surgical concerns are its exact site of entry into the popliteal vein and, with varicose degeneration, the caliber of the vessel and the nature of its tortuosity so that it can be more easily distinguished from other veins in the popliteal fossa. Ultrasound usually cannot provide sufficiently detailed information.

Femoropopliteal Vein

Not named in older anatomic texts, the femoropopliteal vein has assumed practical interest with the development of modern venous surgery. It shows a number of variants relating to diverse patterns of embryologic development.

In the phylogenically oldest form, the small saphenous vein ascends from the foot to the proximal segment of the great saphenous vein, continuing on from there to the vessels of the torso. During development of the popliteal termination of the small saphenous vein, the intermediate segment in the thigh persists as the femoropopliteal vein. The variants derive from variations in

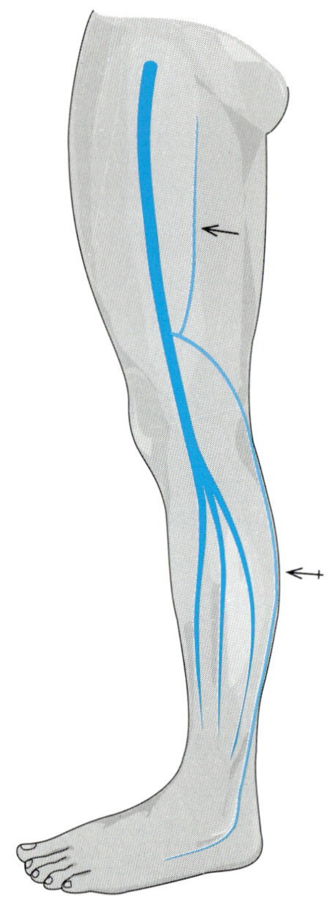

the mode of attachment of the vein to larger trunks proximally and distally.

As a side branch tributary of the small saphenous
trunk, the femoropopliteal vein descends intrafascially on the thigh to the popliteal fossa, where it 29
opens into the small saphenous vein. This variant 30
is the most common. Sometimes the *venous*
valves have an opposite arrangement, however, so
that flow is directed proximally from the small saphenous vein (Schobinger 1975).
Occasionally the small saphenous vein and femoropopliteal vein enter the popliteal vein at *se-* 30

◁

29. Femoropopliteal vein (→) and small saphenous vein (↔) with a common termination

30 a–e. Variations in the course and termination of the femoropopliteal vein (right leg). **a** Side-branch type. **b** Side-branch type with separate termination. **c** Side-branch type with Giacomini's anastomosis. **d** Integrated type with intrafascial course. **e** Integrated type with extrafascial course. *Dark gray,* intrafascial course; *light gray,* extrafascial course

▽

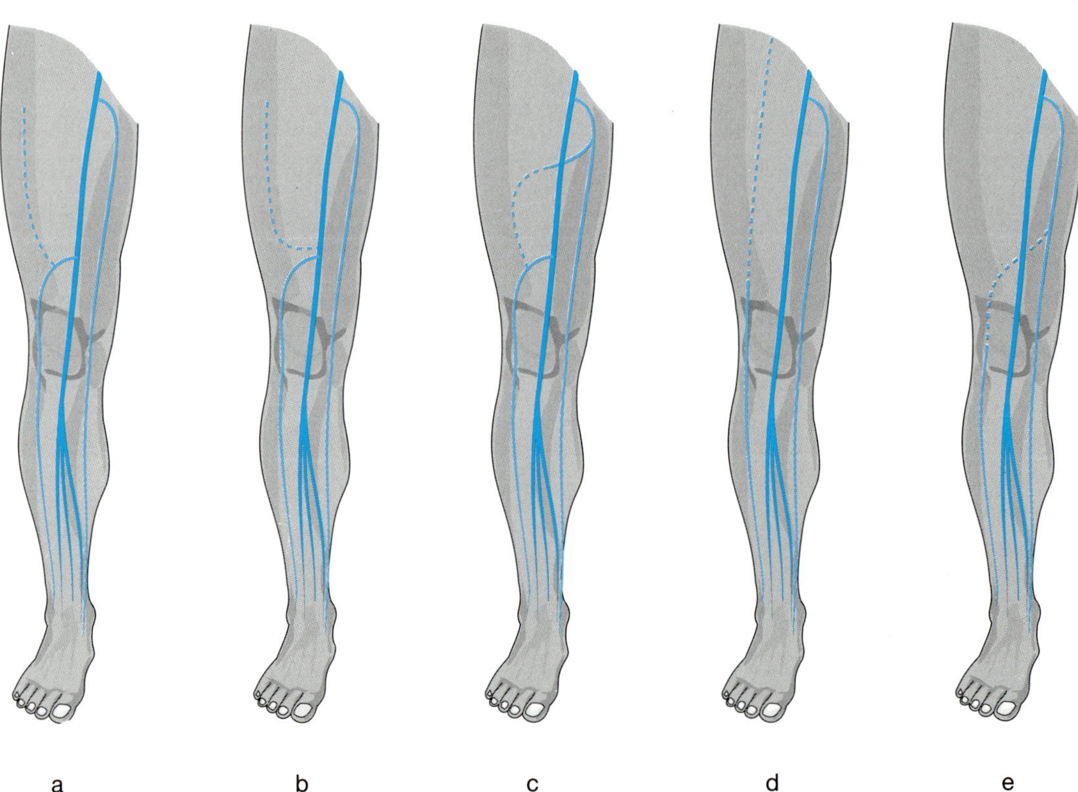

parate sites. Recognition of this variant is important preoperatively because the femoropopliteal vein is not accessible through the standard popliteal approach.

The femoropopliteal vein and medial accessory saphenous vein are sometimes linked by a hemo-
21 dynamically effective connection called ***Giacomi-***
30 ***ni's anastomosis*** (Giacomini 1873). This arrange-
31 ment reflects the embryonic relationship of the vessels. When the terminal valve of the small
177 saphenous vein is incompetent, an incomplete saphenous trunk varicosity of the great saphenous vein can develop via the femoropopliteal and medial accessory veins.

The side-branch type of femoropopliteal termination is
30 distinguished from the *integrated type* in which the vein persists as the femoral portion of an anomalous small saphenous trunk. This may be associated with an intrafascial iliac termination of the small saphenous vein or a high extrafascial union of the great and small saphenous veins.

Variants of the femoropopliteal vein	
Types	Roentgen characteristics
Side-branch type	Vessel caliber small, blood flow directed proximally or distally
Giacomini type	Vessel caliber small, blood flow usually directed peripherally, anastomosis with great saphenous vein
Integrated type	Clinically no separate vessel; directed proximally with - an anomalous iliac termination of the great saphenous vein - a high extrafascial connection of the short saphenous vein with the great saphenous vein

31. Giacomini's anastomosis (→), demonstrated incidentally by ascending pressure phlebography in the antegrade flow direction. ↔ Entrance of medial accessory saphenous vein into the great saphenous vein. External rotation view

Deep Leg Veins

Part of the deep venous system of the leg, the intrafascial trunks drain 90% of the venous blood from the lower extremity, and substantially more during exercise. The assessment of their radiographic morphology and function is of crucial importance in clinical medicine.

Deep Veins of the Lower Leg

The anterior tibial veins, posterior tibial veins,
and peroneal veins accompany their homony- 32
mous arteries within a vascular sheath. Each of
the three venous groups consists of one or two 33
vessels, and rarely of three.

The individual veins are easily identified on roentgenograms by *their positional relationship to the* 34
tibia and fibula. On the standard film with the

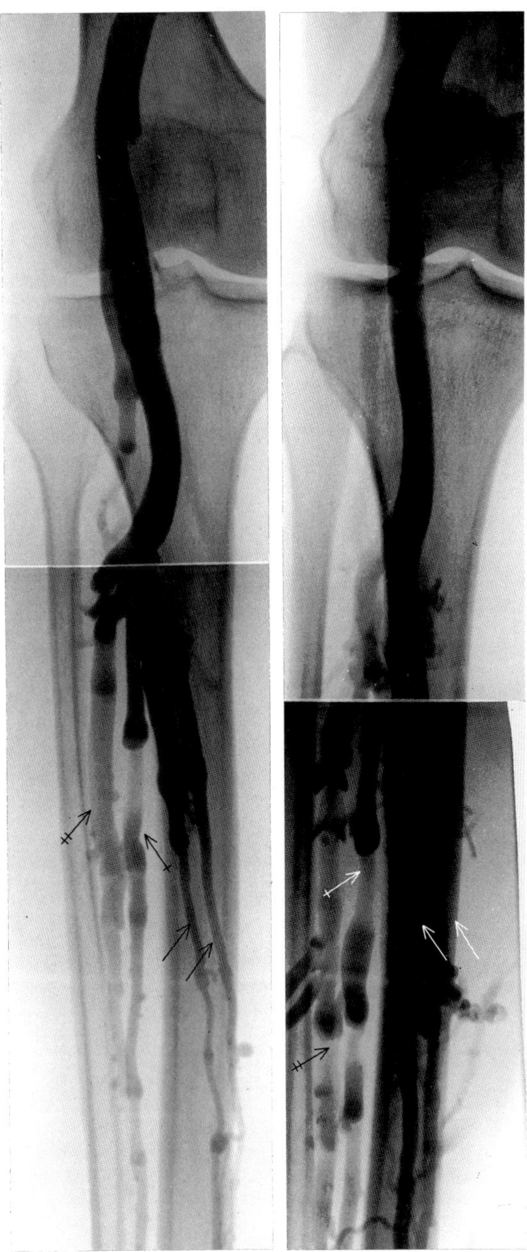

32 *(left).* Crural vessels. Entrance of the peroneal vein (+→) into one trunk of the paired posterior tibial vein (→). Anterior tibial veins (++→), of which only one trunk is filled proximally. Ascending pressure phlebography, internal rotation view

33 *(right).* Crural vessels. Entrance of the peroneal vein (+→) into the anterior tibial vein (++→). Posterior tibial veins (→) with cross-connections ("ladder sign"). Ascending pressure phlebography, internal rotation view

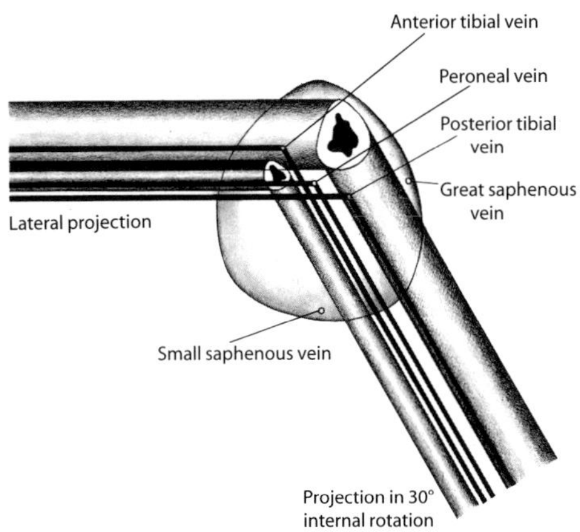

34. Projection of the crural vessels onto the skeletal system for various positions of the lower extremity. To find the topographic relationship of the venous trunks, the observer should turn the drawing so that the bones of the lower leg are pointing toward him. Any projection can be simulated by (mentally) sketching in other positions of the tibia and fibula and turning the picture accordingly. The loop indicates the approximate positions of the saphenous veins

limb internally rotated 30°, the posterior tibial veins overlie the tibia while the anterior tibial veins course just medial to the fibula. In the lateral view the anterior tibial veins overlie the tibia while the posterior tibial veins appear behind the tibia within the posterior soft tissues. The peroneal vein is projected between the other two venous groups. Thus, the posterior tibial veins always appear on the inside of the limb with respect to the trunk axis, while the anterior tibial veins appear on the outside. A knowledge of these topographic relationships permits rapid orientation during fluoroscopic observation. It should be stressed, however, that all the venous groups and trunks do not always spontaneously fill during phlebography; in such cases it is necessary to wait for the overflow effect.

The ***posterior tibial veins*** arise from the plantar 4,5
vein of the foot. They curve behind the medial malleolus as they ascend, so they become somewhat tortuous on plantar flexion of the foot. In the 32
lower leg they course between the deep and superficial plantar flexors, which are very active as muscles of locomotion and posture. This accounts for their importance in the calf muscle pump and the venous return to the heart. They receive numerous muscle veins and perforating veins as tributaries.

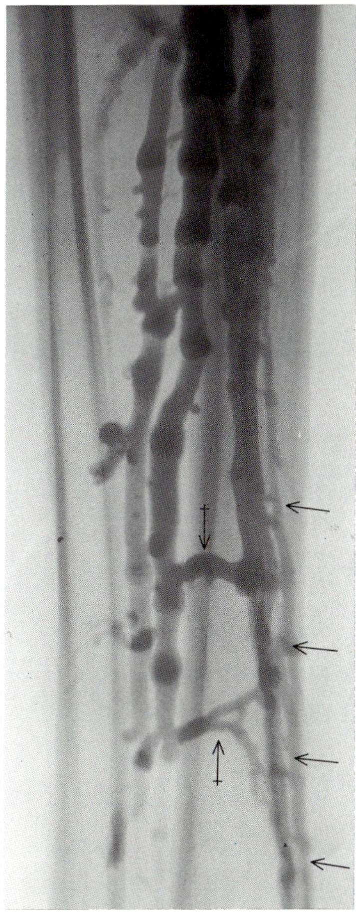

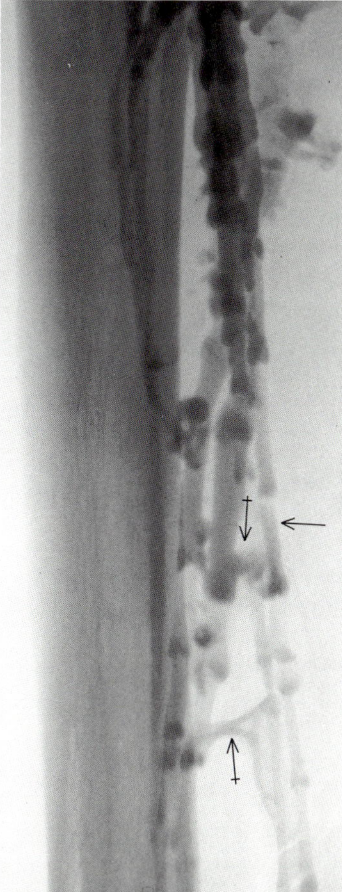

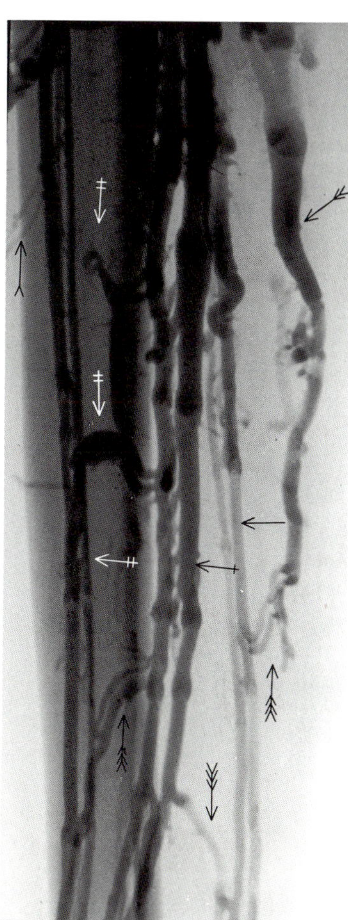

35 *(left, middle).* Rung veins (ladder sign) interconnecting the three trunks of the posterior tibial veins (→), also bridging veins between the posterior tibial veins and peroneal vein (+→). The distal vessel forms a reticulum. Ascending pressure phlebography, internal rotation (*left*) and lateral view (*middle*)

36 *(right).* Crural vessels: posterior tibial veins (→), paired peroneal veins (+→), anterior tibial veins (#→). >→ Perforating veins; »→ muscle veins; ⋙→ bridging veins

Demonstration of the deep venous system by ascending pressure phlebography
Puncture of the dorsal vein of the great toe
Ankle tourniquet
Patient in semiupright position
Leg relaxed and non-weight-bearing for contrast injection
Biplane spot films or delayed films
Valvular function tested by a Valsalva maneuver
Opacification of unfilled vessels by the overflow effect

The paired venous trunks that course with a vascular sheath are interconnected by oblique anastomotic vessels that on phlebograms resemble the
rungs of a ladder. We call this phenomenon the 35
ladder sign, and we call the vessels *rung veins.* 36
These small-caliber vessels can be important in
the development of secondary tibial vein incom- 217
petence (see p. 134) and the collateral circulation
evoked by post-thrombotic occlusion (see p. 179). 240
The ***anterior tibial veins*** originate from the dorsal veins of the foot. They receive small muscle veins from the extensor group and several perforating
veins. Often they merge proximally into a single 32
trunk identifiable by its curved course upon passage through the interosseous membrane. 60

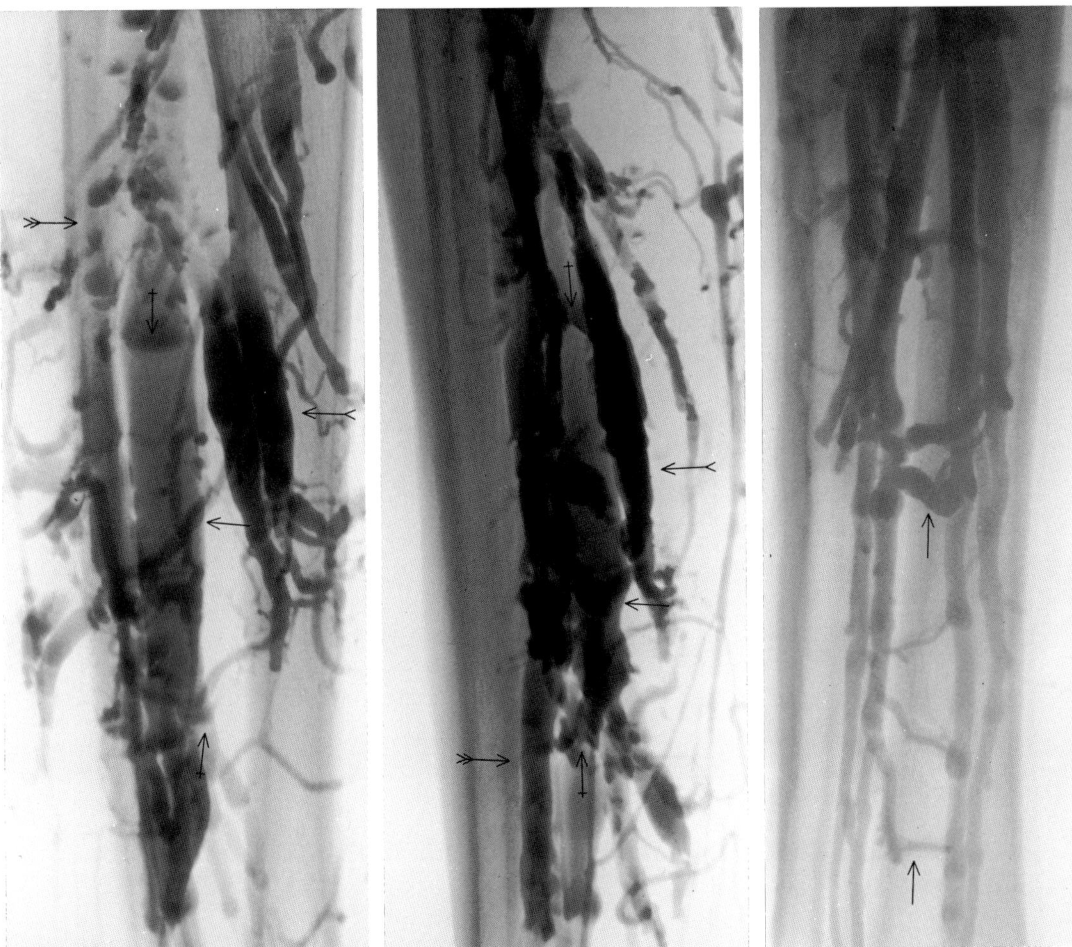

37 *(left, middle).* Regional physiologic ectasia of the peroneal vein (→), bounded by competent venous valves (↔). ↣ Soleus veins; ↠ anterior tibial veins. The posterior tibial veins are not shown. Ascending pressure phlebography, internal rotation (*left*) and lateral view (*middle*)

38 *(right).* Bridging veins (→) interconnecting the posterior tibial veins and the peroneal vein

The ***peroneal vein*** (fibular vein) arises from the most lateral region of the heel. Its tributaries are the perforating vessels and the vessels from the adjacent muscle group. Generally the peroneal vein is single, rarely paired, and it drains proximally into a posterior or anterior tibial vein.

The midportion of the peroneal vein displays a more or less pronounced *regional dilatation* (phlebectasia), which is bounded proximally and
37 distally by competent venous valves. This physiologic dilatation should not be mistaken for a pathologic change. It is so consistently present that it can serve the distinguish the peroneal vein from other vessels. It is not known whether the dilatation may occasionally cause congestive problems or predispose to thrombosis. The ectasia increases with aging and tends to develop regressive changes.

The three deep venous groups are interconnected
by transverse or oblique *bridging veins* of small 35
caliber. Their hemodynamic significance remains
unclear. They may have some role in the develop- 36
ment of the deep collateral circulation. We have 38, 212
detected bridging veins in 28% of subjects with a 281
healthy venous system. Rarely we found persistent
embryonic structures in the form of a plexus-like 39
arrangement of vessels.

The *valves* of the crural veins are spaced at relatively short intervals of 3–5 cm. This serves to distinguish them from the superficial veins, which possess fewer valves. The valves in the trunks of a particular venous group are sometimes located at the same level, which facilitates their identification.

Under normal circumstances the crural vessels usually cannot be positively identified by ***ultrasound examination.*** The duplex procedure offers considerable advantages. The vessels are poorly filled in the recumbent patient and disappear when the slightest transducer pressure is exerted on the calf.

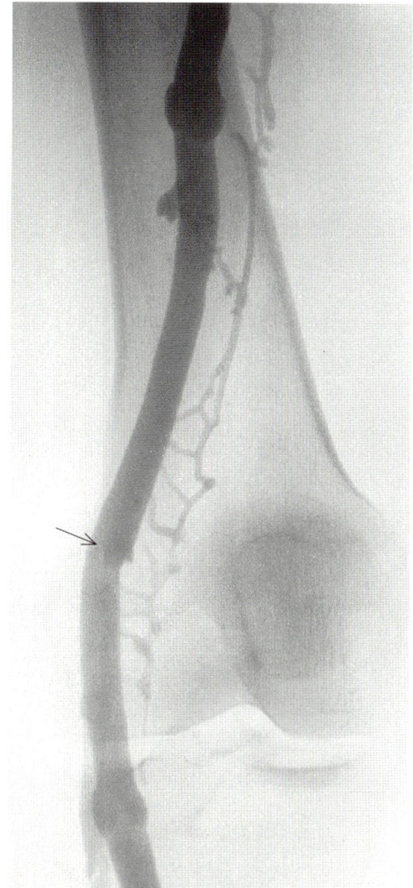

39. Structures of the embryonic vascular plexus alongside the popliteal vein. Competent terminal valve of the small saphenous vein (→)

Popliteal Vein

The popliteal vein is formed by the confluence of the anterior and posterior tibial veins at the distal border of the popliteus muscle, about a hand's width below the knee joint. Accompanying its artery through the popliteal fossa, the vein is flanked on both sides by the heads of the gastrocnemius muscle. Contraction of these muscles compresses
86 the vein to a narrow slit ("popliteal pump") and accelerates centripedal flow. Proximal to the adductor opening, the popliteal vein becomes the superficial femoral vein.

In some cases the deep veins of the lower leg are
27 *doubled or tripled* until they merge at or above the level of the knee joint. These variants play a significant role in the physical diagnosis of venous thrombosis. Doppler sonography and venous occlusion plethysmography are positive only when the vessel is completely occluded. Hence these studies will not detect thrombosis in a branch of the duplicated vessel.

Variations of the popliteal vein	
Origin distal to knee joint	63%
Origin at level of knee joint	15%
Doubled	20%
Tripled	2%

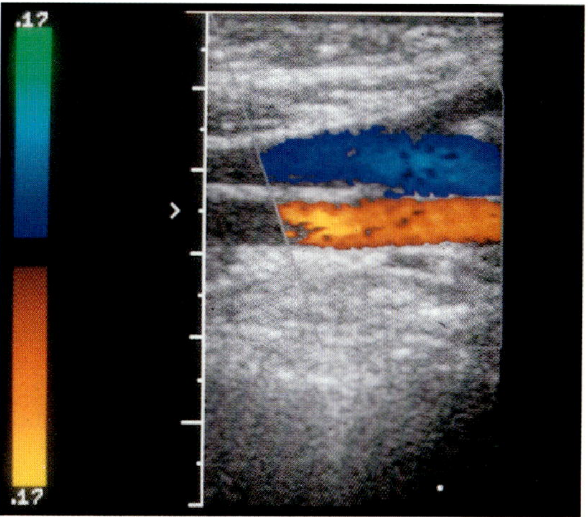

40. Popliteal vein and artery demonstrated by color-coded duplex sonography (Acuson, 7-MHz transducer). The centrifugal flow direction is set to *red* and the centripetal to *blue*

The *tributaries* of the popliteal vein are the small saphenous vein, several perforating veins, and vessels from the adjacent muscles. Generally the gastrocnemius veins drain into the popliteal vein 2–3 cm above the knee joint, entering just below the entrance of the small saphenous vein or termi-

Demonstration of the popliteal vein by sonography
Linear 7-MHz transducer
Patient in prone position
Avoidance of transducer pressure
Scans on transverse and longitudinal planes

nating more proximally in a common sinus with the small saphenous.

39 Occasionally, structures of the embryonic vascular plexus are seen in addition to the popliteal vein. They have no clinical significance.

40 The popliteal vein is plainly demonstrated by ***sonography***. The artery coursing lateral to the vein provides a landmark for identification. The patient is examined in the prone or lateral recumbent position with the leg muscles completely relaxed. Even duplication of the vessel is easily detected if both lumina are of sufficient size. The transition to the adductor canal can be more easily evaluated if the soft tissues are pressed against the head of the transducer manually.

Deep Veins of the Thigh

The ***superficial femoral vein*** begins at the level of the adductor canal as the continuation of the popliteal vein. It receives small tributaries from the adjacent muscles as well as several perforating veins of Dodd's group. It contains an average of one to three venous valves, never more than eight, whose cusps are arranged in a rotary pattern.

At the level of the adductor canal there is often a direct communication between the superficial femoral vein and the profunda femoris vein via the
41-43 ***distal femoral anastomosis***. The anastomosis may be solitary or multiple. The profunda femoris is distinguished from a duplicated superficial femoral vein by its longer course, its increasing proximal caliber, its more plentiful valves, and its many tributaries. With a circumscribed thrombosis in
278 the thigh, the deep femoral veins provide a
288 pathway for the development of a collateral circulation.

Our studies show that a distal femoral anastomosis is present in 1.1% of normal subjects and in 18% of patients with post-thrombotic syndrome. Netzer (1979) estimated a prevalence of 10%. Cockett (1955) observed numerous connecting veins in 72% of cases in his pa-

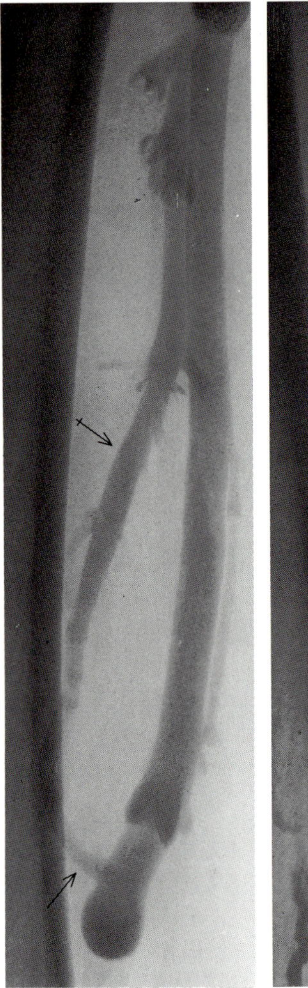

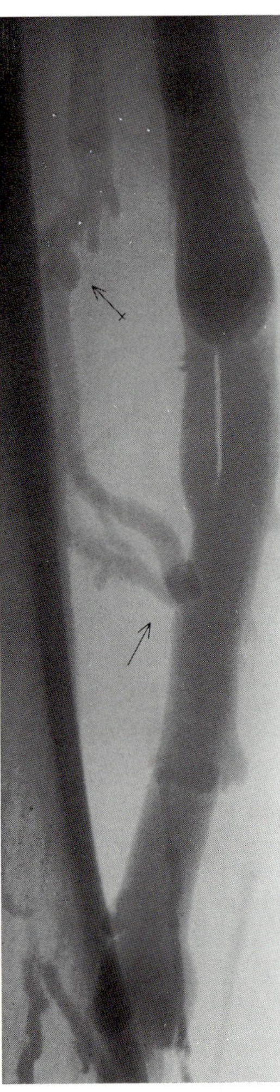

41 *(left).* Distal anastomosis (→) between the profunda femoris vein (↔) and superficial femoral vein. The lumen of the profunda is expanded proximally by numerous muscle vein tributaries, a typical finding

42 *(right).* Duplication of the distal anastomosis (→) between the profunda femoris (↔) and superficial femoral vein

thoanatomic studies, one or more larger veins in 12%, 43
and absence of an anastomosis in 16%.

A knowledge of the variations of the superficial femoral vein can be helpful in clinical phlebography, the most common variant being the presence of two or more trunks.

The trunk is duplicated in 21.2% of cases and is multi- 44
ple in 13.8% (May and Nissl 1973). In 2.78% of cases the 45
duplicated superficial femoral vein arises from a paired
popliteal vein. 52

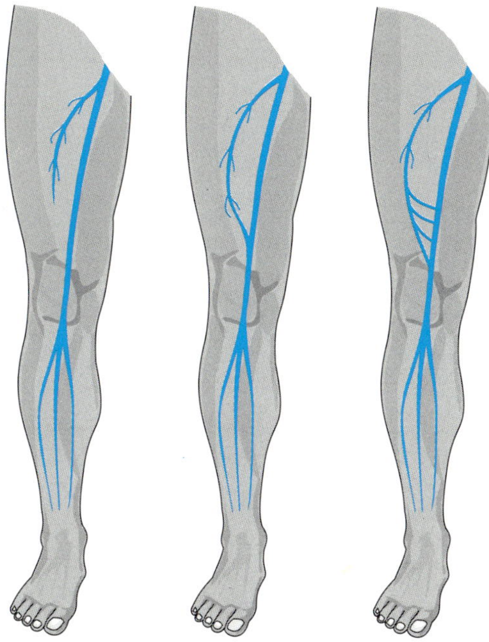

43. Variations of the distal femoral anastomosis. *Left,* no anastomosis; *middle,* single anastomosis; *right,* multiple anastomoses

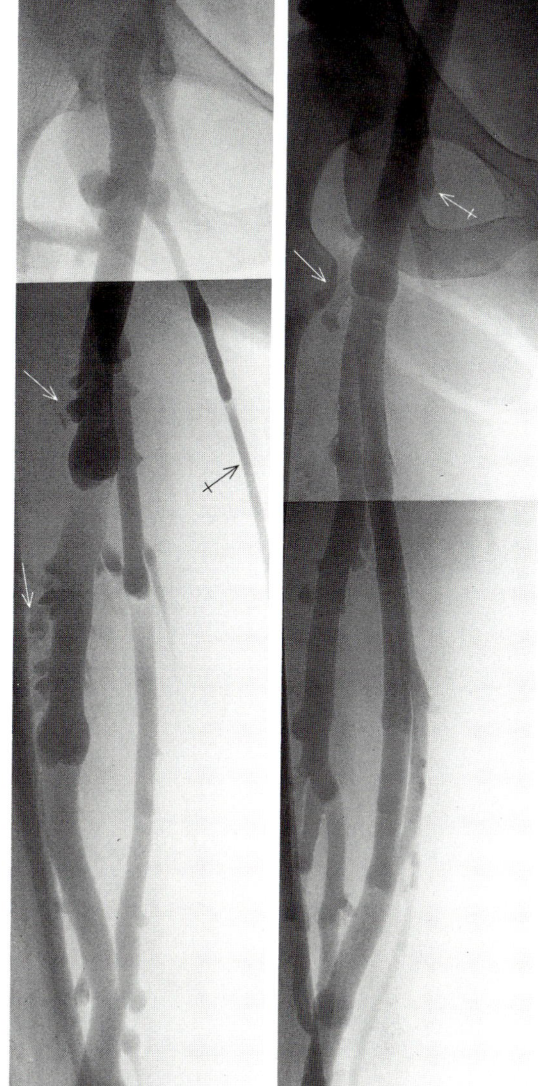

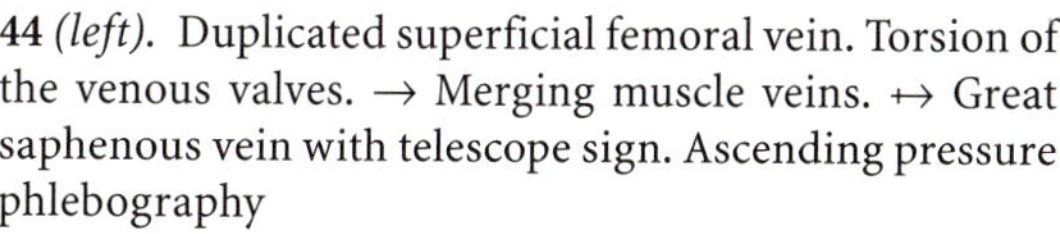

▷

44 *(left).* Duplicated superficial femoral vein. Torsion of the venous valves. → Merging muscle veins. ↔ Great saphenous vein with telescope sign. Ascending pressure phlebography

45 *(right).* Tripled superficial femoral vein. Merging muscle veins (→). Great saphenous vein with sluice valve and telescope sign (↔). Ascending pressure phlebography

Demonstration of the common femoral vein	
by	ascending pressure phlebography retrograde pressure phlebography digital subtraction phlebography

Demonstration of the deep thigh veins by sonography
Linear 7-MHz transducer
Patient in flat supine position
Slight external rotation of the lower limb
Avoidance of transducer pressure
Scans on transverse and longitudinal planes

The superficial and deep femoral veins, which are counted among the muscle veins, converge a hand's width below the inguinal ligament to form
the common femoral vein. The pelvic veins com- 46
mence above the inguinal ligament with the external iliac vein.

The ***common femoral vein*** ascends on the medial side of the homonymous artery and is usually valveless, although it may contain one or two valves.
It receives the great saphenous vein as a tributary 9
at the saphenous opening. Possible variations in the arrangement of the subinguinal venous confluence were previously discussed (see p. 10). 10
The superficial and common femoral veins are
plainly demonstrated by ***sonography.*** The patient 47

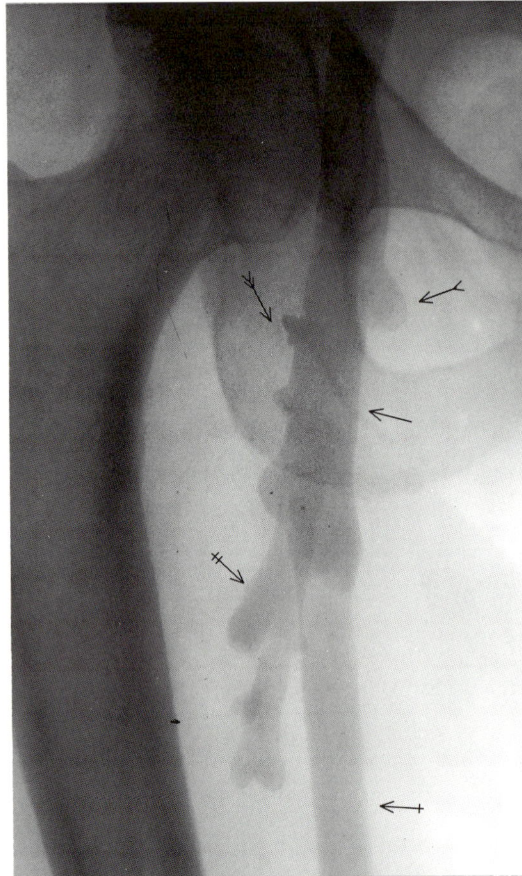

46. Common femoral vein (→) and subinguinal venous confluence. ↦ Superficial femoral vein, ⇸ profunda femoris vein, ↣ terminal valve of great saphenous vein, ⤖ superficial circumflex iliac vein. Ascending pressure phlebography

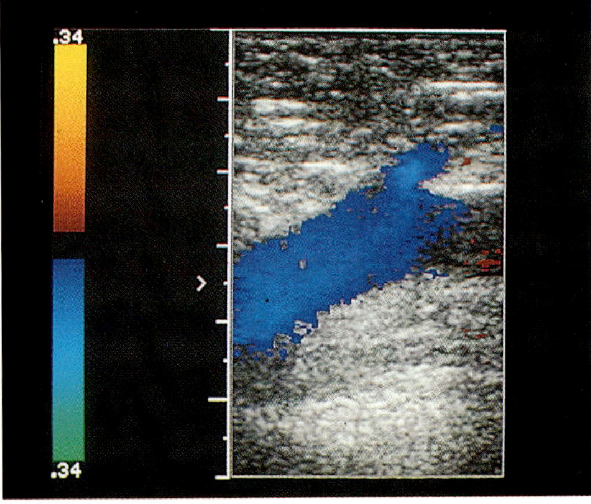

47. Left common femoral vein demonstrated by color-coded duplex sonography (Acuson, 7-MHz transducer). *Top*, cross-section of the terminal region of the competent great saphenous vein. Arteries in *red* and veins in *blue*. *Bottom*, longitudinal section

lies in a relaxed supine position or stands, with a slight external rotation of the lower limb. Towards to adductor canal it is better to bring the soft tissues to the head of the transducer than vice versa.

Perforating Veins

The superficial veins are separated from the deep veins by the large fascial planes of the leg – the fascia lata, crural fascia, and pedal fascia. The perforating veins establish connections between the superficial and deep venous systems.

Formerly a distinction was drawn between communicating veins and perforating veins according to whether they drained into main stem veins or muscle veins. Lanz and Wachsmuth (1972) and Staubesand (1980) speak of deep anastomoses. These anatomic distinctions have no clinical significance, however, so the term *perforating veins* has come to be applied in phlebography to all transfascial connecting vessels.

Proper names are commonly used in phlebographic practice to designate specific perforating 48
veins. For scientific purposes, the nomenclature of 49
van Limborgh (1965) can be used.

Based on anatomic studies, the *number* of perforating veins is estimated to be 95 venous groups (van Limborgh 1965) or 150 individual vessels (Schäfer 1981) in each lower extremity, with 47–55 occurring in the lower leg. An average of only four, or at most 12, paired perforating veins are visualized during ascending phlebography of the crural region. This results from nonuniform drainage conditions in the different vessels and is more or less a random phenomenon. But when a perforating vein becomes incompetent and its blood flow is reversed, the likelihood of its spontaneous opacification increases to 70 %.

According to anatomic descriptions, the perforating veins present numerous *variations* in their
50 course and pattern of branching (Pirner 1957), although these variations are not demonstrated by roentgen examination. The phlebographic appearance of competent perforating veins appears to be quite uniform.

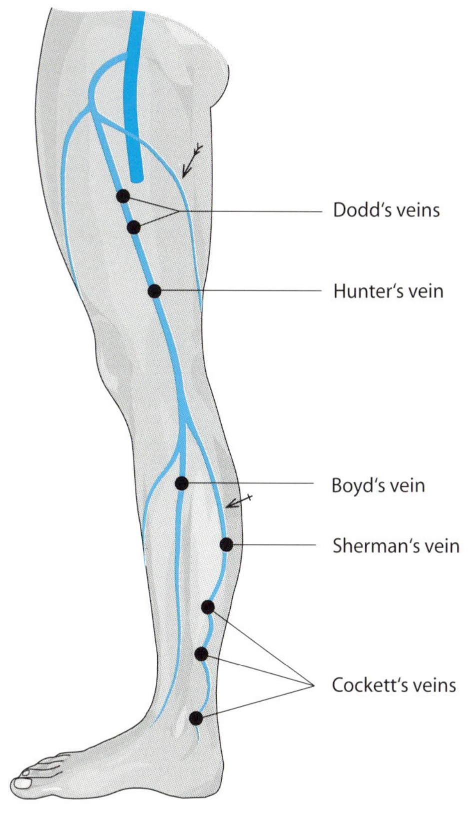

▷

48. Extrafascial veins and sites of the most important perforating veins on the medial side of the lower limb +→. ⪢→ Medical accessory saphenus vein

49. Competent perforating veins in the lower leg. → Upper Cockett's veins, +→ Sherman's veins, ++→ Boyd's veins, +++→ lateral perforating veins. Incidental finding during ascending pressure phlebography, internal rotation view (*left*), close-up view (*right*)

▽

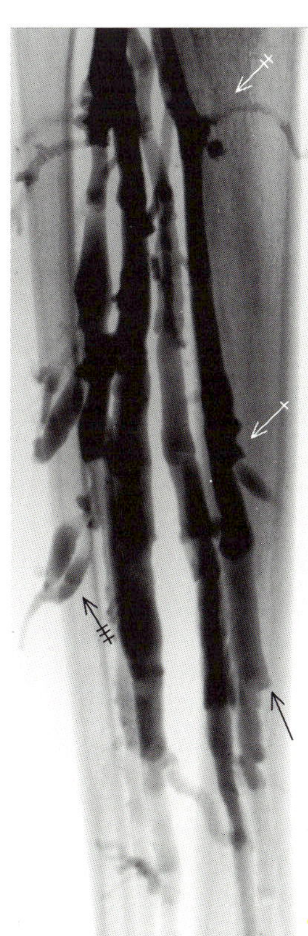

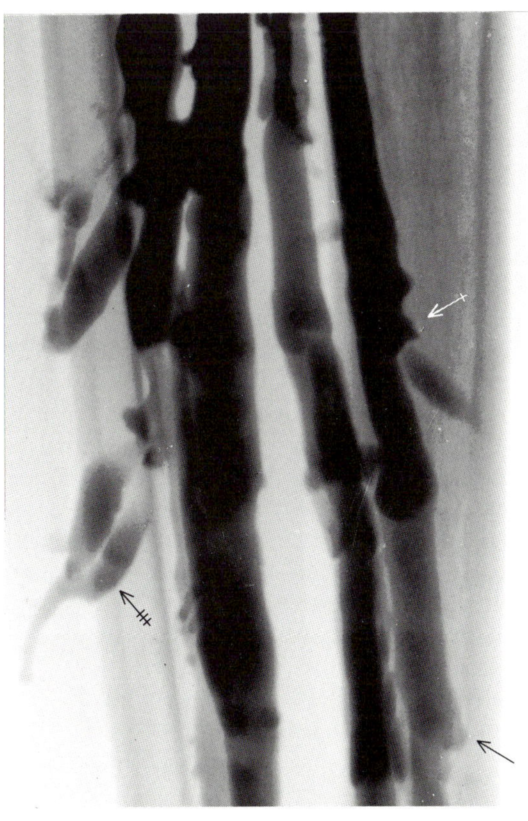

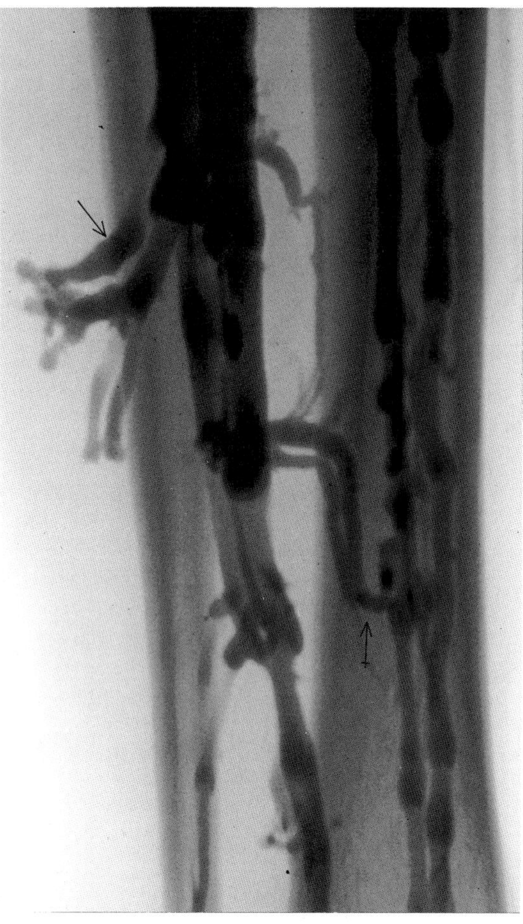
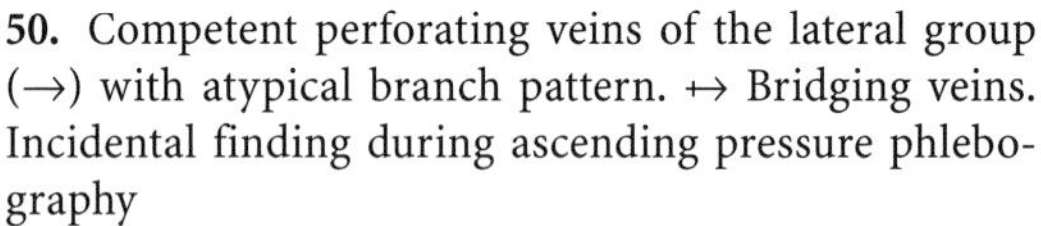

50. Competent perforating veins of the lateral group (→) with atypical branch pattern. ↔ Bridging veins. Incidental finding during ascending pressure phlebography

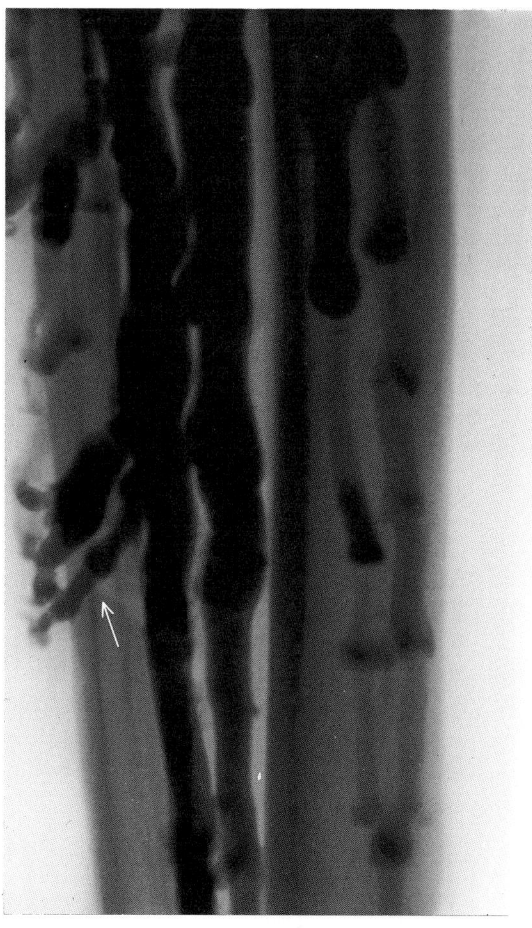

51. Competent perforating veins of the lateral group; → anomaly with three venous valves

The *valvular arrangement* and intravascular pressure gradients in the perforating veins are such that the veins permit blood flow only toward the deep veins. In the region of the foot and popliteal fossa, the perforating veins are valveless and thus permit flow in the opposite direction.

All the perforating veins in the lower leg are *paired*, although a meticulous search may be needed to locate the twin vessel. At its entrance into the deep venous system, the competent perforating vein contains an inward-directed valve that per-
210 mits only a *stump-like opacification* of the vessel
in the presence of retrograde flow. Often, however, the connecting veins are more fully opacified and a pair of subfascial venous valves can be
51 identified (Pirner 1957). In rare cases three valves
are discerned. The segment of vein between the
valves usually shows a *fusiform dilatation* with a 49
maximum diameter of 9 mm and *smooth contours*. The paired arrangement and fusiform 52
shape are not characteristic of Dodd's veins,
which are sometimes observed to communicate 67
with muscle veins. The perforating veins are distinguished by their small caliber and their *oblique ascending course* to the deep trunk, which they enter at an angle that averages 29° and is always less than 60° (Hach 1981). The fascial opening traversed by the vein is usually located at an intermuscular septum but sometimes is directly over the muscle.

Before piercing the fascia, the perforating veins sometimes describe a small *S-shaped* loop, the
purpose of which is to prevent kinking or stretch- 52
ing of the vein when the skin and subcutaneous

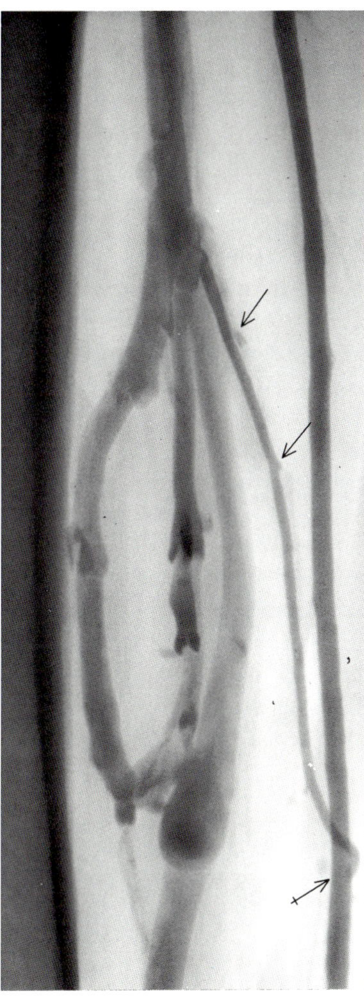

52. Competent Dodd's vein with small muscle vessels (→). Note the loop at the origin from the great saphenous vein (↔). The superficial femoral vein is tripled

Roentgen signs indicating competence of the perforating veins in the lower leg during ascending pressure phlebography
Paired arrangement
Ascends to deep trunk, entering it at <60° angle
Fusiform (spindle) shape
Identifiable venous valves
Smooth outer contours
Antegrade blood flow

tissues shift relative to the fascia during body movements (Gullmo 1964).

Slight retrograde (peripherally directed) contrast filling of the perforating vein and its extrafascial parent vessel should not be interpreted as signifying insufficiency when all other criteria of functional competence are noted. Only a *consistent* reversal of blood flow will cause morphologic distortion of the vessel, which will then display typical radiographic features (see p. 130).

Fusiform expansion and retrograde flow in a competent perforating vein can be explained in terms of the "critical opening and closure phenomenon" of Burton (1961). According to this concept, the vessel can function incompetently even in the absence of pathoanatomic changes. The maximum wall distention produced in a main deep trunk by a retrograde pressure wave is transmitted to the terminal segment of the perforating vein and renders its terminal valve unable to close (*critical opening*). The reflux wave can now enter the vessel and dilate it until the outer venous valve opens as well. The wave flows out into the superficial venous system, and the valves in the perforating vein close (*critical closure*). However, if the diameter of the superficial vein is smaller than the expanded perforating vein and its elastic modulus is greater, the *critical opening pressure* for the superficial veins is not reached. The reflux wave will remain confined to the perforating vessel, distending it like a balloon.

Of the numerous perforating veins in the thigh and lower leg, only a few have clinical significance. They are named after the physicians who studied them.

Of greatest interest to the clinician are ***Cockett's veins***, which are three in number according to anatomic studies. Incompetence of the middle or upper vein – especially when associated with pathologic changes in the deep venous system – underlies the development of chronic venous insufficiency.

The *lower Cockett vein* is adjacent to the medial malleolus and connects the great saphenous vein or a superficial tributary with the posterior tibial veins. It appears to have little clinical significance and rarely fills spontaneously on phlebograms.

Middle Cockett's vein is a collective term applied to a group of three paired veins. The anterior, middle, and posterior vessels can be differentiated clinically and intraoperatively (based on the topography of the muscular septa) but not phlebographically.

The anterior vessel lies directly on the periosteum of the posterior tibial surface, while the middle vessel runs

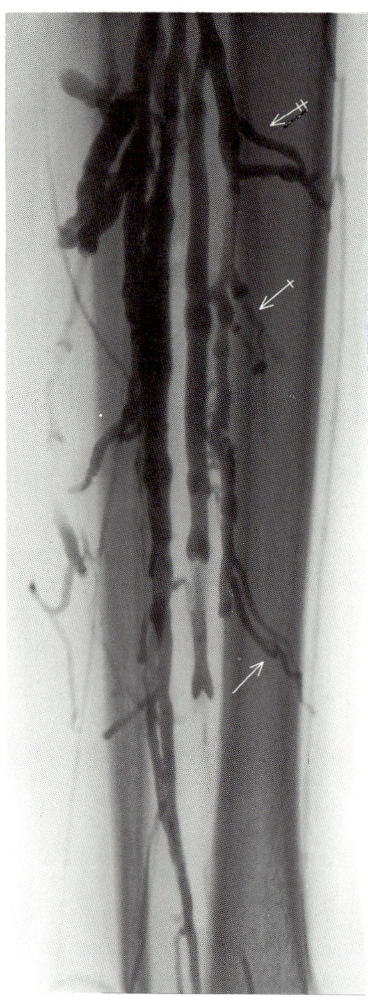

53. Competent perforating veins in the lower leg. Upper Cockett's veins (→) drains directly into the great saphenous vein; +→ Sherman's venous group, ++→ Boyd's veins

past the intermuscular septum. The posterior vein runs obliquely through the muscle; it is distinguished by its longer and slightly tortuous course, which is beneficial in the event of incompetence, as retrograde jet effects have already been slowed down by the time they reach the skin.

53 The anatomy of the *upper Cockett's venous group*
is similar, except that we have never found posterior vessels at operation. The anterior and middle veins are of major clinical importance, however. A topographic differential diagnosis is beyond the capabilities of phlebography.

The upper and middle venous groups usually connect the posterior arch vein with the posterior tibial veins, although in some cases they arise from the great saphenous trunk. The projection of the so-called fascial gaps
on the skin corresponds to the imaginary projection 209
lines (see p. 130).

A fourth group, ***Sherman's veins***, are located at ab- 53
out the middle of the lower leg. These vessels project onto the middle projection line (see p. 130). They are of less practical importance than the upper and middle groups of Cockett's veins.

Formerly, Cockett's and Sherman's veins were designated in terms of their distance from the sole of the heel, i. e., as the 7-cm, 13.5-cm, 18.5-cm, and 24-cm perforating veins. The anatomic studies of Staubesand (1987) refuted this dogma, also weakening the rationale for using a centimeter rule on radiographs.

The ***lateral perforating veins*** (Dodd and Cockett 1956) are posterolateral vessels connecting a side branch of the great saphenous vein with the anterior tibial veins or gastrocnemius veins, passing deeply on an intermuscular septum at the boundary of the middle and distal thirds of the tibia.

May's vein is a perforating vein connecting the 54
small saphenous vein with the gastrocnemius
veins at the midcalf level (gastrocnemius point). 55

Demonstration of competent perforating veins by combined ascending pressure phlebography and noncompression phlebography
Puncture of the dorsal vein of the great toe
Ankle tourniquet
Patient in semiupright position
Leg relaxed and non-weight-bearing for contrast injection
Tourniquet released
Reinjection of contrast medium (noncompression phlebography)
Manual direction of the contrast medium
Biplane spot films

The ***midcrural veins*** (Green et al. 1958) connec- 56
ting the anterior arch vein with the anterior tibial veins enter the intrafascial space on the anterolateral side of the lower leg between the tibialis anterior and extensor digitorum longus muscles. A lower, middle, and upper group have been identified (Fegan 1967).

Boyd's vein courses between the great saphenous 48
vein and the posterior tibial vein a hand's width 57
below the knee joint on the medial side of the calf.

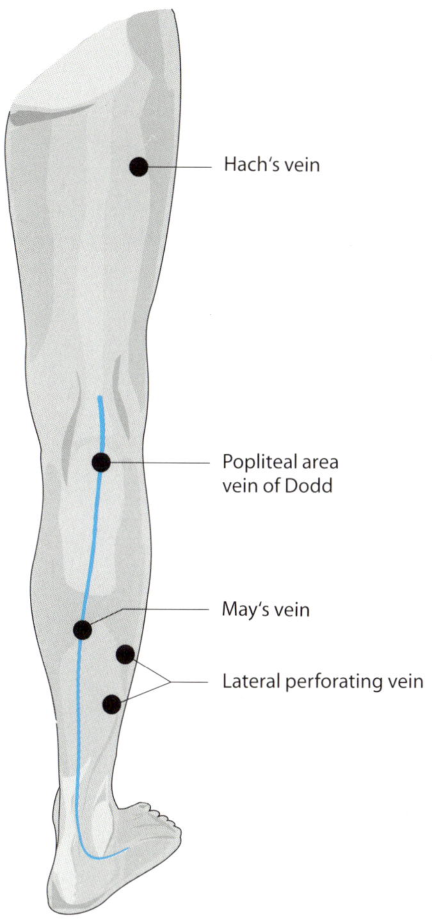

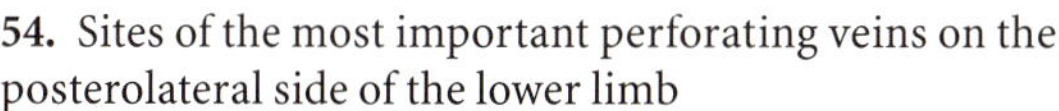

54. Sites of the most important perforating veins on the posterolateral side of the lower limb

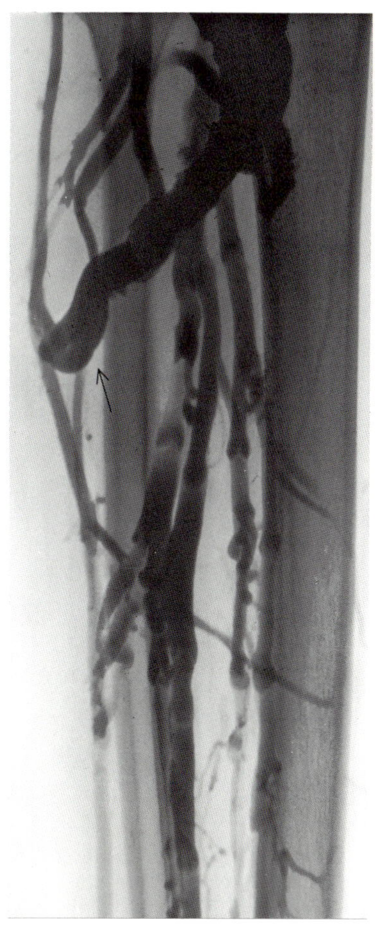

55. Competent May's perforating vein (→) connecting the small saphenous vein with the gastrocnemius veins, which show regressive changes

8 ***Dodd's venous group*** consists of three to five pair-
48 ed or single vessels coursing between the great
saphenous vein and superficial femoral vein in the
48 lower third of the thigh. *Hunter's perforating vein*
is at the level of the adductor canal.
54 The ***popliteal area vein*** of Dodd connects superficial vessels with the poplieal vein at the center of
the popliteal fossa.
54 The ***profunda perforating vein,*** first investigated
59 by us using varicography (Hach 1985), is the most
proximal of the perforating veins. This posterolateral thigh vessel drains blood from the extrafascial veins into the profunda femoris vein (see p. 136).

Muscle Veins

The muscle veins are regarded as a separate group owing to the special hemodynamic function that is associated with muscular exertion. The muscle
veins are clearly demonstrated by spot radio-
graphs. They differ from other veins in their 68
numerous, closely spaced valves and the rapid expansion of their vascular trunk by many small tributaries.
The ***soleus veins*** enter the peroneal vein by one, 60
two or three trunks in the middle third of the lower leg. Perforating veins connect them with the superficial venous system, most notably the small saphenous vein and its tributaries. Frequently there are connections between the distal end of the soleus vein and the posterior tibial veins. These connections are established by bridging

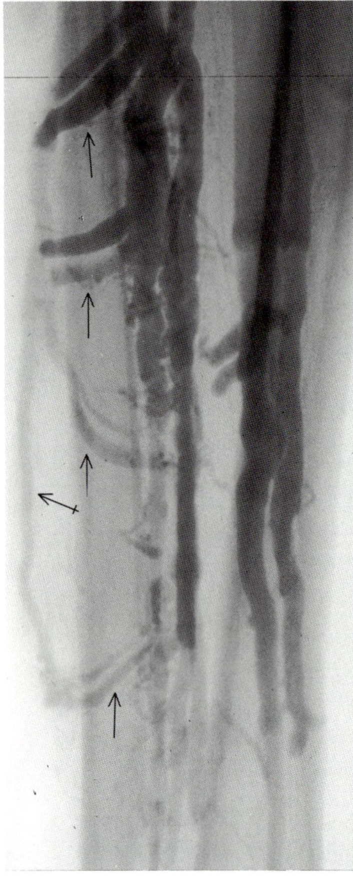
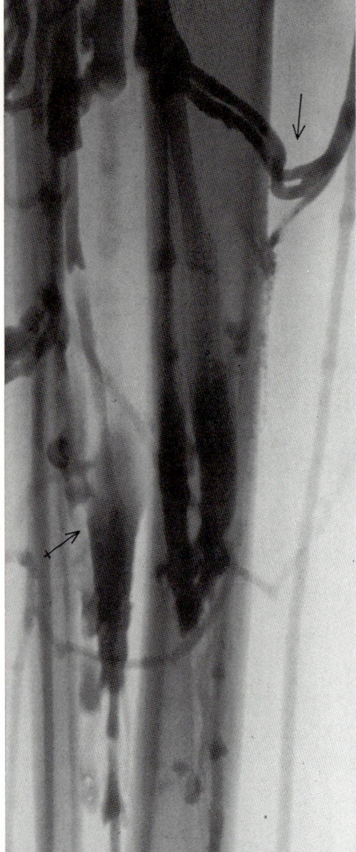
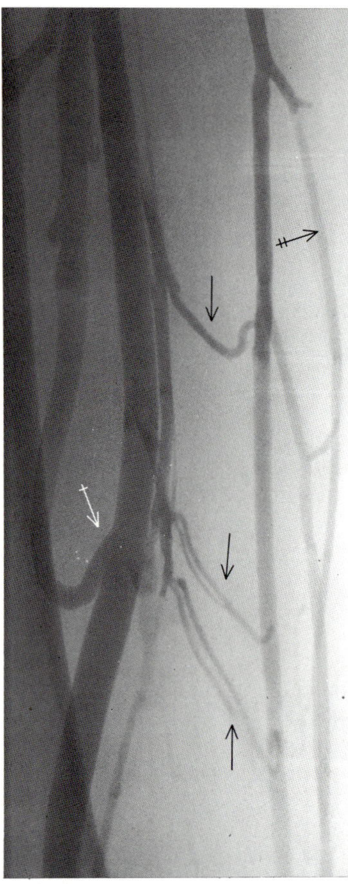

56 *(left).* Midcrural veins, perforating veins of the anterolateral group (→) that connect the anterior arch vein (↔) with the anterior tibial veins. Ascending pressure phlebography and strong internal rotation

57 *(middle).* Competent Boyd's vein (→) connecting the great saphenous vein and posterior tibial veins. Regional ectasia of the peroneal vein (↔)

58 *(right).* Perforating veins of Dodd's group (→). A distal femoral anastomosis (↔) is incidentally shown. The great saphenous vein (⇸) is multiple

62 veins that carry a proximally directed flow. The
61 soleus veins are best appreciated on a lateral film.
62 They are opacified by retrograde settling and
overflow of contrast medium with the patient relaxed and semiupright on a steeply tilted table. By about 25–30 years of age the veins begin to develop *regressive changes* characterized by irre-
362 gular dilatation and tortuosity with a decrease in
the number and competence of the valves. Sites of
363 pronounced fusiform dilatation look like varices
("muscle varices") and can cause congestive problems.

Real-time sonography poorly demonstrates normal muscle veins. Severe regressive changes in the soleus veins with marked luminal enlargement can sometimes be detected in the prone patient

Demonstration of the muscle veins by ascending phlebography
Puncture of the dorsal vein of the great toe
Ankle tourniquet
Patient inclined 30°–60°
Leg relaxed and non-weight-bearing for contrast injection
Manual direction of the contrast medium
Utilization of overflow effect
Internal-rotation and lateral spot films

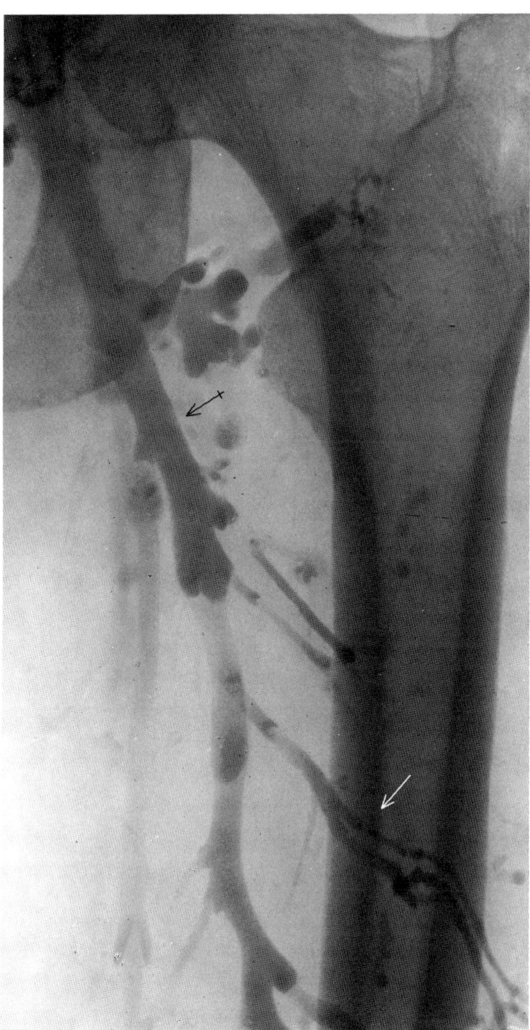

59. Competent profunda perforating vein of Hach (→) connecting lateral thigh veins with the profunda femoris vein. Incidental finding during ascending pressure phlebography in a 35-year-old woman with post-thrombotic syndrome of the leg and pelvic veins

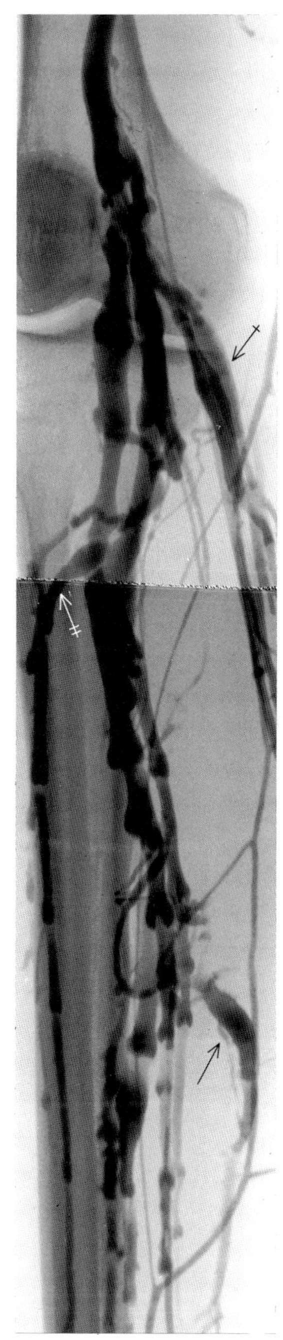

60. Soleus veins (→) and gastrocnemius veins (+→). The paired popliteal vein each empty into a separate anterior tibial venous trunk through a curved terminal segment (++→). Ascending pressure phlebography, lateral view

when the transducer is placed on the skin without pressure.

The ***gastrocnemius veins*** enter the popliteal vein by a common trunk 2–3 cm above the knee joint.
24 Usually there are two vessels in each muscle head,
25 sometimes several. The veins in the medial head are often somewhat larger than in the lateral head, and they display better contrast filling. The
63 gastrocnemius veins are distinguished from the small saphenous vein on lateral views chiefly by
64 their valvular density, which decreases proximally, and on internal-rotation views by their oblique medial-to-lateral, distal-to-proximal course.

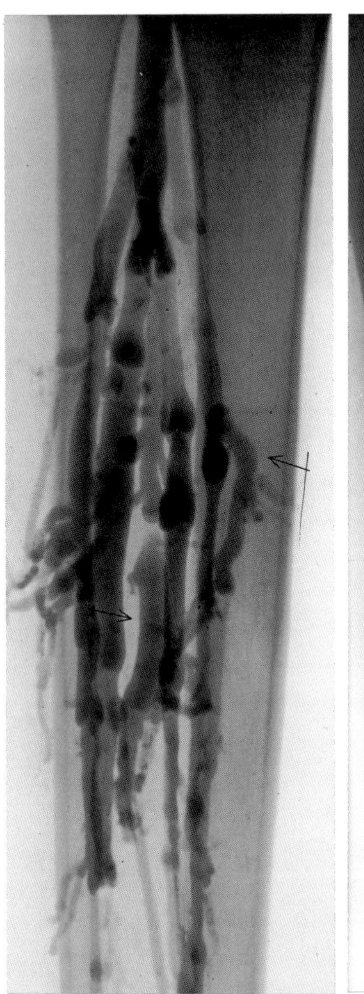

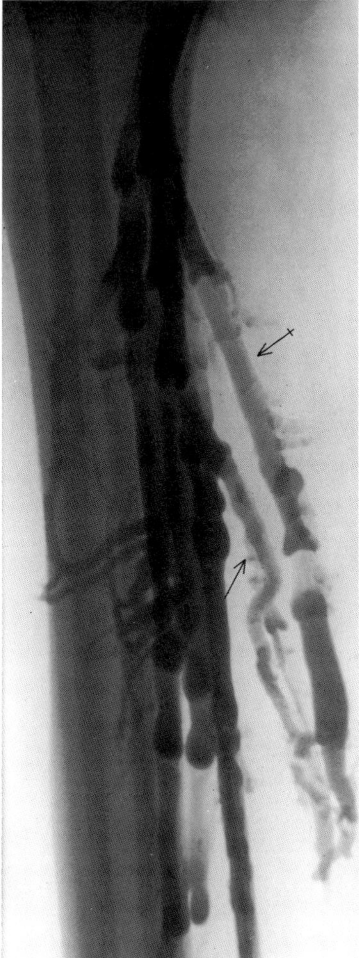

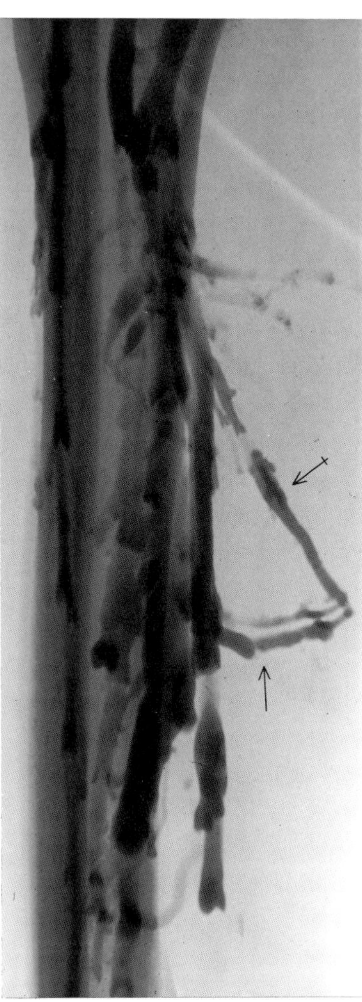

61 *(left, middle).* Soleus veins. The lower vessel opens into the posterior tibial vein (→) and the upper vessel (↔) into the peroneal vein, recognized by its mild physiologic ectasia. Ascending pressure phlebography, internal rotation (*left*) and lateral view (*middle*)

62 *(right).* Bridging veins (→) connecting the posterior tibial vein and soleus veins (↔), demonstrated by ascending pressure phlebography

May's perforating vein at the midcalf level connects
the small saphenous vein with the gastrocnemius
55 veins. Its projection onto the skin corresponds
roughly to the static "gastrocnemius point," or the
attachment of the Achilles tendon to the two heads
219 of the gastrocnemius muscle. Incompetence of the
perforating vein can lead to isolated varicosity in
this area and in rare cases to incomplete varicosity
of the small saphenous trunk.

The gastrocnemius veins, too, frequently undergo
361 severe regressive changes with fusiform dilata-
364 tions and a reduction in valve number. This condition is easily mistaken for varicosity of the small
saphenous trunk.

The ***vastus medialis muscle*** veins are sometimes 65
demonstrated in the distal thigh by ascending
phlebography. They have a tufted appearance and 66
drain directly into the superficial femoral vein, the 67
profunda femoris, or one of Dodd's perforating
veins.

The ***profunda femoris vein*** is included among the
muscle veins of the thigh. It drains blood from the 68
adductors and flexors and a portion of the exten-
sors. Like all muscle veins it is more densely valved than the main stem veins, and its trunk shows a
rapidly expanding caliber due to its numerous
tributaries. In 1.1% of patients with a competent
venous system, an anastomosis with the superfici-

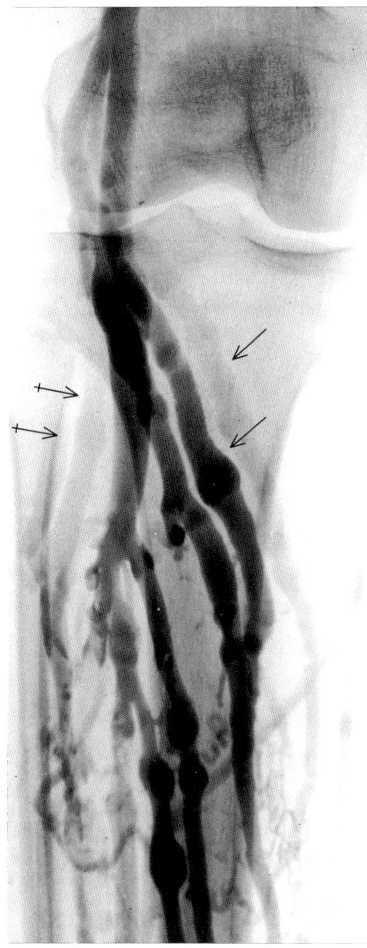

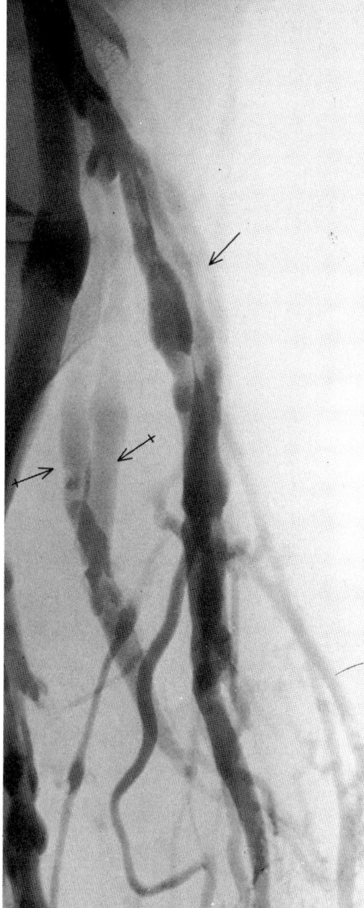

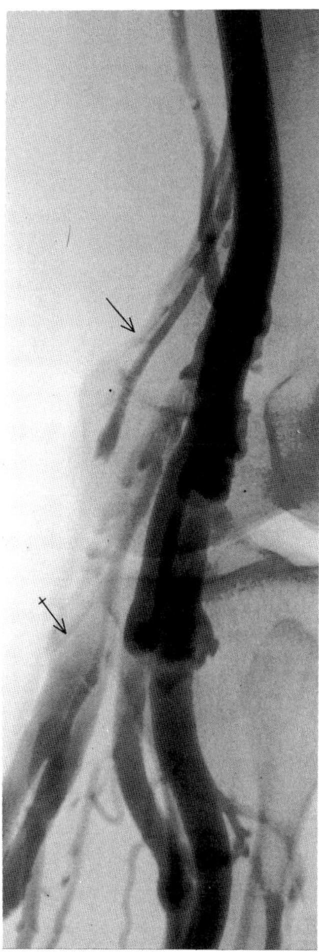

63 *(left, middle).* Gastrocnemius veins with a common termination in the popliteal vein. The vessels of the medial gastrocnemius (→) are larger and better opacified than those of the lateral head (↔). Ascending pressure phlebography, internal rotation (*left*) and lateral view (*middle*)

64 *(right).* Separate terminations of the small saphenous vein (→) and gastrocnemius veins (↔) in the popliteal vein. The vessels are distinguished by their luminal size and number of valves

al femoral vein, the *distal femoral anastomosis*
41 (see p. 24) can be demonstrated at the level of the adductor canal.
The profunda femoris is not usually demonstrated
43 by ascending phlebography. Sometimes its proximal segment is opacified by a retrograde overflow
46, 288 effect. Conditions are most favorable when contrast medium can enter the profunda system
59 through a distal femoral anastomosis.
There are several connections on the lateral side of the proximal thigh which drain blood directly from the extrafascial vessels to the profunda femoris. These are the profunda perforating veins described by the authors. A typical syndrome can
222 result from varicose degeneration of these vessels (see p. 136). Under normal conditions they are not demonstrated by phlebography.

References

Burton AC (1961) Hemodynamics and the physics of the circulation. Med Physiol Biophys 18: 643

Cockett FB (1955) Venous ulcers of the leg. Brit J Surg 43: 260

Dodd H, Cockett FB (1956) The pathology and surgery of veins of the lower limb. Livingstone, Edinburgh

Fegan WG (1967) Varicose veins. Heinemann, London

Giacomini C (1873) Osservazioni anatomiche per servire allo studio della circulazione venosa dell estremita inferiore Parte I–III. Giornale R Acad Med (Torino) 1: 109

Gillot C (1975) Die intraoperative Phlebographie der V. sa-

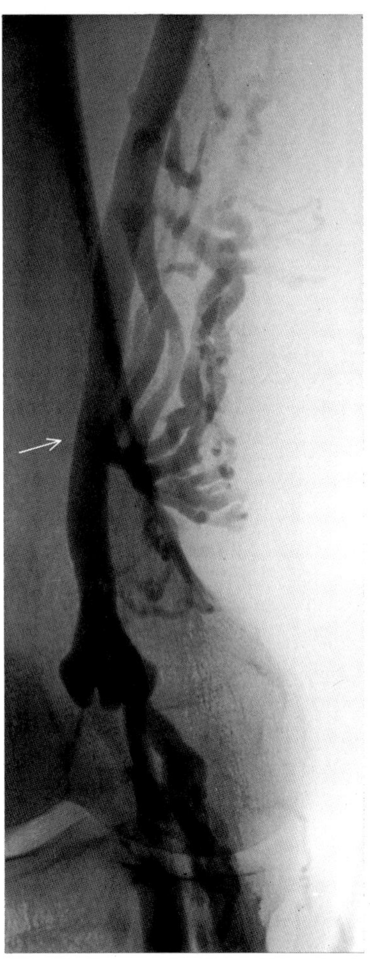

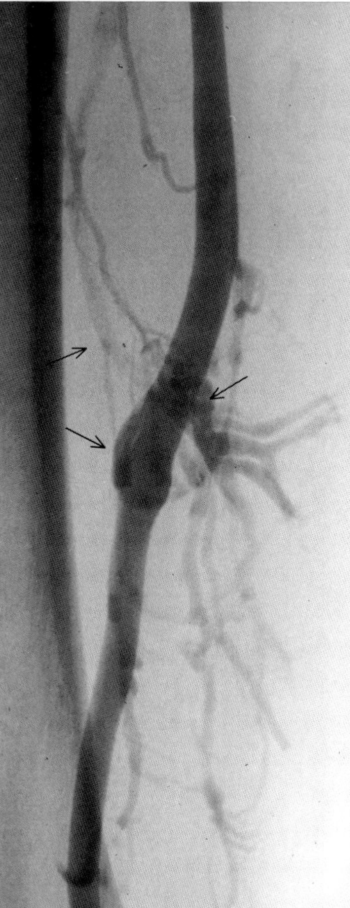

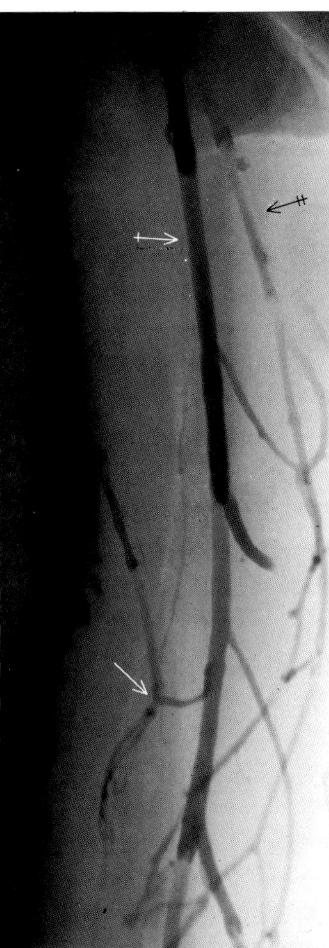

65 *(left).* Vastus medialis muscle veins enter the superficial femoral vein by a common trunk (→). Incidental finding during ascending pressure phlebography

66 *(middle).* Some vastus medialis veins enter the superficial femoral vein (→) by large trunks, others drain directly into the profunda femoris (↔). Incidental finding during ascending pressure phlebography

67 *(right).* Vastus medialis veins (→) entering Dodd's perforating vein. ↔ Great saphenous vein, ↮ medial accessory saphenous vein. Incidental finding during ascending pressure phlebography

phena parva. In: Brunner U (Hrsg) Die Kniekehle. Huber, Bern

Green NA, Griffiths JD, Lavy GA (1958) Venous drainage of anterior tibio-fibular compartment of the leg, with reference to varicose veins. Brit Med J 1: 1209

Gullmo AL (1964) Phlebographie der peripheren Venen. In: Diethelm L (Hrsg) Röntgendiagnostik des Herzens und der Gefäße. Springer, Berlin Göttingen Heidelberg New York (Handbuch der medizinischen Radiologie, Bd X/3)

Hach W (1981) Spezielle Diagnostik der primären Varikose. Demeter, Gräfelfing

Hach W (1985) Die Varikose der Profunda-Perforans – ein typisches phlebologisches Krankheitsbild. Vasa 14: 155

Haeger K (1962) The surgical anatomy of the saphenous-popliteal functions. Cardiovasc Surg 3: 420

Jecht EW (1983) Crosse oder Krosse; zur Etymologie des Wortes. Phlebol Proktol 12: 64

Kosinski G (1926) Observations on the superficial venous system of the lower extremity. J Anat 60: 131

Lanz T von, Wachsmuth W (1972) Praktische Anatomie I/4. Bein und Statik. Springer, Berlin Heidelberg New York

Limborgh J van (1965) Anatomie der Venae communicantes. Zbl Phlebol 4: 268

May R, Nissl R (1973) Die Phlebographie der unteren Extremität. Thieme, Stuttgart

Moosmann A, Hartwell Jr W (1964) The surgical significance of the subfascial course of the lesser saphenous vein. Surg Gynec Obstet 118: 761

Netzer CO (1979) Anatomie. In: Ehringer H, Fischer H, Netzer CO, Schmutzler R, Zeitler E (Hrsg) Venöse Abflußstörungen. Enke, Stuttgart

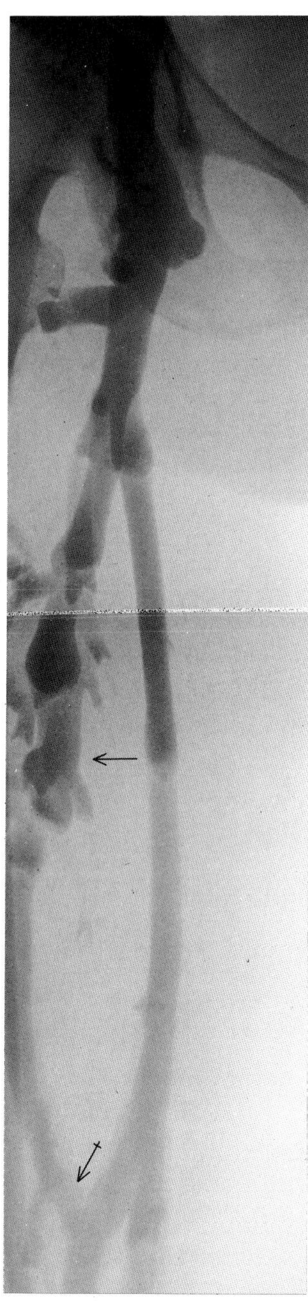

68. Profunda femoris vein (→), filled spontaneously through a distal femoral anastomosis (↔) during ascending pressure phlebography. The vein is distinguished by its rapidly increasing caliber and its numerous valves and tributaries

Pirner F (1957) Der variköse Symptomenkomplex. Enke, Stuttgart

Schäfer K (1981) Verlauf, Fasziendurchtritte und Einteilung der Vv. perforantes. In: May R, Partsch H, Staubesand J (Hrsg) Venae perforantes. Urban & Schwarzenberg, München

Schobinger RA (1975) Bedeutung einer persistierenden V. femoropoplitea. In: Brunner U (Hrsg) Die Kniekehle. Huber, Bern

Sherman RS (1949) Varicose veins, further findings based on anatomic and surgical dissections. Ann Surg 130: 218

Staubesand J (1980) Anmerkungen zur vaskulären Anatomie der Knöchelregion. In: Brunner U (Hrsg) Die Knöchelregion. Huber, Bern

Staubesand J (1987) Kleiner Atlas zur systematischen und topographischen Anatomie der Venae perforantes. In: Cockett F, Klüken N (Hrsg) Die klinische Bedeutung der Venae perforantes. Schattauer, Stuttgart

Extraperitoneal Venous Systems of the Pelvis and Abdomen

A comprehensive assessment of venous hemodynamics in the lower extremity should include visualization of the venous systems of the pelvis and retroperitoneum.

Pelvic Veins

The pelvic veins commence above the inguinal li- 69
gament with the ***external iliac vein,*** the continuation of the common femoral vein. At first the vein is medial to the external iliac artery. On the right, it is crossed by the artery a hand's width above the
inguinal ligament, and this can sometimes pro- 70
duce a slight indentation.

An important tributary of the external iliac vein is the *deep circumflex iliac vein,* which runs along the iliac crest and anastomoses with the lumbar veins.

The external iliac vein unites with the internal
iliac vein to form the ***common iliac vein,*** which lies 69
above and behind the homonymous artery. At the 385
level of the fifth lumbar vertebra, it joins with the
opposite common iliac vein to form the inferior 71
vena cava. Shortly before its termination, the common iliac vein receives the ascending lumbar vein, which enters the common iliac from above; it is one of the valveless vessels of the paravertebral system. Just before it ends in the inferior vena cava, the left common iliac vein shows a band-shaped
lucency (see p. 244) caused by indentation by the 74

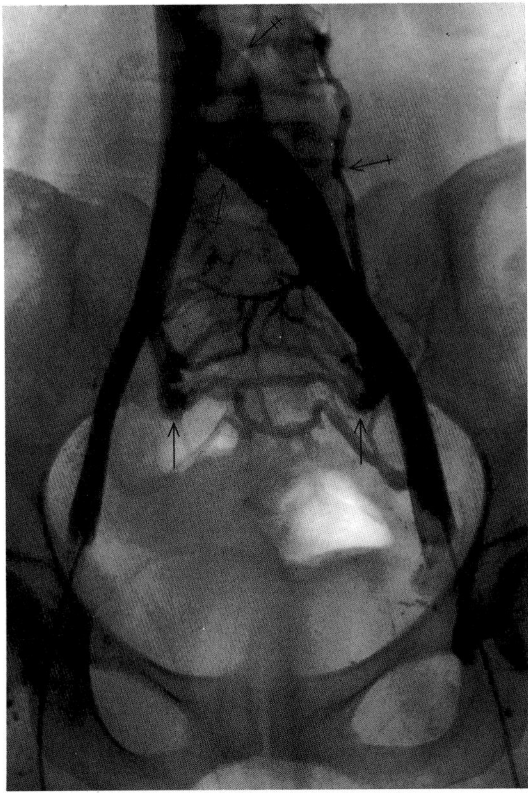

69. Pelvic veins demonstrated by pelvic phlebography using the Seldinger technique. → Internal iliac vein and presacral plexus, ↦ ascending lumbar vein, ⇸ compression of left common iliac vein by right common iliac artery

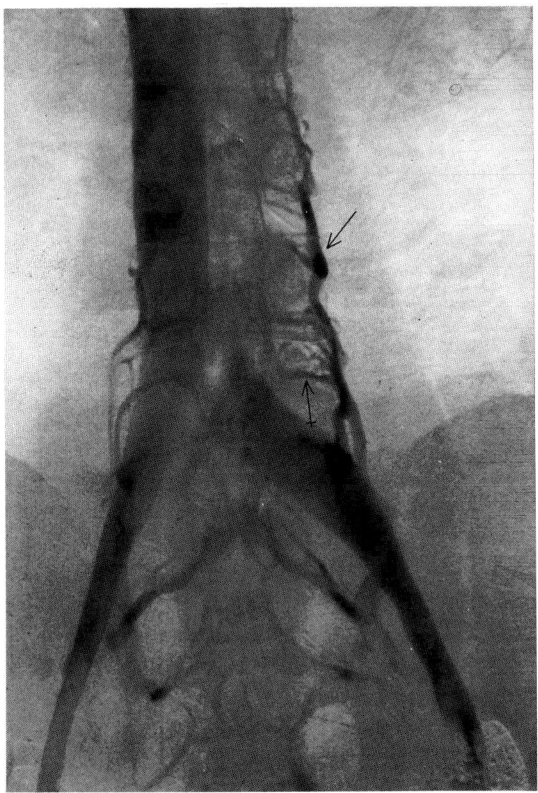

71. Inferior vena cava and paravertebral veins in the lumbar region, demonstrated by pelvic phlebography with the Seldinger technique and photographic subtraction. → Ascending lumbar vein, ↦ lumbar veins

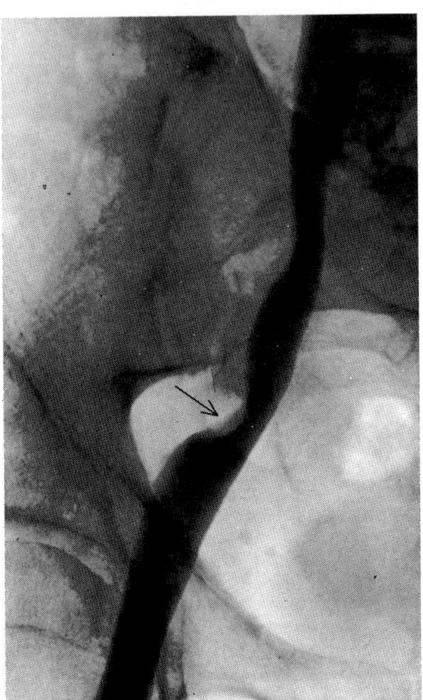

70. Arterial impression (→) of the right external iliac vein

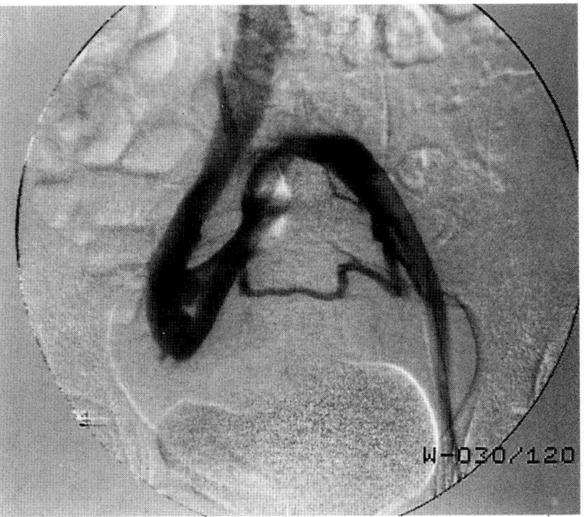

72. Agenesis or atresia of the left common iliac vein in a 52-year-old woman, demonstrated by digital subtraction phlebography

385 right common iliac artery. An intravascular spur
72 is often present at that site.
73 The ***internal iliac vein*** drains the capacious venous plexus of the pelvic organs. Its trunk is 3–7 cm long. In projection, its union with the external iliac vein is level with or caudal to the sacroiliac
74 joint. The principal anomalies are entry of the right internal iliac vein into the left pelvic veins and vice versa.

Five groups of veins drain into the internal iliac trunk. The *sacral veins* form an anastomotic network with the opposite side. The internal iliac receives *visceral veins* from the rectum, bladder, vagina, and uterus. Its most caudal tributaries are the obturator veins, the internal pudendal veins at the level of the femoral head, and farther laterally the glutal veins.

To a degree, the territory of the internal iliac vein
293 is already within the province of special organ anatomy and pathology. Owing to its numerous anastomoses with the opposite side, it can figure prominently in the development of collateral
294 pathways following occlusion of the common iliac vein and inferior vena cava.
75 ***Sonography*** can delineate the external and common iliac veins in thin patients, and the terminal portion of the internal iliac vein can usually be evaluated. The value of the study is limited by obesity and intra-abdominal gas.

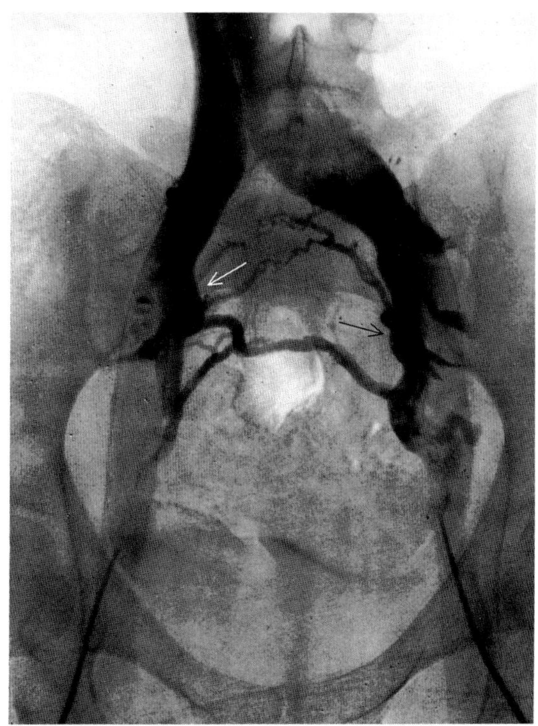

73. Internal iliac vein (→) and presacral anastomoses, demonstrated by pelvic phlebography using the Seldinger technique

Inferior Vena Cava

On the right the inferior vena cava ascends in front of the vertebral column to the vena caval aperture of the diaphragm. Its tributaries are the renal and adrenal veins, the right ovarian vein, the hepatic veins, and several parietal vessels. It communicates with the vertebral plexuses through the segmentally disposed lumbar veins. The inferior vena cava does not contain valves.

Ultrasound is useful for assessing both the morphology and function of the inferior vena cava.
76 The vessel can be traced from its bifurcation to the diaphragm. The entry points of the renal and hepatic veins can be identified. Normal hemodynamics is confirmed by demonstration of the typical "double stroke phenomenon."

The *ontogenic development* of the inferior vena cava from paired vessels accounts for the diversity of anatomic variants and anomalies. The paired cardinal veins are formed in the third week of embryonic develop-

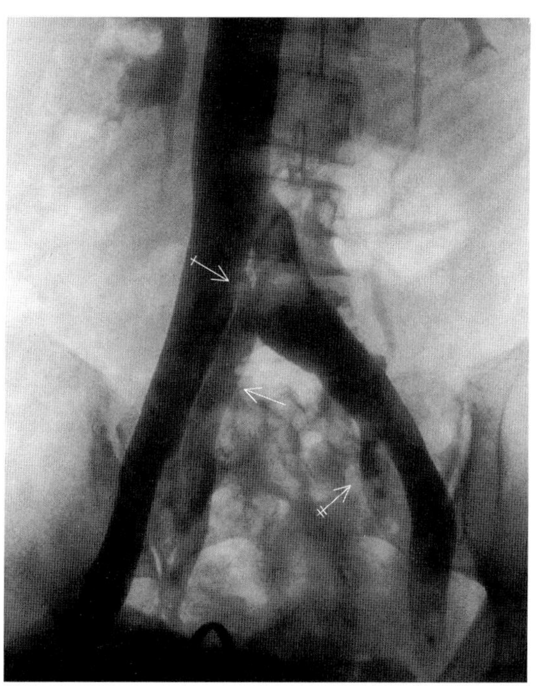

74. Anomalous entry of the right internal iliac vein (→) into the left common iliac vein. ↔ Pelvic venous spur, ⇸ left internal iliac vein

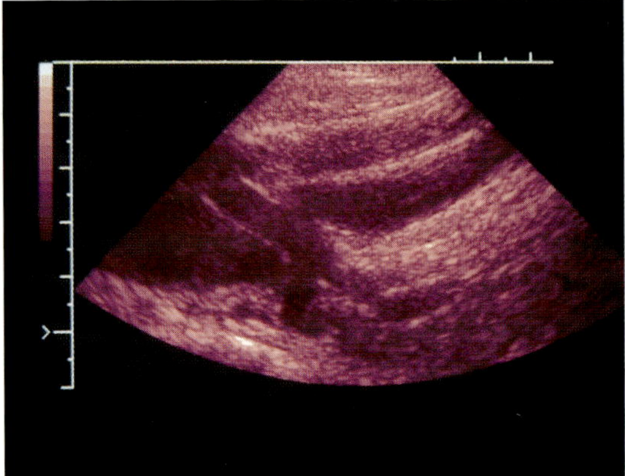

75. External and common iliac veins at the level of the junction of the internal iliac vein, demonstrated by real-time sonography with color coding. Accompanying arteries above the veins in each case. (Acuson, 3.5-MHz sector transducer)

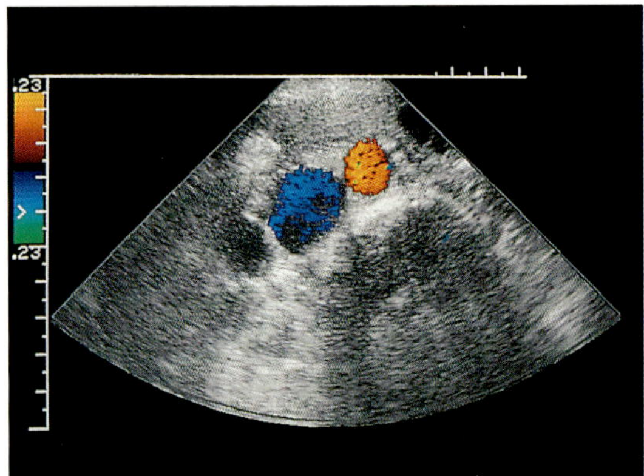

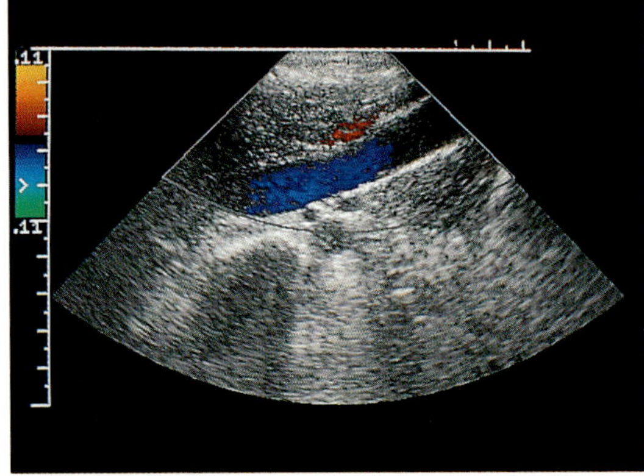

76. Cross-section of the abdominal aorta and inferior vena cava (*top*) and longitudinal section of the inferior vena cava (*bottom*), demonstrated by color-coded duplex sonography. (Acuson, 3-MHz sector transducer)

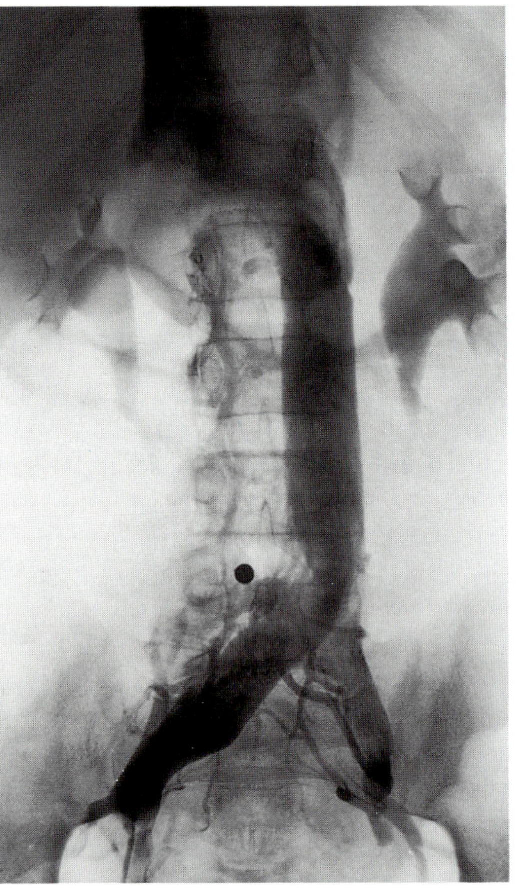

77. Infrarenal leftward inferior vena cava. (By courtesy of Prof. J. Weber, Hamburg)

ment, followed shortly thereafter by the subcardinal veins. Various segments then fuse to form the unpaired vena cava. Most anomalies result from an isolated error or arrest of development. The most common is duplication of the infrarenal caval segment, with an incidence
of 1% (Luzsa 1972) to 3% (Milloy et al. 1962). The inci- 77
dence of a left-sided inferior vena cava is approximately 0.2% (Luzsa 1972).

Vertebral and Paravertebral Venous Systems

The veins of the vertebral column form *external* 78
and internal vertebral venous plexuses (Clemens 1961). The external venous plexuses are located in front of the vertebral body (anterior external plexuses) and also behind the ligamentum flavum that bounds the vertebral canal posteriorly (posterior external plexuses). The capacious internal venous plexuses show an essentially vertical ar-

Demonstration of the pelvic veins and inferior vena cava
By pelvic phlebography or digital subtraction angiography (DSA)
Puncture of the femoral vein
Manual injection of contrast medium
Serial angiography or DSA
By ascending phlebography
Puncture of the dorsal vein of the great toe on each side
Ankle tourniquet
Patient in horizontal position
Bilateral injection of 50 ml contrast medium
Manuál direction of contrast medium into the pelvic region
Spot films
Photographic or digital subtraction

rangement along the anterior and posterior walls of the vertebral canal (anterior and posterior internal plexuses). The venous plexuses form a functional unit with the paravertebral system through the segmentally arranged lumbar veins in the lumbar region and through the intercostal veins in the thoracic region.

The paravertebral system includes the two
79 ***ascending lumbar veins,*** longitudinal vessels that lie upon the transverse processes adjacent to the vertebral column. They drain into the common iliac veins at their lower end. They also communicate with the sacral venous plexus, the portal vein, and the visceral plexuses. Cranially the ascending lumbar vein joins the subcostal vein and enters the thorax as the ***azygos vein*** on the right, and as the
315 ***hemiazygos vein*** on the left. At the level of the 12th thoracic vertebra the vessels turn forward and ascend on the anterior side of the vertebral bodies. The hemiazygos and accessory hemiazygos veins enter the azygos vein jointly or by separate trunks, the azygos vein in turn entering the superior vena cava from behind. The azygos system also receives numerous tributaries from the organs of the posterior mediastinum. A detailed description of its radiographic anatomy may be found in Bücheler (1971).

In 24% of cases the azygos vein contains competent valves, which regress with aging and cease to be demonstrable on phlebograms (Bücheler 1971). The vertebral plexuses and the paravertebral vessels are devoid of valves and permit drai-

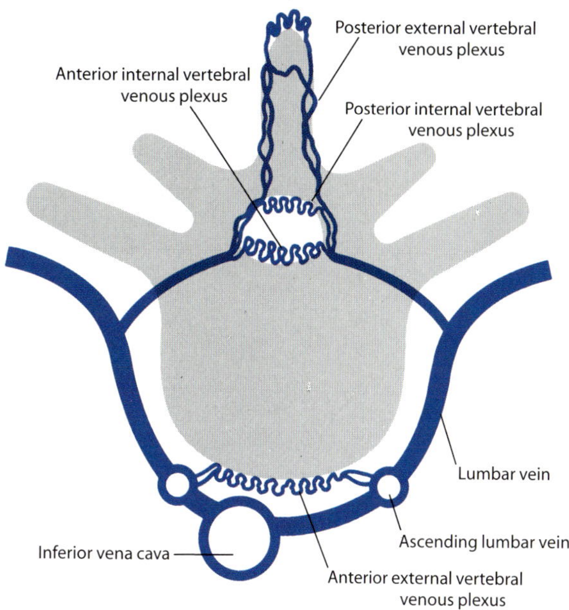

78. Vertebral plexus

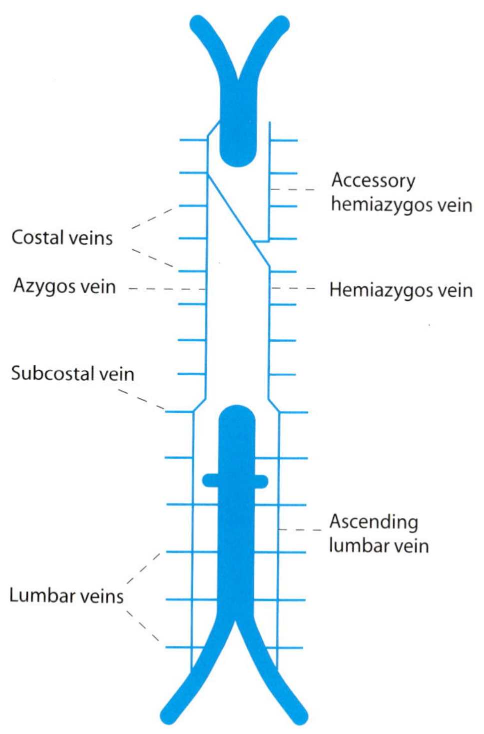

79. Vena cava inferior and superior and the paravertebral venous systems nage in any direction. The only exception is the radicular veins, whose valves prevent reflux into the spinal cord (Clemens 19961), and also the terminal portion of the azygos vein. With occlusion of the inferior or superior vena cava, the vertebral and paravertebral vessels are available as important *collateral channels*; they extend from the pelvic plexus to the cranial veins. They also serve as blood reservoirs, assist in pressure regulation, and contribute to the hematogenous spread of metastases (Batson 1964).

Under normal hemodynamic conditions, the vertebral and paravertebral venous systems are not filled by pelvic phlebography. Their evaluation requires special methods such as selective injection of the ascending lumbar vein (Clemens 1961). Occlusion phlebography (Weber 1978) and intraosseous phlebography (Clemens a1961; Fischgold et al. 1952) are no longer employed. The diagnostic procedures of choice for suspected disease of the retroperitoneal and paravertebral vessels are digital subtraction angiography and magnetic resonance imaging.

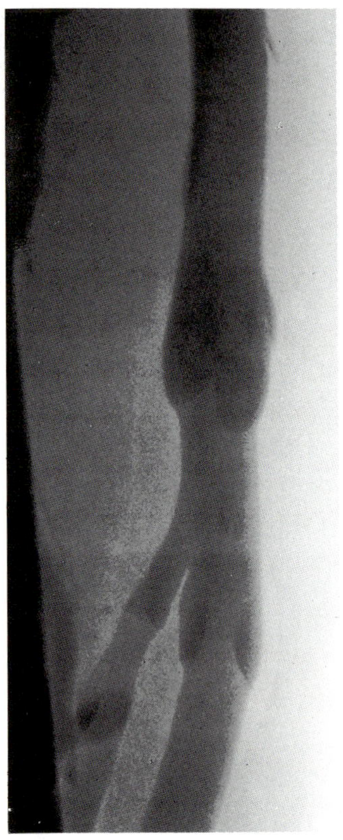

80. Valves of the superficial femoral vein in the open and closed state, demonstrated by ascending pressure phlebography. Valves usually occur distal to the sites of merging veins

References

Batson OV (1964) Vertebral phlebography. In: Schobinger RA, Rudzicka FF (eds) Vascular roentgenology. McMillan, New York

Bücheler E (1971) Die direkte Angiographie der Vertebralplexus, der lumbalen Venen und des Azygosvenensystems. Röntgenanatomie und klinische Anwendung. Ergebn Med Rad, Bd III. Thieme, Stuttgart

Clemens HJ (1961) Die Venensysteme der menschlichen Wirbelsäule. De Gruyter, Berlin

Fischgold H, Clement JC, Talairach J, Ecoiffier J (1952) Opacification des systemes veneux rachidiens et crâniens par voie osseuse. Press Med 60: 599

Luzsa G (1972) Röntgenanatomie des Gefäßsystems. Barth, Frankfurt/M

Milloy FJ, Anson BJ, Cauldwell EW (1962) Variations in the inferior caval veins and their renal and lumbal communications. Surgery 115: 131

Weber J (1978) Phlebographie und Venendruckmessung im Abdomen und Becken. Witzstrock, Baden-Baden

Venous Valves

The venous valves are arranged so as to prevent
the reflux of blood toward the periphery. Often,
80 though not always, they are located distal to the
81 entry point of a small tributary. They consist of
two or occasionally three delicate *cusps* whose
82 convex border projects into the lumen of the vessel. The venous wall proximal to the valve cusps is frequently dilated into a sinus.

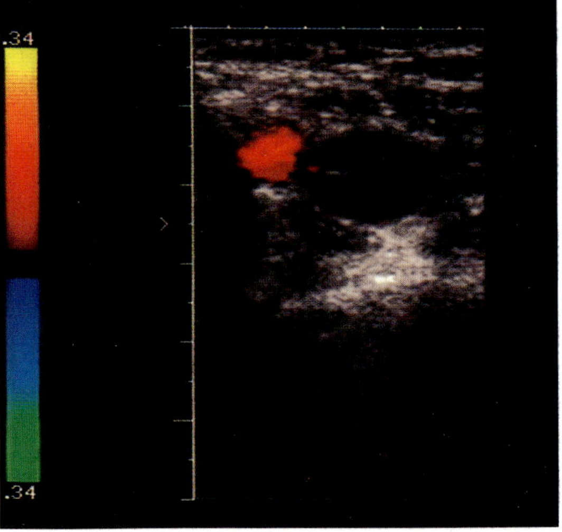

81. Closed venous valves demonstrated by color-coded duplex sonography (Acuson, 7-MHz transducer). Arteries coded *red*, veins *black* (due to lack of flow) with a diagonal valve cusp

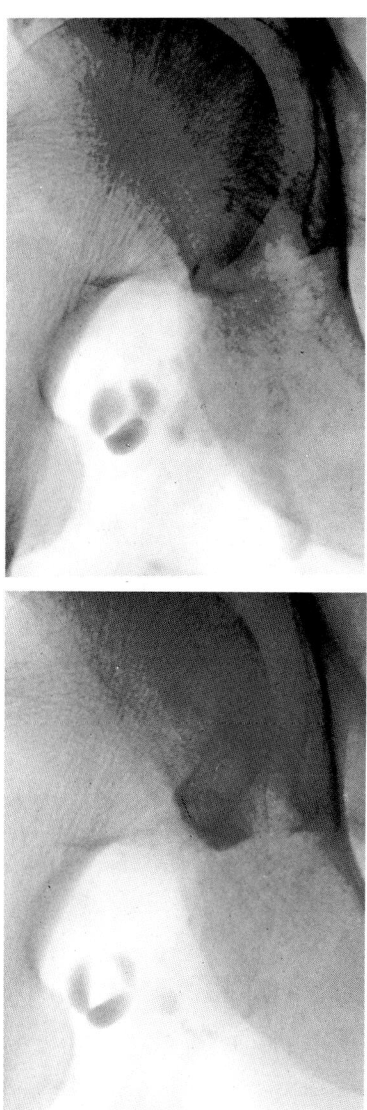

82. Terminal valves of the profunda femoris vein in the closed (*top*) and open state (*bottom*). Antegrade projection of three equivalent and symmetrically arranged valve cusps. Incidental finding in a 70-year-old man with femoral vein thrombosis

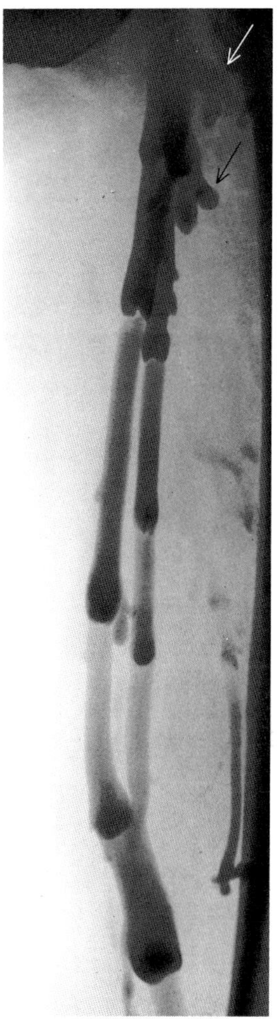

83. Torsion of the valves in paired superficial femoral veins. The profunda terminates by two separate, large trunks (→)

Unlike the muscle veins, which receive numerous
tributaries, the main stem veins of the leg usually
do not show significant caliber changes proximal
11 and distal to their valves. An exception is the ter-
12 minal portion of the great saphenous vein, whose
caliber increases significantly above the two sluice
valves and culminates in the large ostial sinus at
the saphenofemoral junction. The small saphenous vein shows similar caliber changes in its terminal segment. This phenomenon, called the *tele-* 23
scope sign, is useful for confirming valvular com- 44, 131
petence on phlebograms.

During the phase of slow steady blood flow, in
which ascending phlebography is performed, the
venous valves are open and appear radiographically as a slight bulging of the vessel wall. When
the patient inhales deeply or performs a Valsalva
maneuver, the valves close, appearing phlebogra- 83

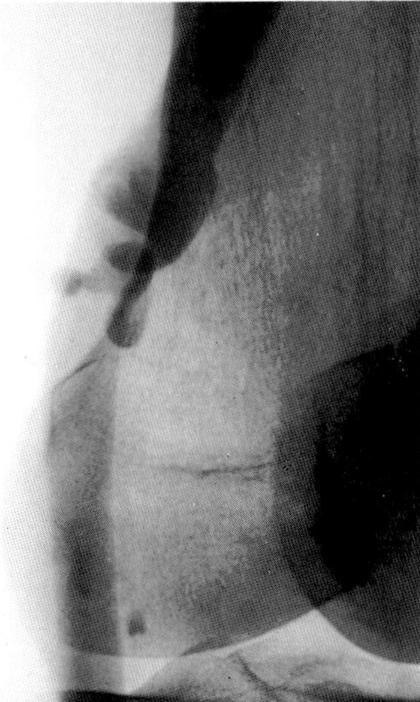

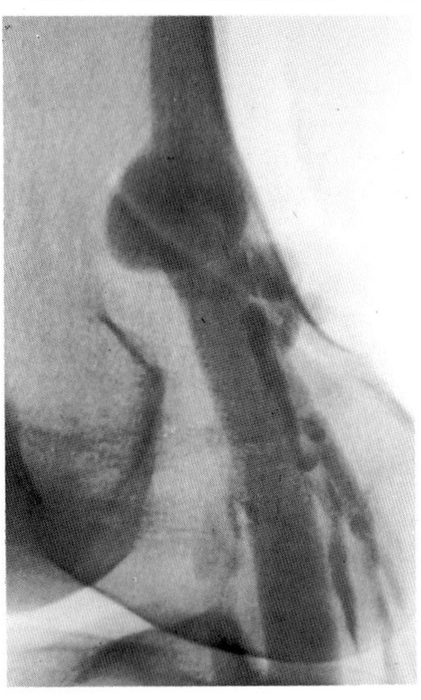

84. Asymmetric valve in Hunter's canal, demonstrated by ascending pressure phlebography, internal rotation (*top*) and lateral view (*bottom*)

Number of valves in selected veins (Lodin et al. 1961)	
Superficial femoral vein	4 (1– 9)
Popliteal vein	2 (1– 5)
Posterior tibial vein	10 (7–20)
Anterior tibial vein	10 (9–12)
Peroneal vein	10 (6–12)
Great saphenous vein	10 (7–20)
Small saphenous vein	8 (5–15)

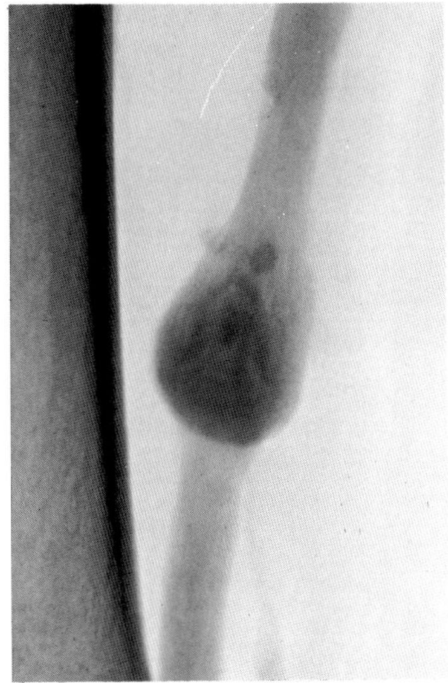

85. Abnormally enlarged venous valves in Hunter's canal with zones of turbulent flow. Incidental finding during ascending pressure phlebography

phically as a nodular thickening in the course of the vein. Having a higher specific weight than blood, the contrast medium tends to settle in the pouches of the valve cusps, so it can clearly delineate valvular anatomy in the semiupright patient.

When a Valsalva maneuver is initiated, a slight degree of reflux can occur even through competent valves. Thus, the demonstration of retrograde contrast flow alone should not be interpreted as valvular incompetence. In the case of the *overflow effect* (see p. 59), this phenomenon can be utilized 96
to fill specific vascular regions.

Venous valves are most numerous during the fetal period. Normally their *number* decreases steadily from birth to 70 years of age, by which time there are only 19% of the original fetal complement (Kubik 1982).

Venous valves are more plentiful in the peripheral part of the circulation than centrally. The average number of valves in selected veins are shown in the table on p. . Muscle veins are relatively densely valved.

Corresponding vessels in both extremities or in particular venous groups, such as the posterior tibial veins, often contain valves sited at *corresponding locations*. Occasionally this fact can be utilized diagnostically. A spiral arrangement of 83
the valves can be demonstrated in the larger venous trunks.

Selective delineation of the venous valves by ascending phlebography
Patient inclined 30°
Leg relaxed and non-weight-bearing for contrast injection
Manual direction of the contrast medium
Valsalva maneuver
Wait for settling of contrast medium
Spot films in two planes

Occasionally a venous valve may show congenital
84 *deformities*. The valve in Hunter's canal is affected
with some frequency. Asymmetric development
85 of the valve cusps or abnormal enlargement of the
valve sinuses is commonly observed.

The essential ***function*** of venous valves is to block the transmission of retrograde pressure waves (Netzer 1979). The lower the flow rate and flow pressures in the antegrade direction, the greater the need for these protective barriers. A single valve is not fully competent in this situation, and a series of valves are needed to damp a retrograde pressure wave with complete efficiency. The muscle pumps can perform optimally only when valvular function is intact (Schneider and Fischer 1969).

Another task of the valves is to intercept retrograde flow waves. This function is hemodynamically significant during the change from a recumbent to an upright position.

Ultrasound can occasionally demonstrate a ve- 81
nous valve under favorable conditions, but it does not allow a detailed morphologic assessment of the valves in an extremity vein.

References

Kubik S (1982) Die Anatomie des Fußes unter besonderer Berücksichtigung der Faszien, Faszienräume und der Gefäßversorgung. In: Brunner U (Hrsg) Der Fuß. Huber, Bern

Lodin A, Lindvalla N, Gentele H (1961) Congenital absence of valves in the deep veins of the leg. Acta Derm Venerol (Stockholm) 41: 45

Netzer CO (1979) Die Physiologie des Niederdrucksystems. In: Ehringer H, Fischer H, Netzer CO, Schmutzler R, Zeitler E (Hrsg) Venöse Abflußstörungen. Enke, Stuttgart

Schneider W, Fischer H (1969) Die chronisch-venöse Insuffizienz. Enke, Stuttgart

Hemodynamics of Venous Return

The functions of the veins in the circulatory system are to return blood to the heart and provide for temporary storage of blood that is not immediately needed by the circulation. Venous function is regulated by the transmural pressure, which determines the vascular cross-sectional area, and by the flow pressure. The flow resistance in the venous system is very low compared with the arterial system and capillaries (Netzer 1979).

In the supine position, the pressure gradient from the postcapillary region to the heart is adequate to sustain a slow central venous flow through the *vis a tergo mechanism*. The corresponding flow pressures are 15–25 mmHg in the venules, 8–20 mmHg in the common femoral vein, and 5–7 mmHg in the right atrium (Burton 1960).

Respiration acts like a pressure-suction pump (*vis a fronte*) through the reciprocal generation of opposite intrathoracic and intra-abdominal pressure fluctuations. *Cardiac activity* accelerates venous flow in two ways: by the passage of blood collected in the atrium and pericardial vessels into the relaxed right ventricle, and during the ejection phase by the displacement of the closed valve planes. Both events can be detected sonographically by noting the double-stroke effect in the inferior vena cava.

In a recumbent posture, the *cutoff effect* is observed in the inferior vena cava; if the subject takes a deep breath, the vessel closes at the level of the diaphragm, and during this period the blood flows away via the azygos system (Gardener and Fox 1989). The cutoff phenomenen occasionally leads to a wrong diagnosis being made.

In an upright posture, the *hydrostatic pressure* is added to the postcapillary flow pressure. This pressure, ranging from 80 to 90 mmHg depending on body size, acts on both the arterial and venous sides of the circulation of the lower extremity. Thus, the arteriovenous pressure difference remains constant at rest but increases during muscular exercise (Pentecost et al. 1963).

During sitting and standing, a blood volume of 300–350 ml is shifted from the thorax to the periphery, causing dilatation of the venous capacity vessels (Kappert 1976). When the lower extremities are relaxed and dependent, the venous pool in the legs is greater than during active standing. This fact influences the appearance of the veins during ascending phlebography.

Various peripheral mechanisms with synergistic actions can promote venous return to the heart. Scientists now attribute a certain hemodynamic effect to the *arteriovenous coupling* again, i. e., the transferral of arterial pulsations to the accompanying veins within the adventitia (Gardener and Fox 1989). Considerably more important are the muscle pumps, especially the *calf muscle pump* (Schneider and Fischer 1969). The pressure within the soleus muscle rises from 13 to 87 mmHg during contraction, squeezing the blood from the muscle veins as from a sponge. The pressure within the gastrocnemius muscle rises from 11 to 23 mmHg during exercise, while that in the quadriceps femorus, the activator of the muscle pump in the thigh, rises from 0 to 15 mmHg (Ludbrook 1966).

The increase in the girth of the muscle bellies during contraction compresses the intrafascial venous trunks, exerting an estimated pressure of 70 mmHg in the lower leg (Netzer 1970). The soleus muscle is believed to produce the greatest compressive effect.

The vascular calibers are expanded distal and proximal to the compressed venous segments as blood is ejected from the limb. During relaxation of the muscles, the deep veins refill with blood drawn from the superficial system via the perforating veins. This mechanism, combined with the function of the venous valves, leads to a marked acceleration of venous return during walking.

Of the various venous pumps in the lower extremity, only the contraction of the calf muscles affects the radiographic assessment of the popliteal vein. We discovered the phenomenon in phlebographic studies and called it the *popliteal pump*. When the subject contracts his leg muscles, the lumen of the popliteal vein is compressed to a narrow slit by the expanding gastrocnemius muscle bellies. When the muscles relax, the vessel immediately reassumes its original caliber. The popliteal pump appears to exert a significant hemodynamic effect during cyclical motor activities such as walking and bike riding.

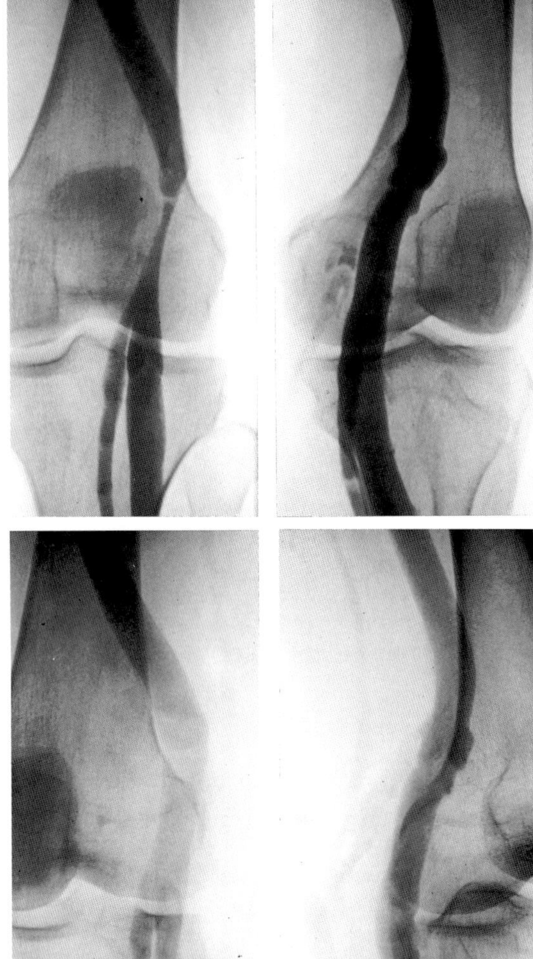

86. Popliteal pump. *Top,* the popliteal vein is compressed from both sides to a narrow slit by the contracting gastrocnemius muscles. Ascending pressure phlebography, internal rotation and lateral view. *Bottom,* normal popliteal vein caliber in the relaxed leg

A compression effect on the popliteal vein dependent on the subjects *position*, on the other hand, has long been recognized (Rabinow and Paulin 1972) and was attributed to the pressure of the femoral condyle or the popliteal muscle by Britton (1964) and Thomas and Carty (1975) and to the position of the knee-joint by Robertson et al. (1974). The effects of other peripheral venous pumps cannot be documented by changes in X-ray morphology. A knowledge of these effects is important, however, because they can interfere with the conduct of the examination.

The *foot muscle pump* is based on compression of the plantar veins by the contracting plantar muscles of the foot (Pegum and Fegan 1967). When the main stem veins of the lower leg are closed due to contraction of the calf muscles, the blood first drains through valveless perforating veins into the venous network on the dorsum of the foot, passing from there to the great and small saphenous trunks (Netzer 1979; Ochsner et al. 1951). According to phlebographic studies (Gardener and Fox 1989), the plantar veins are stretch liked a bowstring during weight bearing, thus being emptied without any active contribution from the foot muscles.

Heel-to-toe rocking of the foot during walking assists the muscle pump by expelling the contents of the plantar venous network. Also, the expansion of the intermetatarsal spaces during weight bearing creates a suction in the plantar veins that facilitates drainage from the surrounding tissues and from the toes (Netzer 1979).

Anatomists (Braune and Müller 1889; Staubesand 1980) have drawn attention to the efficacy of the *ankle pump*. With each movement of the ankle joint, tension exerted on the skin, fasciae, and ligaments expels blood from the venous plexuses of the malleolar, tarsal, and metatarsal regions. Meanwhile, the stress exerted on the ankle joint by motion of the fasciae and tendons causes an expansion of the intrafascial tissue spaces ("aeration"), leading to filling of the venous plexuses within them and dilatation of the small saphenous vein.

The *large fasciae* in the leg also contribute to the acceleration of centripetal venous flow. The change in the direction of the obliquely oriented fibers acts much like an elastic stocking on the lower leg, tightening when the knee joint is extended and loosening when it is flexed (O. Askar, cited from Schneider and Fischer 1969).

The *popliteal suction mechanism of Knauer* functions during both active and passive flexion of the knee joint (Lanz and Wachwmuth 1972). Stretching of the popliteal fascia creates a suction effect in the popliteal fossa, causing blood to be aspirated from the popliteal vein. In the same way, stretching of the crural fascia over the contracted calf muscles relaxes the fascia above the malleoli and aspirates blood from the distal veins of the lower leg.

In the upper leg, the superficial femoral vein is compressed by contraction of the *quadriceps muscle* of the thigh, which leads to an increase in the velocity of bloodflow. However, the *sartorius muscle pump* is even
more effective. It is thought to be particularly pro- 87
nounced in professional cyclists due to hypertrophy of the muscle (Gardener and Fox 1989).

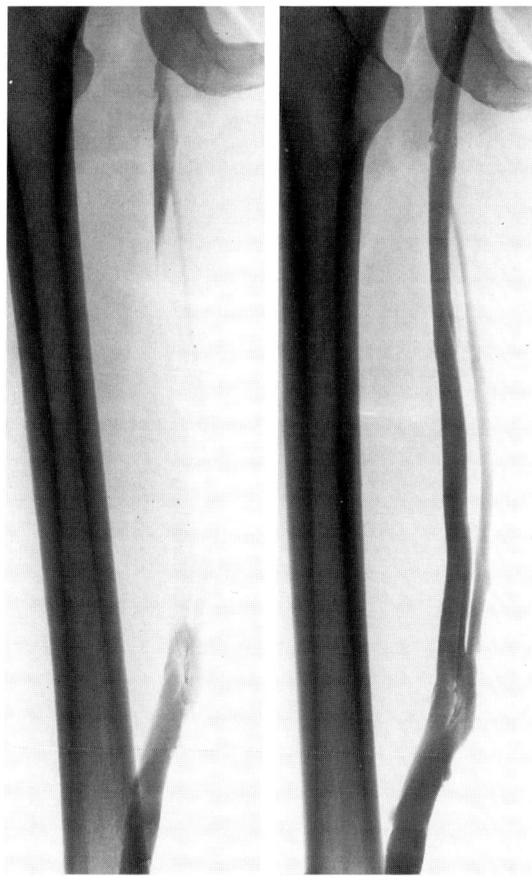

87. Sartorius muscle pump. Impression of the superficial femoral vein around the junction between the mid- and upper thirds medially, during strong contraction of the leg muscles (*left*). Normal lumina of the duplicated superficial femoral vein in the relaxed leg (*right*). Incidental observation in an active 29-year-old woman

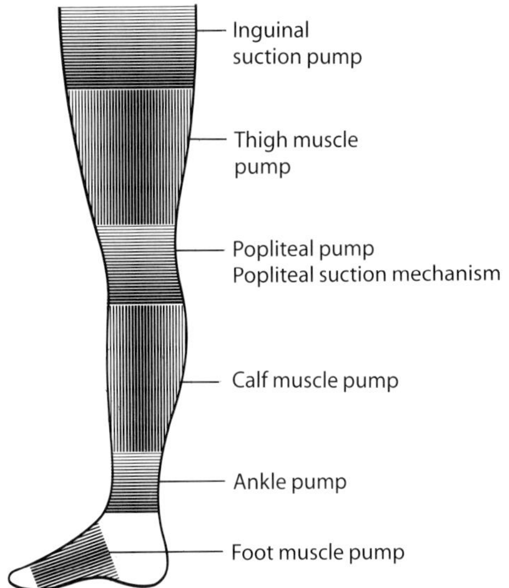

88. Pressure-suction pumps in the lower extremity

A similar suction pump mechanism exists in the *region of the saphenous opening* (Staubesand 1980), where connective tissue tension is transmitted to the femoral vein below the inguinal ligament and within the iliopectinate fossa in such a way that active and passive hip movements expand the lumen of the vein, producing a suction effect.

An increase in *flow resistance* has the opposite effect on centripetal venous flow. Normally this resistance is very low, not exceeding 4.5 mmHg along the pathway from the foot to the heart (Ochsner et al. 1951). Blood flow in the pericardiac vessels is reduced by contraction of the right atrium and by deep respiration; it is reduced in the peripheral veins by inhalation and by the Valsalva maneuver.

88 Whether desired or not, the foregoing mechanisms can accelerate blood flow during phlebography and thus can affect the *course of the examination*. In ascending pressure phlebography, even gentle finger pressure on the sole of the foot or on the soleus pressure point will promote contrast filling of the more proximal venous channels. The major importance of active and passive movements of the foot and ankle joints for the prevention of thrombosis also derives from physiologic principles.

The *flow velocity* of the blood depends on the blood volume and the cross-sectional area of the vein. As a result, blood flow toward the heart is more rapid in a horizontal position than in an upright posture. An average flow velocity of 7.7 cm/s has been measured in the thigh veins of recumbent subjects, 1.6 cm/s in a relaxed hanging position, and 2.1 cm/s during active standing (Rieckert 1970). These findings suggest that a relaxed, dependent position of the lower extremity is the most favorable for contrast radiography of the venous system.

References

Britton RC (1964) Phlebography. In: Schobinger RA, Rudzicka FF (eds) Vascular roentgenology. McMillan, New York

Braune W, Müller P (1889) Die Venen des Fußes und des Unterschenkels. In: Braune W (Hrsg) Das Venensystem des menschlichen Körpers. Veit, Leipzig

Burton AC (1960) Medical physiology and biophysics, 18th edn. Saunders, Philadelphia

Gardener AMM, Fox RH (1989) The return of blood to the heart. Libbey, London

Kappert A (1976) Lehrbuch und Atlas der Angiologie. Huber, Bern

Lanz J von, Wachsmuth W (1972) Praktische Anatomie, Bd I/4. Bein und Statik. Springer, Berlin Heidelberg New York

Ludbrook J (1966) Aspects of venous function in the lower limbs. Thomas, Springfield

Netzer CO (1979) Hämodynamik des Niederdrucksystems. In: Ehringer H, Fischer H, Netzer CO, Schmutzler R, Zeitler E (Hrsg) Venöse Abflußströmungen. Enke, Stuttgart

Ochsner A, Colp Jr R, Burch GE (1951) Normal blood pressure in the superficial venous system of man at rest in the supine position. Circulation 3: 674

Pegum JM, Fegan WG (1967) Anatomy of the venous return from the foot. Cardiovasc Res 1: 241

Pegum JM, Fegan WG (1967) Physiology of the venous return from the foot. Cardiovasc Res 1: 249

Pentecost BL, Irving DW, Shillingford JP (1963) The effects of posture on the blood flow in the inferior vena cava. Clin Sci 24: 149

Rabinov K, Paulin S (1972) Roentgendiagnosis of venous thrombosis in the leg. Arch Surg 104: 134

Rieckert H (1970) Die Hämodynamik des venösen Rückflusses aus der unteren Extremität. Arch Kreislaufforschung 62: 293

Robertson K, Bergquist D, Hallböök T (1974) Constriction of the popliteal vein related to the position of the knee-joint. Vasa 8: 329

Schneider W, Fischer H (1969) Die chronisch-venöse Insuffizienz. Enke, Stuttgart

Staubesand J (1980) Die anatomischen Grundlagen der sog. Sprunggelenkspumpe. Swiss Med 2: 48

Thomas ML, Carty H (1975) The appearance of artefacts on lower limb phlebograms. Clin Radiol 26: 527

Methods and Techniques of Phlebography

Radiographic examination of the lower extremity veins must allow for a *comprehensive assessment* of venous hemodynamics and provide the attending physician with detailed information that can guide the formulation of an appropriate treatment plan. Several phlebographic techniques are available for this. The selection of a particular technique depends on the type of information required and the nature and location of the disease, and so is determined mainly by clinical considerations.

The basic methodology of peripheral phlebography was essentially perfected with the introduction of low-risk nonionic contrast media and a refined roentgenographic technique. Digital image processing and peripheral image intensification avoid the problem of unsuccessful exposures. Basic problems relating to the anatomy of the venous system cannot be resolved. A major disadvantage is the uncontrolled contrast filling of certain vascular regions, especially parallel venous pathways. It must be realized that the phlebographic medium is injected into the peripheral root of a widely arborizing vascular tree, so that antegrade blood flow tends to keep contrast medium from entering
89 parallel veins. This differs fundamentally from arteriography, where contrast filling proceeds outward from a vascular trunk.

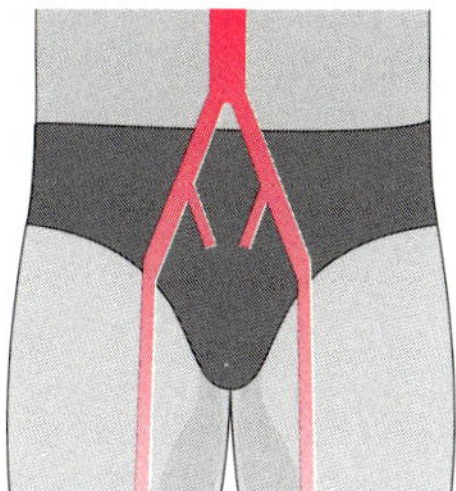
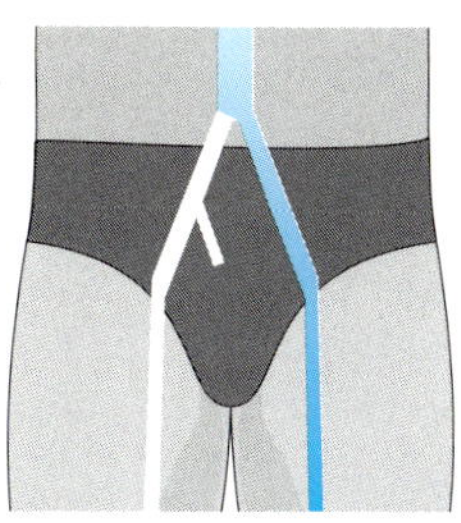

89. Basic differences in the contrast filling of arteries and veins. *Left,* in arteriography, all the vessels are opacified as contrast medium is carried from the main trunk into smaller branches. *Right,* in phlebography, the contrast medium directly opacifies only vessels in the direct path of flow; shunt regions are not demonstrated

The advent of digital subtraction angiography has established new indications for the radiographic examination of the major proximal veins and visceral veins. Computerized sonography and magnetic resonance imaging also have expanded our diagnostic capabilities in these areas. Substantial progress has resulted from the use of ultrasound techniques such as real-time B-mode sonography and especially color-coded duplex scanning, which not only demonstrate the morphology of a vessel and its surroundings but also provide functional information.

General Guidelines

Prior to the examination, the patient is questioned concerning previous X-ray examinations and allergic conditions. According to Katayama et al. (1990), patients with allergic disorders are almost three times more likely to suffer a mild or severe contrast reaction than healthy subjects.

Particular attention is given to any *previous reactions* the patient may have had to contrast injections. The risk of intolerance is five times higher in patients with a known history of reactivity. The incidence of adverse reactions appears to decline markedly after 60 years of age.

Contrast media with fewer side effects have been developed in recent years, so it may be wise to elicit details on the type of agent previously used. An adverse reaction to cholangiography or urography 20 years ago is of far less concern than a reaction to a more recent phlebography. It should be noted, moreover, that allergic reactions to ionic contrast media reportedly are about four times more frequent than reactions to nonionic media (Katayama et al. 1990).

Pregnancy should be excluded in female patients; if doubt exists, the study should be postponed until after the next menstrual period. If phlebography is urgently indicated during pregnancy, selection can be decided on a case-by-case basis, taking into account the therapeutic benefit to be derived. Informed consent begins by having the patient read an *information sheet* on the nature and risks of the phlebographic procedure. This is supplemented as needed by verbal instructions from the physician, and signed consent is secured. If the study is done for disability assessment, the patient should be advised that the procedure is not compulsory. It is helpful to have a radiology technician present while the patient is counseled.

Routine phlebography includes visualization of the deep leg veins and pelvic veins and an assessment of the terminal valves of the saphenous veins. In a preoperative evaluation of varicose veins, the pelvic films may be omitted to reduce radiation exposure. The experienced examiner should have no difficulty incorporating the fluoroscopic impression of venous function into his findings, with no additional expenditure of time.

The *X-ray request sheet* should indicate the particular vascular region that is of interest to the requesting physician. In addition, the radiologist should familiarize himself briefly with the patient's complaints, local findings, and any proposed therapeutic measures; this can be done easily without loss of time. The patient should always be questioned about any previous episodes of thrombosis. Generally the layperson will be unaware of the important distinction between superficial and deep venous involvement, so the history will have to be supplemented by specific questions on disease symptoms.

Radiographic Equipment

A fluoroscopy unit with a *television monitor* is essential for phlebography of the lower extremity. Since the route of contrast drainage through the venous system cannot be predicted, there is no justification for the use of blind, nonfluoroscopic techniques in the lower extremity.

Any room equipped with a *tilting table* is satisfactory. For imaging of the lower leg, the patient must be positioned high on the table. Adequate head support in this situation may require attaching an *extension plate*, which may have to be specially made, to the tabletop.

The small *focus-film distance* of the fluoroscope leads to a slight distortion of relative sizes on the image, but in practice this is not a significant problem, and a distractor is not required. Nor do we believe that an X-ray ruler with radiopaque markers is necessary or advantageous for preoperative interpretation of the phlebograms.

The *remote control technique* has not proven satisfactory for peripheral phlebography. When a steep table tilt is used for the procedure, there is always the danger that the patient may slip from the hand grips, requiring an immediate response by the physician. Moreover, the immediate presence of the radiologist is necessary for the manual examination technique.

Phlebography of the large proximal veins and visceral veins is performed in the supine patient, following the technique for arteriography. After the needle or catheter has been inserted, the contrast medium is injected by hand or with an automatic injection pump with determined flow.

When the digital subtraction technique is used, images are *documented* on magnetic or video tape; with conventional apparatus, a cut film changer is used. Some centers already have facilities for digital recording with a "picture archiving and communication system" (PACS). Interventional procedures on the venous system can be documented with a spot film device.

Radiation Exposure and Protection

Tube voltages of 65–70 kV are required for ascending phlebography in the lower leg, 80–90 kV in the thigh, and 100 kV in the pelvic region. Mellmann (1979) calculated surface dose products of 650–2000 R $\times$ cm^2 (approximately 565–1740 cGy $\times$ cm^2) for fluoroscopic times of $^1/_2$ to $1^1/_2$ min, and 140–400 R $\times$ cm^2 (approximately 122–350 cGy $\times$ cm^2) for an X-ray film of the pelvic vessels. This corresponds to a *gonad dose* of 30–100 mrem (0.03–0.1 mSv). Omitting the pelvic exposure reduces the gonad dose by half. For this reason phlebography performed exclusively for preoperative assessment of the extrafascial venous system routinely proceeds no higher than the femoroiliac junction.

The most effective *radiation protection* consists in minimizing the fluoroscopic time and making the filming sequence as efficient as possible.

The main purpose of *fluoroscopy* is to help the radiologist position the spot films and assess contrast filling in the region of interest. He or she can also gain a useful impression of venous hemodynamics; an experienced radiologist needs only seconds to detect secondary popliteal and femoral vein incompetence and quantify its severity by the stem vein function test. Similar information can be obtained in post-thrombotic syndrome. The importance of the "second look" in the diagnosis of primary varicose veins is additionally noted. With these facts in mind, the fluoroscopic time for a routine lower-extremity examination consisting of six phlebograms is 30–50 s when the procedure is performed by an experienced examiner.

Contrast Media

Nonionic contrast media have greatly reduced the risk of phlebography to the patient (see p. 261), and in recent years they have largely superseded the use of ionic media throughout the world.

Ionic contrast media are triiodinated benzoic acid derivates. They include substances such as iothalamate (Conray), ioxithalamate (Telebrix), and diatrizoate (Angiografin). The media have a relatively high osmolality of 1500 mosm/kg H_2O, which is seven times that of plasma (300 mosm). A number of side effects have been attributed to this physical property alone. Ioxaglate (Hexabrix) is a low-osmolality medium (490 mosm), but its dimer structure gives it a relatively high viscosity.

90 *Nonionic contrast media* cannot dissociate owing to the structural transformation of the carboxyl group of the triiodinated benzoic acid derivative. Consequently they do not possess an electric charge, so they have low protein-binding and enzyme-inhibiting properties, resulting in better tolerance at biologic membranes. With an equal iodine content to that of the ionic media, the nonionic media are more hydrophilic and show substantially better tolerance. It should be noted that the nonionic media are slightly nephrotoxic, so a creatinine level of 2 mg% would constitute a relative contraindication to their use.

Owing to their low osmotic pressure, the nonionic media cause only minimal *biochemical changes* in the endothelium; this is considered to be a major factor in the declining incidence of postinjection pain during phlebography. Also, superficial and mild deep vein thrombosis after phlebography is becoming so infrequent as to be clinically insignificant. This is consistent with findings on endothelial damage and endothelial permeability in experimental rats. Nonionic media are also thought to produce less chemotoxic effects on the endothelium, which accounts for differences in the reactivity of certain nonionic media that have equal osmolalities (bibliography in Weber and May 1990).

Osmolality and iodine content of comparable contrast media

Chemical name	Trade name	Osmolality at 37 °C (mosm/ kg H2O	Iodine content (mg/ml)	Viscosity (mPa.s)
Ionic contrast media				
Iothalamate	Conray 60	1540	282	3.5
Diabrizoate	Angiografin	1530	306	
Ioxithalamate	Telebrix 300	1600	300	5.5
Amidotrizoate	Peritrast	1500	300	
Ioxaglate	Hexabrix	490	320	7.0
Nonionic contrast media				
Metrizamide	Amipaque	470	300	6.2
Iohexol	Omnipaque	720	300	5.7
Iopromide	Ultravist	610	300	4.9
Iopamidol	Solutrast 300	616	300	4.5
Iomeprol	Imeron 300	521	300	4.5
Comparison				
Blood	–	300		

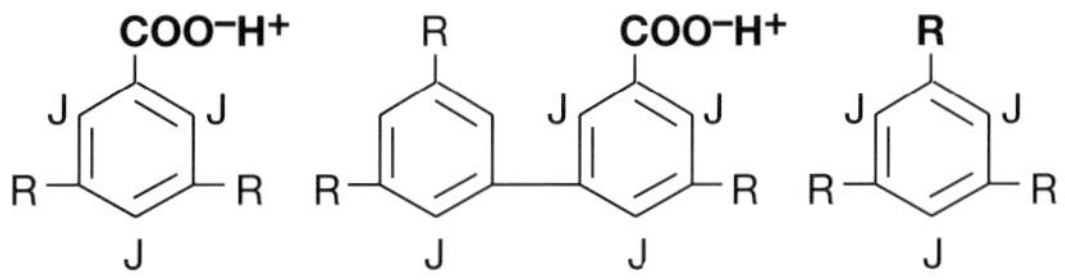

90. Basic chemical formulas of contrast media. *Left,* basic formula of ionic contrast media of the triiodinated benzoic acid type (monomer). *Middle,* basic formula of ionic contrast media of the ioxaglate type (dimer). *Right,* basic formula of nonionic contrast media of the iopamidol, iohexol , and iopromide type (monomer)

The largest *comparative study* of ionic and nonionic contrast media was published in 1990 by the Japanese Committee for Contrast Media Safety (Katayama et al. 1990). The study encompassed a total of 337 647 patients who received contrast injections for urography, computed tomography, or digital subtraction angiography. Ionic media were used in 50.1 % of cases, nonionic media in 49.9 %. The prevalence of side effects was 12.6 % in the first group and 3.13 % in the second group, of which 0.22 % and 0.04 %, respectively, were classified as severe. The one death in each group was not clearly referable to the injected medium.

Regarding the effects of contrast injections in patients with a *known allergic diathesis*, a comparison of published reports by Schmiedel (1989) indicated allergic side effects in 52 % of subjects receiving ionic media and 5 % of subjects receiving nonionic compounds.

Side effects of ionic and nonionic contrast media according to symptoms; each case includes one or more episodes (Katayama et al. 1990)

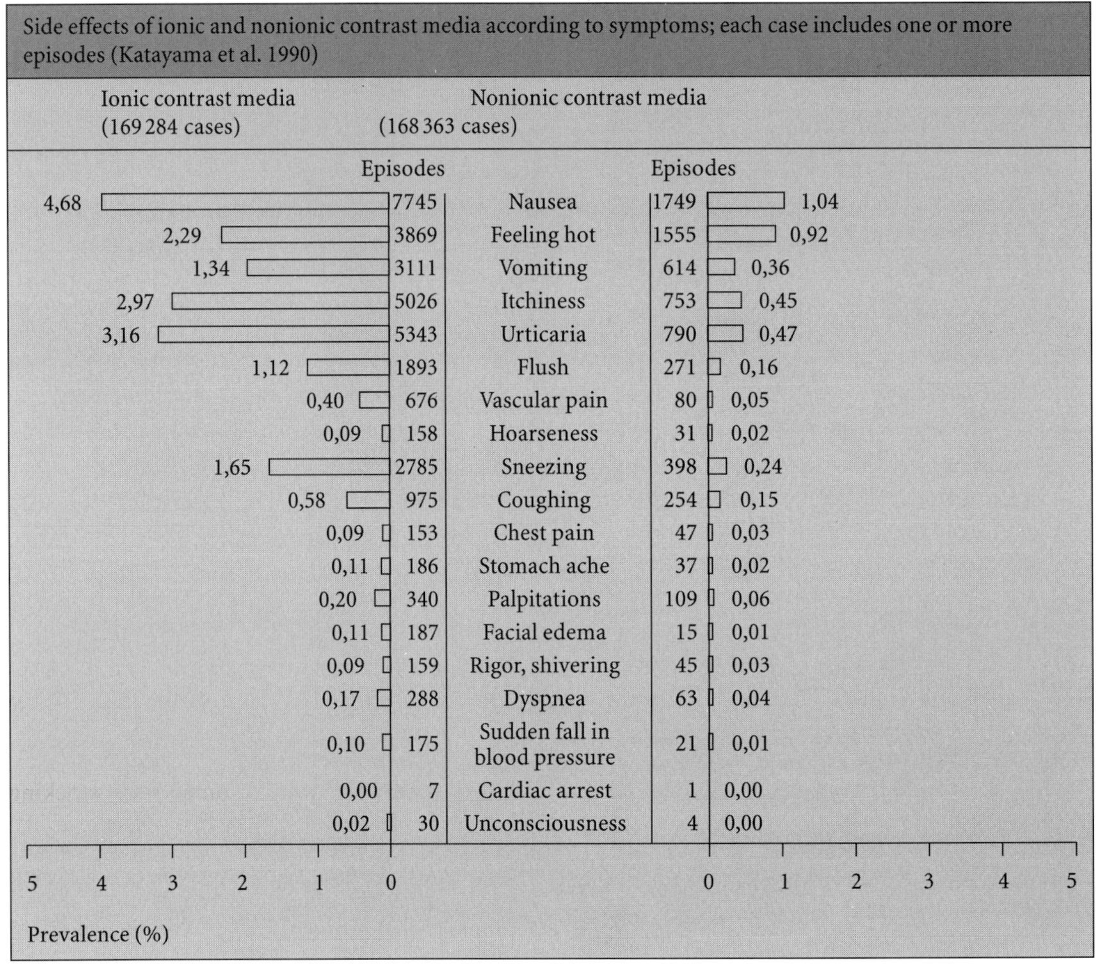

In a series of 119621 patients, Benness and Fischer (1989) identified high-risk subgroups that experienced a 0.3% incidence of serious complications with ionic contrast media versus only a 0.3% incidence with non-ionic media. One death was recorded in the first group. Bettmann et al. (1987) used the iodine-125 fibrinogen uptake test to study the effect of contrast medium on the deep leg veins following phlebographic examinations. The test was positive in 26% of cases where ionic medium was used, as opposed to only 4% of patients receiving the nonionic medium iopamidol.

In ascending pressure phlebography, routine visualization of the intra- and extrafascial vessels requires an average of *30 ml of a 60% contrast solution.* When a selective manual compression technique is used, different grades of dilution can be produced in different vessels, providing for optimum delineation of even subtle lesions. The relatively high concentration of contrast medium in the popliteal vein and common femoral vein also provides good transfascial filling of varicose saphenous veins and their tribu-taries.

Mellmann (1979) and Schmitt (1977) prefered a *40%–45% contrast solution* for phlebography, injecting up to 150 ml. This technique routinely provides good delineation of very small wall changes or thrombi in the deep venous system, although it cannot opacify extrafascial primary varicosities. Concentrations of 32% and 20%, as employed by Alison et al. (1985), are too dilute for ascending pressure phlebography. The recommended *method of choice* would be to use a *larger* volume of contrast medium with a *lower* iodine content for selective imaging of the deep veins, while a *smaller* volume of a *more* concentrated medium would be advantageous for the comprehensive evaluation of *all* venous systems including the extrafascial vessels.

Prophylaxis of Postphlebographic Thrombosis

The routine use of phlebography for a wide range of indications under outpatient conditions is feasible only if undesired side effects can be largely eliminated through prophylactic measures. The intravenous injection of a concentrated solution, such as phlebographic contrast medium, will cause *endothelial damage* if it remains in contact with the vessel wall for too long (Gottlob and Zinner 1959). In varices, blood may remain stagnant for several minutes under unfavorable conditions. McLachlin et al. (1960) even reported finding residual contrast medium in valve pockets for up to 27 min post injection. Spontaneous clearance is also significantly delayed in the presence of severe postthrombotic syndrome.

The potentiating effect of contrast medium on the risk of iatrogenic thrombosis of the deep leg veins has been documented in numerous studies. Generally, however, these episodes have no clinical significance.

The collective statistics of Hach, Helmig, May, and Schmidt (Hach 1985) in a population of 86000 showed that thrombotic complications arose in four patients injected with ionic contrast media (see p. 261). However, several authors have reported noteworthy findings with the iodine-125 fibrinogen uptake test (bibliography in Weber and May 1990), which indicated thrombosis rates of 21%–53% following the use of ionic media. When nonionic media were used, the risk fell below 5% in almost all studies.

A meaningful risk profile cannot be established for contrast medium-induced venous thrombosis. It is difficult to take into account such factors as impaired venous drainage, decreased motility, inadequate thromboprophylaxis, and especially lack of examiner experience with high contrast doses and correct technique. As a result, the use of *nonionic contrast media* is now routinely recommended as the *leading principle* in the prevention of postphlebographic thrombosis.

Phlebothrombosis can develop in the deep veins of the leg and pelvis, producing severe associated symptoms. Occasionally, thrombosis is observed in the superficial veins of the foot, where the contrast medium was injected. Mechanical irritation at this site can incite a cordlike thrombophlebitis or varicophlebitis. One cause is direct endothelial damage by the needle, but a more important cause is *distention* of the delicate vessel by high-pressure instillation of the fluid. The examiner can prevent this kind of damage by placing his fingertips over the vein to keep it from overdistending. This will also give the examiner a "feel" for how forcibly he may inject the solution, and any paravascular complications can be quickly recognized.

The best way to prevent thrombotic complications is to perform the phlebography swiftly and purposefully. The total time of contact between the contrast medium and vein wall should not exceed 2 min. Use of the bolus technique (see p. 60) limits the contact times to *less than 1 min* for individual venous segments.

Residual contrast medium is eliminated immediately following the examination. The table is moved to the horizontal position, and the limb is
elevated and forcibly stroked toward the heart to 91
clear the superficial veins of contrast material. Then the patient repeatedly extends the flexed
knee against the resistance of the examiner's hand 92
and performs alternating, forcible dorsiflexion and plantar flexion of the elevated foot until the
needle is removed. When these precautions are 93
taken, it is unnecessary to check the valve pockets for residual contrast medium by fluoroscopy.

We recommend applying a compression stocking or an *elastic pressure bandage* from the foot to the knee following phlebography. If the venous system is normal and the examination has been swift, the bandage may be waived or removed in 2 h; if venous disease is present, it should remain in place for 24 h or more.

The compression bandage may consist of two elastic short-tailed bandages 10 cm wide (Ideal, Rhena-Varidress, Comprilan). Poorly fitting bandages or the use of long-tailed bandages cause furrows and may incite a phlebitis that is falsely attributed to the phlebography. The bandages are applied in three overlapping turns, encompassing the heel but leaving the toes free. If acute thrombosis is detected radiographically, the compression bandage should extend to the groin, using three 12-cm-wide bandages on the thigh. The hold in this area can be made more secure by placing a foam layer (Autosana) beneath the compression bandage or by fixing the bandage with adhesive tape (Acrylast).

Finally the patient is told to walk at a brisk pace for 10 min. The *walking exercises* can be initiated in the corridor of the radiology department.

Local phlebitic reactions usually occur only in patients with post-thrombotic syndrome or severe varicose disease, which apparently lead to increased reactivity of the previously damaged vascular system. This has led some authors (May and

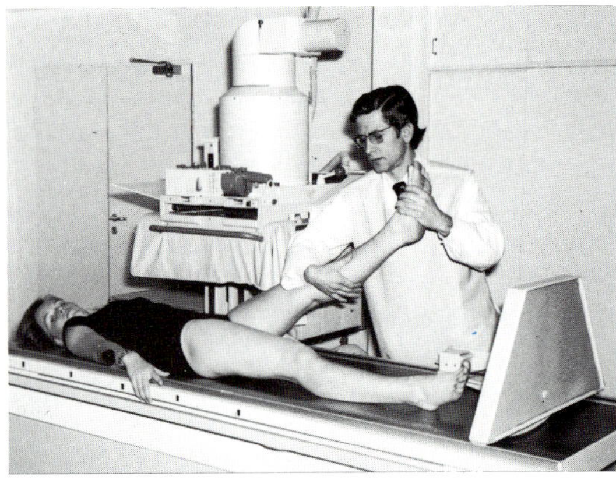

91. The examiner clears the superficial veins of contrast medium by stroking the elevated limb proximally

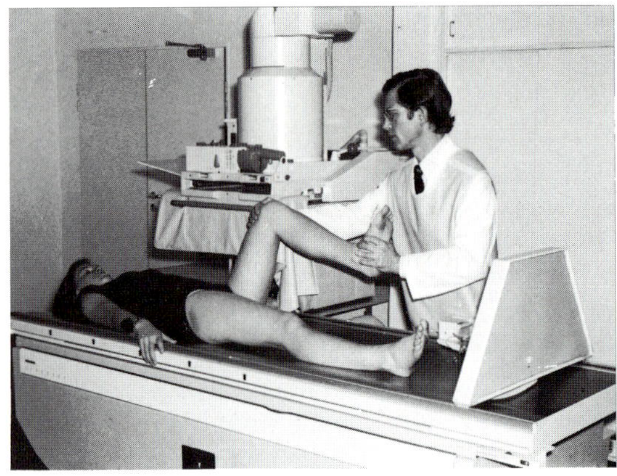

92. The patient extends the leg against the resistance of the examiner's hand to accelerate venous drainage

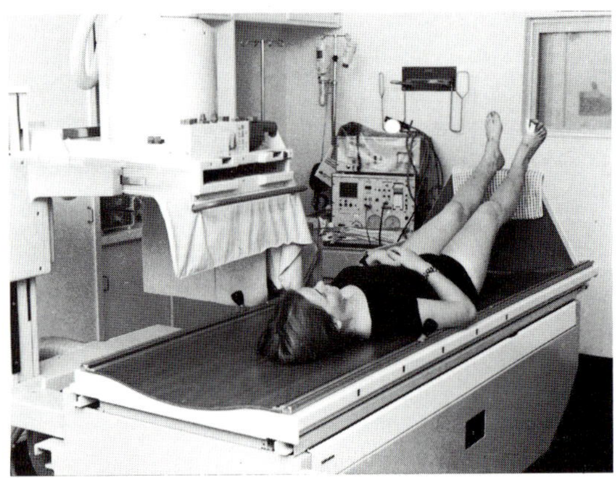

93. The feet are actively flexed and extended with the legs elevated to accelerate venous outflow

Nissl 1973; Schmitt 1977) to recommend the injection of 5000 units of *heparin* in 100 ml physiologic saline to reduce the risk of thrombosis. We reserve this prophylaxis for cases in which the examination lasted an unusually long time due to unfavorable outflow conditions or when multiple contrast injections were required. Otherwise a swift examination technique offers the best safeguard against thrombosis. Special antithrombotic medication is contraindicated in anticoagulated patients taking a *coumarin derivative.*

Discoveries in thrombotic research have shown that *platelet aggregation inhibitors* of the acetylsalicylic acid or pyramidamol type do not afford adequate protection against venous thrombosis (Breddin 1974). Thus they appear to have only a limited role in postphlebographic prophylaxis.

If *acute thrombosis* is diagnosed during the roentgen examination, specific treatment should be instituted *without delay.* In an outpatient setting, 5000 units of heparin diluted in physiologic saline is injected into an arm vein through the phlebographic needle, and the affected limb is wrapped from heel to groin with compression bandages. If the thrombi extend into the common femoral vein or pelvic veins, the risk of embolization is increased, and the patient must be immobilized at once and transferred by ambulance to an appropriate center.

Prevention of postphlebographic thrombosis
Stroking the veins proximally in the elevated leg
Active leg exercises against a resistance
Dorsiflexion and extension of the elevated foot
Walking for 10 min
Compression bandage
Intravenous injection of 5000 U heparin (only in selected cases)

Iodine-Induced Hyperthyroidism Following Contrast Injection

The healthy thyroid gland can adapt in various ways to a large iodine load: increased hormone retention, blockage of iodine uptake, decreased hormone secretion, and neutralization of the iodine (bibliography in Steidle 1989). If these autoregulatory mechanisms are impaired, there is a danger of decompensated hyperthyroidism or thyrotoxic crisis. This requires the presence of autonomous tissue structures or functional analogs like those commonly encountered in endemic nodular goiter.

Steidle (1989), in a retrospective study, reported on 89 cases of hyperthyroidism in a series of 663 patients who received contrast injections. The disease appeared from 6 to 12 weeks after administration of an ionic contrast medium; 63 % of those affected had a struma nodosa.

Patients with overt *hyperthyroidism* are not acceptable candidates for a radiographic contrast study. But even persons with normal biochemical parameters of thyroid function can develop hyperthyroidism in response to contrast injection. A high risk is signaled by decreased thyroid-stimulating hormone (TSH) secretion in response to thyrotrophin-releasing hormone (TRH) stimultion in older individuals and by the detection of antimicrosomal and antithyroid antibodies. Although the iodine atom is firmly bound to the molecules of commercially available contrast media, small amounts of iodine can apparently be split off by the organism and produce side effects. Before phlebography is performed, a careful *thyroid history* should be taken. All patients with known hyperthyroidism or thyroiditis should be excluded. Latent hyperthyroidism in older individuals does not present typical symptoms and is very difficult to diagnose, so a careful endocrinologic workup may be prudent before contrast medium is administered. This particularly applies to patients with struma nodosa in endemic iodine-deficient regions.

References

Albrechtsson U, Olsson CG (1979) Thrombosis following phlebography with ionic and non-ionic contrast media. Acta Radiol Diagn 20: 46

Benness GT, Fischer HW (1989) Reactions to ionic and nonionic contrast media. Radiology 170: 282

Berge T, Bergquist D, Efsing HO, Hallbook T, Lindblad D, Lindhagen A (1981) Complications of phlebography. A randomized comparison between an ionic and non-ionic contrast medium. Clin Radiol 32: 595

Bettmann M, Robbins A, Braun SD, Wetzner S, Dunnik NR, Finkelstein J (1987) Contrast venography of the leg: Diagnostic efficacy, tolerance, and complication rates with ionic and nonionic contrast media. Radiology 165: 113–116

Breddin K (1974) Medikamentöse Thromboseprophylaxe nach Operationen am Venensystem. Phlebol Proktol 3: 284

Gottlob R (1980) Lokale Kontrastmittelschäden – Ursachen, Testmethoden, Ergebnisse. Krankenhausarzt 53: 549

Gottlob R (1990) Kontrastmittel und Venenschäden. In: Weber J, May R (Hrsg) Funktionelle Phlebographie. Thieme, Stuttgart

Gottlob R, Zinner G (1959) Über die Schädigung des Venenendothels durch verschiedene Noxen. Wiener Klin Wochenschr 71: 482

Hach W (1985) Phlebographie der Bein- und Beckenvenen. Schnetztor, Konstanz

Hagen B (1983) Unerwünschte Nebenwirkungen bei und nach der Bein-Beckenvenenphlebographie. Ergebnisse kontrollierter Untersuchungen mit ionischen und nichtionischen Kontrastmitteln. Röntgenpraxis 36: 382

Holtas S, Almen T, Tejler L (1976) Proteinuria following nephroangiography. Acta Radiol Diagn 19: 401

Katayama H, Yamaguchi K, Kozuka T, Takashima T, Seez P, Matsuura K (1990) Adverse reactions to ionic and nonionic contrast media. Radiology 175: 621–628

Laerum F, Holm HA (1981) Postphlebographic thrombosis. A double blind study with Methylglucamine, Metrizoate and Metrizamide. Radiology 140: 651

May R, Nissl R (1973) Die Phlebographie der unteren Extremität. Thieme, Stuttgart

Mellmann J (1979) Technik der aszendierenden Beinphlebographie. Radiol Praxis 2: 51

Raininko R (1979) Endothelial permability increase produced by angiographic contrast media. Fortschr Röntgenstr 131: 433

Schmiedel E (1989) Reduzieren nicht-ionische Kontrastmittel das Untersuchungsrisiko? Röntgenpraxis 42: 335–337

Schmitt HE (1977) Aszendierende Phlebographie bei tiefer Venenthrombose. Huber, Bern

Steidle W (1989) Iodine-induced hyperthyreoidesm after contrast-media: Animal experimental and clinical studies. In: Taenzer V, Wende S (eds) Recent developments in nonionic contrast-media. Thieme, Stuttgart

Törnquist C, Almen T, Gohman K, Holtas S (1980) Proteinuria following nephroangiography. Acta Radiol 362 [Suppl]: 49

Weber J, May R (Hrsg) (1990) Funktionelle Phlebographie. Thieme, Stuttgart

Phlebography of the Lower Extremity

Numerous techniques have been devised for the radiographic visualization of the leg veins, but only a few have general practical importance today. The most frequently performed examination is ascending pressure phlebography. Therefore greater space is devoted to this technique from a theoretical and practical standpoint. The other roentgen techniques are occasionally used for special inquiries.

Ascending Pressure Phlebography (Hach 1974)

Ascending pressure phlebography is suitable for the *comprehensive evaluation* of the deep stem veins and muscle veins, the detection of incompetent perforating veins, and the special evaluation of saphenous and side-branch varicosities. Use of the overflow effect in the relaxed, semiupright patient provides reliable filling of parallel channels, especially the important muscle veins, in both normal and diseased venous systems. This has caused ascending pressure phlebography to become the "reference standard" among all phlebographic techniques.

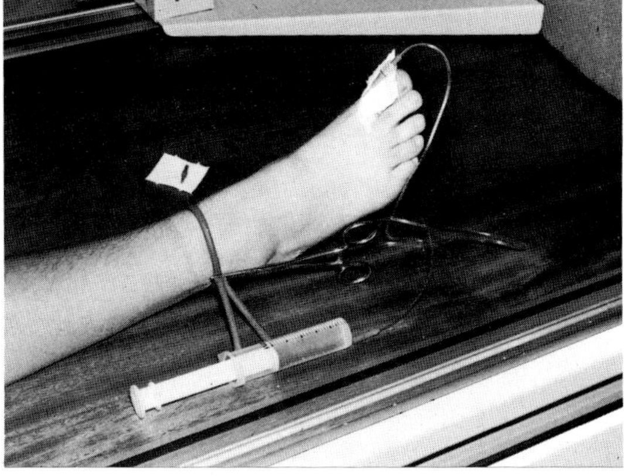

94. A connecting tube is attached to the needle; an ankle tourniquet is in place above the malleolus

Technique of Examination

Preparation of the patient begins with a warm *foot bath* of 5 min duration to bring the veins into prominence and facilitate needle insertion. A no. 2-gauge disposable needle, slightly curved with a sharp bevel, is satisfactory.
If combined examinations such as digital subtraction phlebography of the pelvic veins and inferior vena cava or phlebodynamometry (Weber 1978) are proposed, it is better to use a butterfly needle with a short bevel.
The venepuncture can be made painless by first raising a mepivacaine *wheal* with a vaccination gun (Dermojet). The dorsal vein of the great toe is generally easy to locate even on an edematous foot and guarantees uniform drainage of the contrast medium into the three deep veins of the lower leg. The higher the level of the injection, the less complete the filling of the crural vessels, and the greater the chance of misinterpreting the phlebogram.
94 After a connecting tube (perfusor infusion line) has been attached to the needle hub and secured with adhesive tape, the patient lies flat on the X-ray table, which is then brought to a 20°–40° tilt. The patient does not actively stand on a foot rest, but supports himself on *lateral hand grips* while
95 the legs are *completely relaxed and dependent.* To prevent hypotensive or vagovasal circulatory reactions, the patient's head and entire body must rest against the tabletop. In that position the patient can watch the examination on the television monitor while listening to explanatory comments from the radiologist.

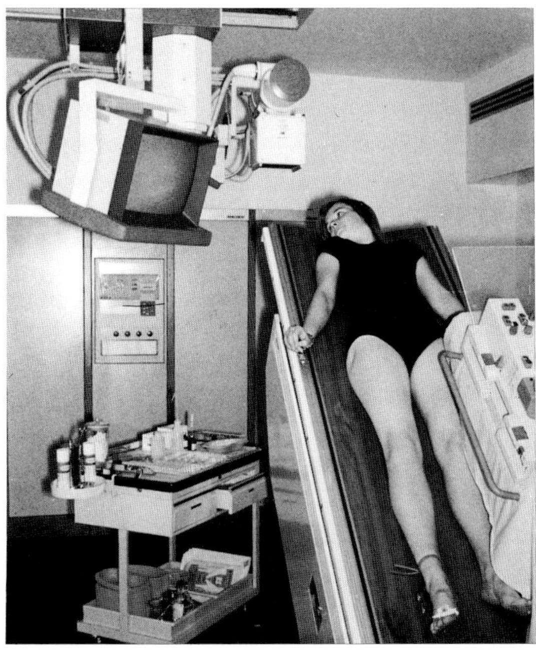

95. Relaxed semiupright position for ascending pressure phlebography. A plate has been inserted to extend the X-ray table

In the *relaxed semiupright position*, it is rare for the venepuncture needle to become dislodged and perforate the vein wall. The contrast bolus is not propelled out of the leg by involuntary movements, which are unavoidable if the patient is actively standing on a hard surface. The vessel lumina appear optimally dilated, so the injection of the contrast medium is likely to be painless. The venous valves are open but will close at once in re-

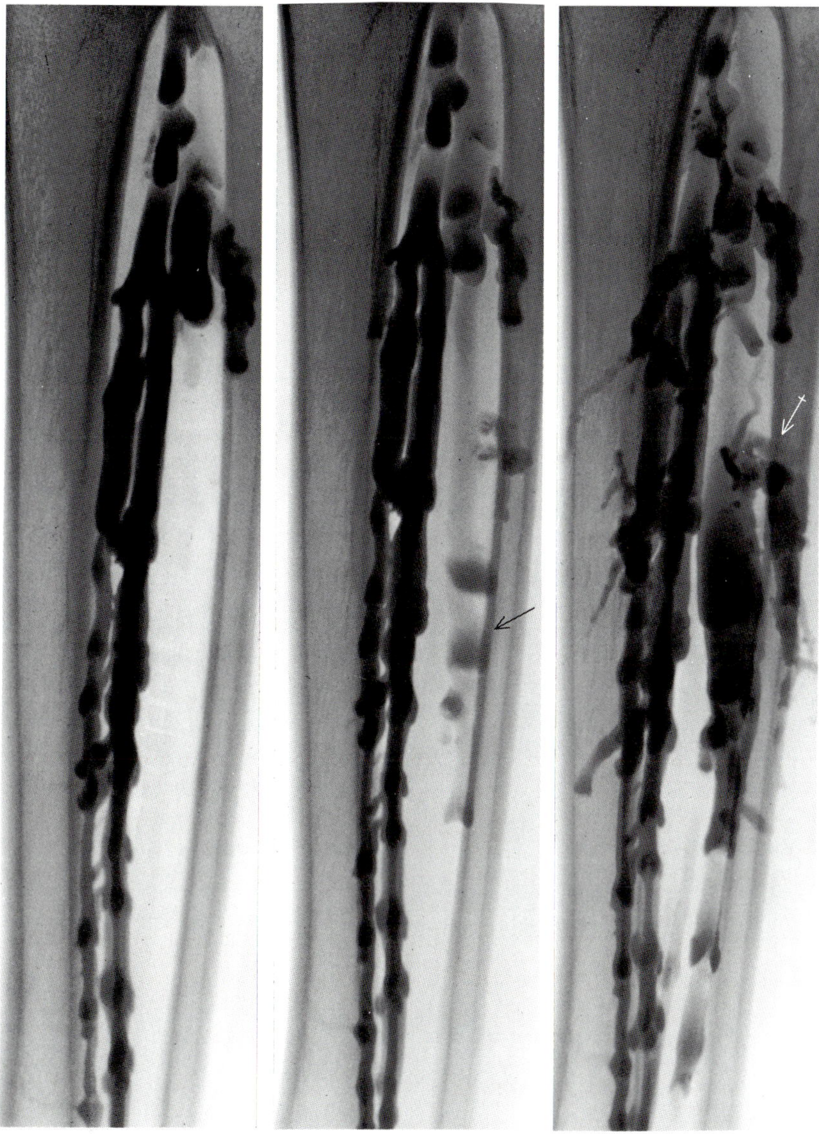

96. Overflow effect during ascending phlebography in the relaxed, dependent limb with a 20°–60° table tilt, using 30 ml of a 60% contrast solution. *Left,* filling of the posterior tibial veins at the start of the examination. *Middle, right,* increasing retrograde filling of the fibular vein with regional ectasia (→) and of the soleus veins (↔). The anterior tibial veins are not yet opacified

Measures for a painless examination
Warm foot bath
Local anesthesia (Dermojet)
Sharp-beveled venepuncture needle
Light fingertip pressure on the injected vein
Leg relaxed and non-weight-bearing
Swift, purposeful examination technique
Compression bandage

sponse to a brief Valsalva maneuver (straining). Layering of contrast material beneath the blood, a potential source of misdiagnosis, does not occur. With its higher specific gravity, the contrast medium settles back through the open venous valves against the slow centripetal outflow and enters parallel venous tributaries, producing an *overflow effect* that allows for retrograde filling of all vascular regions. 96

In patients who are generally debilitated or have an arm disability that prevents safe use of the

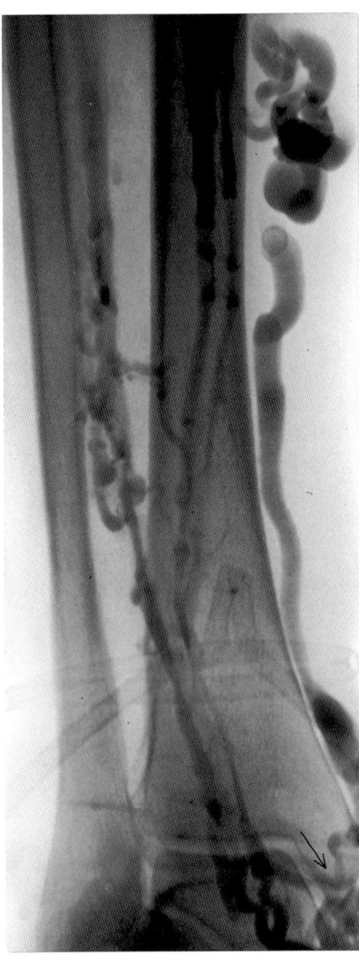

97. Inadequate ankle compression results in poor filling of the deep stem veins due to contrast runoff through the varicose great saphenous vein. → Internal malleolar vein

hand grips, a *10° table tilt* may be used. This is sufficient to achieve contrast sedimentation on the venous valves and avoid artifacts due to layering. Under these conditions the examination can be done in the presence of virtually any severe coexisting disease.

An *ankle tourniquet* is placed tightly above the malleolus to direct the contrast medium into the deep veins of the lower leg. Fluoroscopic observation at this time will demonstrate whether the great and small saphenous veins are totally oc-
97 cluded. Some additional tightening of the tourniquet may be needed to obtain nonsuperimposed views. The best tourniquet for phlebography is a rubber tube held in place with a large Kocher forceps. If there is severe ankle swelling, adequate occlusion generally cannot be obtained.

The contrast medium is injected by hand as rapidly as possible to produce a dense *bolus*. During the injection the radiologist places light digital pressure on the needle and injected vein with his left hand. This protects the vein wall from mechanical overdistention by the injectate, and the patient feels no pain. Also, the radiologist will immediately note any extravasation and correct the needle placement before significant injury occurs. Another safety advantage of the manual technique is that the injection pressure is easily adapted to the individual case; an overvigorous injection is recognized at once by the palpable distention of the vessel.

In the relaxed dependent extremity, the contrast medium flows very slowly or not at all into the deep crural veins under normal conditions. The flow can be accelerated by applying *light* digital pressure to the sole of the foot or by careful *manual compression* of the transverse pedal arch. Contrast medium expelled from the fusiform plantar veins and muscle veins enters and opacifies the stem veins of the lower leg. An *appropriate* amount of pressure applied to the soleus point, a pressure point over the tendinous insertion of the soleus muscle at the mid-calf level, selectively empties the calf muscle sinuses, causing the venous blood to drain to the thigh. As soon as the pressure is released, the blood flow velocity decreases again. This allows sufficient time for obtaining the desired radiographic views. By the alternate application of selective compression with antegrade blood flow, by utilizing the overflow effect (retrograde settling of contrast medium into parallel tributaries), and by arresting venous flow by having the patient inhale deeply or perform a brief Valsalva maneuver to close the valves, all vascular regions can be selectively visualized. 98

This selectivity is the essential advantage offered by the manual examination technique. Diluted by the blood, even a 60% contrast medium can delineate very fine morphologic details. Through the selective opacification of adjacent venous segments, 30 ml contrast medium is adequate for overall delineation of the leg veins and, if desired, can provide a general impression of venous outflow in the pelvic region.

The *venous valves* can be evaluated only in the closed condition. The patient is told to take a deep breath or perform a Valsalva maneuver. The X-ray table can be moved temporarily to a somewhat steeper tilt to promote rapid sedimentation of contrast material in the valve sinuses.

Technique of ascending pressure phlebography
Puncture of the dorsal vein of the great toe or other dorsal foot vein
Ankle tourniquet
Patient in semiupright position
Limb relaxed and non-weight-bearing for contrast injection
Manual direction of the contrast medium
Use of overflow effect to extend contrast filling
Fluoroscopic assessment of hemodynamics
Spot films of the deep venous system
Valsalva maneuver during passage of contrast medium through the popliteal and common femoral veins
Spot films of terminal and sluice valves of the saphenous veins
Final fluoroscopic assessment (second look)

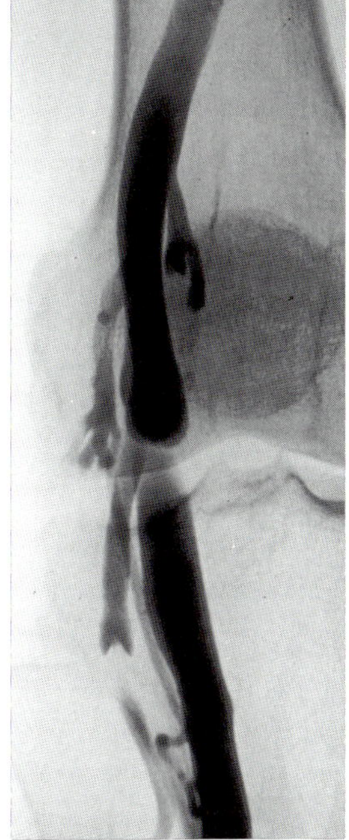
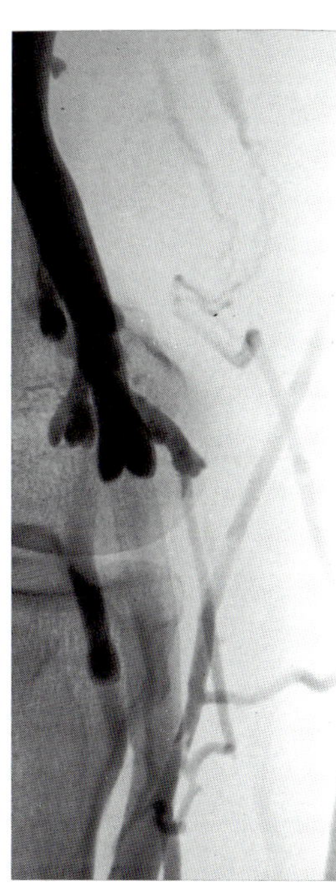

98. Evaluation of fine morphologic details by individual application of the dilution effect with the manual compression technique. Popliteal vein demonstrated by ascending pressure phlebography. *Left,* internal rotation; *right,* lateral views

In patients with primary varicose veins due to *incompetent transfascial communications,* the focus of the examination is on the terminal valves of the great and small saphenous veins or the perforating veins. Once the contrast bolus has passed through the terminal region of the saphenous veins, the patient is told to perform a Valsalva maneuver while keeping the muscles of the lower extremity completely relaxed.

Routine use of the *Valsalva maneuver* is the key to a successful examination in ascending phlebography. It leads to closure of all the venous valves in the lower extremity, allowing the contrast medium to settle on the valve cusps; this provides an optimum definition of fine morphologic details in the relaxed semiupright patient. The Valsalva maneuver is contraindicated in patients with thrombosis of the deep leg and pelvic veins due to the danger of pulmonary embolism. However, the effect can be simulated by having the patient inhale deeply.

In patients with *varicose saphenous veins,* contrast medium will reflux into the superficial vein through the incompetent transfascial communication when a Valsalva maneuver is performed. Retrograde flow will fill the great saphenous vein past the knee with continued straining, while retrograde flow in the small saphenous vein may extend to the distal part of the lower leg. This makes it possible to identify the distal site of incompetence in the varicose saphenous system and determine the stage of the disease, which are essential considerations for preoperative planning.

Radiographic examination of the deep leg veins and muscle veins is generally performed on *two planes* to allow for positive differentiation between pathologic changes and flow phenomena. Even the small saphenous vein should be imaged in a second projection to avoid confusion with the gastrocnemius veins. For radiography of the thigh veins, it is usually sufficient to take one film with the leg rotated slightly outward; flow phenomena are more easily excluded by taking a second *delayed film* in the same projection.

All *limb position changes* are performed by the examining physician with no active assistance from the patient, since leg muscle contraction would immediately expel the contrast medium from the regions of interest.

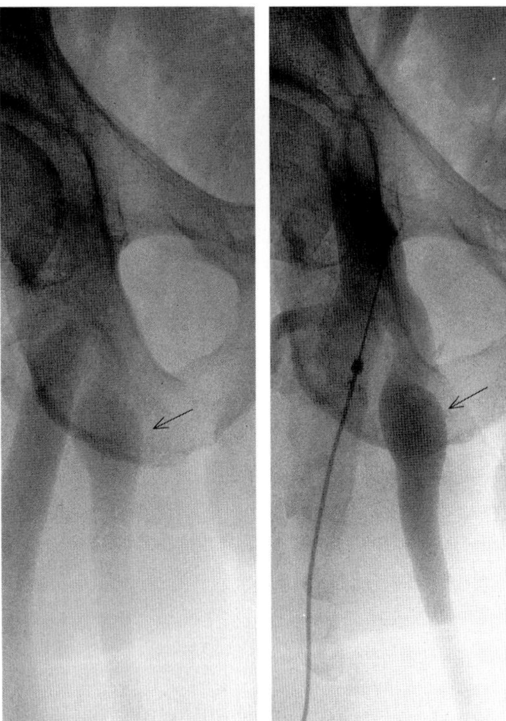

99. Secondary incompetence of the popliteal and femoral veins with severe (stage III) great saphenous varicosity. *Left,* ascending phlebography with a Valsalva maneuver. Washed-out effect or inadequate visualization of the common femoral vein during the calf compression test with a Valsalva maneuver. Great saphenous vein enlarged to the thickness of a thumb (→). *Right,* retrograde pressure phlebography. Clear demonstration of the great saphenous vein, but only minimal return into the superficial femoral vein

Phleboscopy

Although prolonged phleboscopic monitoring of lower extremity venous flow is contraindicated due to radiation hazard, the radiologist should still form an impression of venous hemodynamics and incorporate it into his evaluation. With secondary popliteal and femoral vein incompetence, the calf compression test will no longer produce rapid expulsion of the opaque column, signifying an antegrade flow deficiency that differs from the predominantly retrograde deficiency seen in post-thrombotic syndrome. The secondary incompetence can be approximately quantified by the femoral vein function test (see p. 64).

With severe deep-vein circulatory impairment in the setting of secondary popliteal and femoral vein incompetence or post-thrombotic syndrome, the contrast medium becomes diffusely mixed with the blood during the course of the examination. The vessels are not clearly delineated, and the phlebogram presents a faded or washed-out appearance. The study may be repeated if neces- 99
sary using a larger contrast bolus and a more rapid examination technique. Compression bandaging of the lower leg can further improve the quality of the evaluation.

The purpose of fluoroscopy, besides conveying an impression of flow dynamics, is to guide the radiologist in obtaining optimum radiographic views of selected regions. The diagnosis is based chiefly on an evaluation of the X-ray films.

Filming Sequence

The standardized technique of ascending pressure phlebography permits us to define a standard,
routine filming sequence consisting of three 100
24/30-cm films divided into two or 35/35-cm films divided into three. Following injection of the contrast medium, a view is obtained of the deep lower-leg veins with the leg internally rotated 30° (*exposure 1*). Then the contrast medium is directed into the popliteal vein, and the patient is told to strain. Fluoroscopic observation will readily disclose incompetence of the small saphenous vein, which is projected onto the fibula lateral to the popliteal vein in the internally rotated extremity (*exposure 2*). While the patient continues straining to prevent premature outflow of the contrast medium, the physician rotates the limb externally and obtains a lateral view of the popliteal vein (*exposure 3*). A film is also taken of the deep lower-leg veins in the lateral view, which may additionally show the retrograde filling of a varicose small saphenous vein (*exposure 4*); the vessel may be projected onto the fibula. With severe perforator incompetence the phlebograms of the crural vessels are taken successively in both planes (exposures 2 and 4 are interchanged) to avoid excessive superimposition of the extrafascial veins.

The patient may breathe normally until the next phase of the examination. The leg remains in external rotation. After the spot film device has been centered on the inguinal region, the examiner compresses the calf muscles with his hand, applying moderate pressure, until the contrast bolus passes into the common femoral vein. The patient

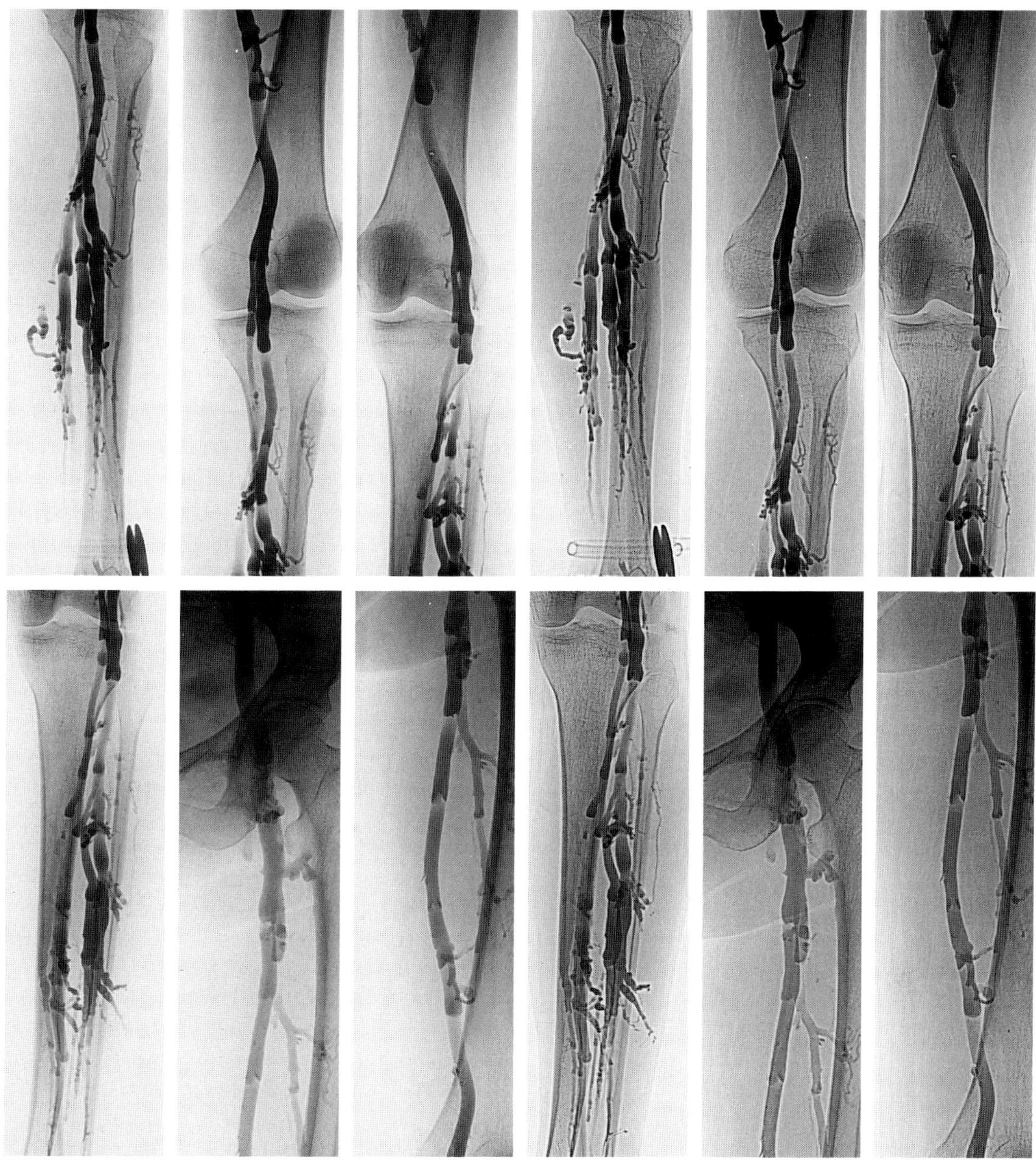

100. Normal filming sequence in ascending pressure phlebography. The images on the left were obtained using a conventional technique, and those on the right using electronic peripheral intensification. (For the imaging sequence, see text)

is again told to perform a Valsalva maneuvr. Competent terminal valve function of the great saphenous vein as well as contrast reflux into the incompetent vessel are easily detected by fluoroscopic observation (*exposure* 5). The last film (*exposure 6*) is then taken of the thigh veins, demonstrating antegrade filling of the superficial femoral vein and any simultaneous retrograde filling of an incompetent great saphenous vein. Fluoroscopy is used a final time to locate the distal site of incompetence and check for incompetent transfascial communications at atypical sites.

The standard filming sequence can be supplemented if necessary by *special views*. For example, an intermittent Valsalva maneuver may be performed to better evaluate the venous valves, or the ankle tourniquet may be removed to permit contrast flow into the superficial venous system (non-

compression or superficial phlebography). In patients with thigh vein disease, *additional views* should be taken after changing the rotational position of the limb or after a brief delay.
The *venous valves* are of particular interest during interpretation of the phlebograms, so we routinely have the patient inhale deeply or perform a brief Valsalva maneuver to close the valve cusps before each exposure is taken.
At the conclusion of the procedure, the table is returned to a horizontal position so that thromboprophylactic leg and foot exercises can be initiated.

Phlebographic Femoral Vein Function Test of Hach

The *femoral vein function test* is a semiquantitative procedure used during phlebography to assess the severity of secondary popliteal and femoral vein incompetence. It requires the use of a *standardized technique*. With the table tilted 30°, the relaxed, dependent lower limb is externally rotated. A 30-ml bolus of 60% contrast solution is injected within 25 s. First the opaque column is manually directed into the lower leg vessels under fluoroscopic control. Then the examiner grasps the patient's calf from behind with his ipsilateral hand (right leg of patient and right hand of examiner) and applies a *brief*, forceful compression. Normally the deep thigh veins fill spontaneously or immediately after the initial compression. If two compressions are required to fill the thigh veins, the incompetence is graded as mild; if three or more repetitions are required, the incompetence is graded respectively as moderate or severe. The calf compressions are performed in rapid succession, no more than 2 s apart, to shorten the duration of X-ray exposure.

Stem vein function test
Table tilted 30°
Lower limb completely relaxed and non-weight-bearing
Contrast medium in 60% concentration
Injection of 30-ml bolus within 25 s
Manual direction of bolus into lower leg vessels
Calf compression test
Fluoroscopic observation of thigh veins

The femoral vein function test is used mainly to evaluate the recirculating flow patterns that develop in association with saphenous vein varicosity. Secondary popliteal and femoral vein incompetence is associated with *antegrade outflow*. Similar findings are seen with severe regressive changes. Post-thrombotic syndrome and venous dysplasia also present an antegrade component in addition to the predominantly retrograde flow.

Special Problems and Pitfalls

Deviations from the standard technique can distort the phlebographic picture in various ways, leading to errors of interpretation and diagnosis.
In most techniques of peripheral venous radiography, the patient *stands passively* on the affected leg and, when cued by the examiner, *actively* changes the leg position. The active muscular contraction and weight bearing on the injected leg lead to an *uncontrolled acceleration of blood flow*, causing incomplete deep venous filling. Active muscular effort also has a *compressive effect on the popliteal vein* from the expanding gastrocnemius muscle bellies (see p. 47). Standing on a rotating platform (Grollmann and Straede 1977) or small box (Rabinov and Paulin 1972) with the opposite foot offers no advantages over the totally non-weight-bearing position; in fact, most patients find it more difficult to maintain a one-legged stance than to support themselves on hand grips.
The dependent, non-weight-bearing limb position permits the use of a sharp-beveled venepuncture needle that is easy to insert and causes no pain (Hach 1976). A short-beveled butterfly needle is preferred if phlebography is to be followed by venous pressure measurement or digital subtraction angiography.
The radiologist can detect *extravasation* at once by placing his fingertip over the tip of the needle. Generally he will be able to resume the examination by slightly adjusting the needle position and buttressing the vein with his fingertips (see p. 60).
The *venepuncture site* is significant in terms of achieving satisfactory contrast filling of the deep veins of the lower leg. Injecting the medium into a lateral marginal foot vein sometimes leads to deficient filling or nonfilling of the posterior tibial vein group, because the lateral foot veins drain mostly into the anterior tibial veins. The ideal puncture site is the dorsal vein of the great toe.

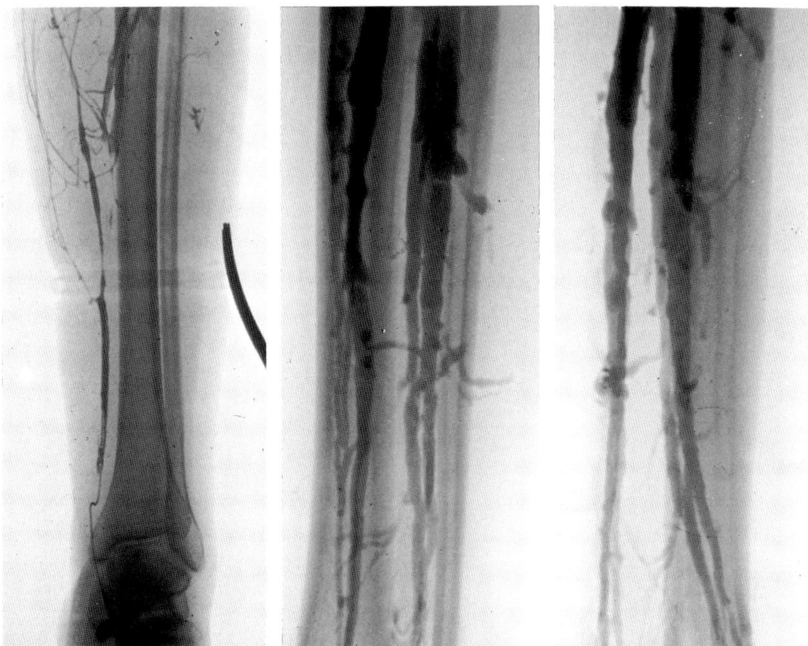

101. Faulty phlebographic technique. *Left,* nonopacification of the intrafascial veins following direct injection of contrast medium into the great saphenous vein through an intravascular catheter. The tourniquet is positioned too high. Misdiagnosis: acute deep leg vein thrombosis. *Middle, right,* normal-appearing deep venous system in ascending pressure phlebography. *Middle,* internal rotation view; *right,* lateral view

Contrast medium injected at that site drains into the dorsal venous arch of the foot, is evenly distributed among the metatarsal veins, and passes readily into the main outflow channels. Another advantage of the toe vein is its thick wall, which can tolerate a relatively high injection pressure.

If filling of the deep lower leg veins is unsatisfactory, the examiner must wait until they are opacified by the *overflow effect* in a later phase of the examination. Occasionally this effect is useful in cases where the dorsal foot venepuncture is unsuccessful and the study cannot be rescheduled; in this case retrograde filling of the peripheral deep venous segments can often be achieved by injecting contrast medium into a varix in the lower leg. At this time the patient is brought to a nearly vertical position, the legs still relaxed and dependent, to promote more rapid settling of the contrast bolus.

The *ankle tourniquet* directs the contrast flow into the deep veins. Except in special inquiries, runoff of the contrast medium through the superficial venous system is not desired and would cause confusion due to overlapping venous opacities. Moreover, vascular incompetence, even in the extrafascial vessels, is diagnosed best by the *detection of retrograde flow.*

The superficial veins are effectively occluded by compressing them against the bone proximal to the ankle mortise. If contrast medium is injected directly into the great saphenous vein, its passage
through the deep vessels may be greatly delayed or 101
incomplete, especially if the medial malleolar vein is absent or rudimentary. This technique also increases patient discomfort.

If the ankle tourniquet is too tight, its occlusive effect may be transmitted to the intrafascial vessels through compression of the muscles and tendons.
Fortunately this error is easily recognized and cor- 102
rected during the examination.

Some authors (Höjensgard 1949; Thomas and Lea 1972) place a *second tourniquet* above or below the knee in the belief that it enhances deep venous filling. But comparative studies with and without a second tourniquet have shown no significant differences (Rabinov and Paulin 1972). Use of a second tourniquet, moreover, prevents the radiographic diagnosis of saphenous varicosity, and the annular constriction of a floating thrombus in the

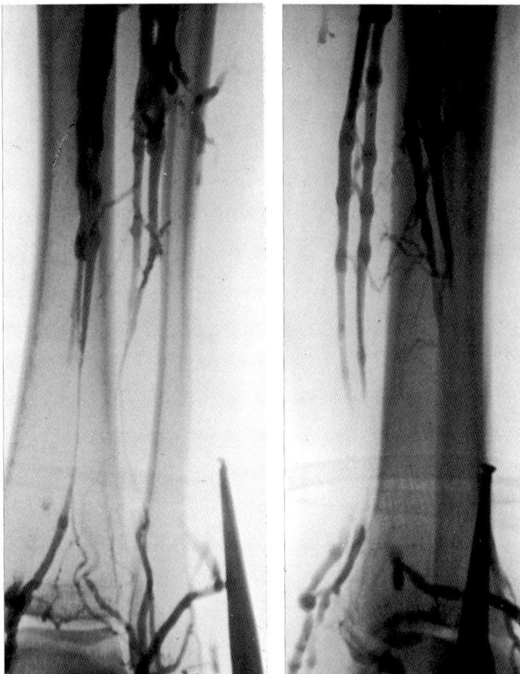

102. Undesired deep venous compression by too tight an ankle tourniquet. Ascending pressure phlebography: *left*, internal rotation view; *right*, lateral view

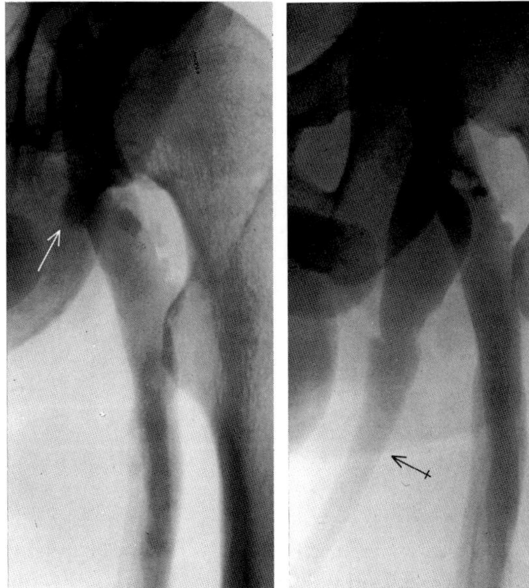

103. Faulty technique of ascending pressure phlebography. *Left*, incomplete Valsalva maneuver. Apparent (!) delineation of the terminal valve of the great saphenous vein with indistinct contours (→). *Right*, a more forceful Valsalva maneuver demonstrates severe great saphenous varicosity (↔)

deep venous system may pose a risk of detachment and pulmonary embolism.

Normal venous outflow from the relaxed, dependent lower extremity proceeds at a very slow rate, if at all. Applying digital pressure to the sole of the foot or the calf pressure point as well as gentle compression of the transverse pedal arch or calf will augment the blood flow velocity in a controlled manner. A frequent source of error is misunderstanding how to perform the Valsalva maneuver: instead of *straining*, the patient contracts his leg muscles. This immediately expels the opacified blood from the lower extremity. The terminal portions of the saphenous veins are not visualized, and severe incompetence of the great or small saphenous vein may be missed. The venous surgeon cannot profit from phlebograms that do 103
not assess valvular competency in the terminal part of the saphenous system.

During fluoroscopic observation on the monitor screen, it is easy to miss an incomplete varicosity of the long saphenous trunk that does not fill through incompetent sluice valves but through an incompetent Dodd's perforator or varicose side branch. An incomplete varicosity of this type usually is not detected until the end of the examination. The radiologist should thus make it a practice to screen the medial soft tissues of the thigh for *abnormal vascular connections.* Sometimes this region shows poor image contrast on the monitor or lies outside the image frame.

Usually the muscle veins do not appear until a later phase of the examination, when they are filled by the overflow effect. Thus, a *delayed film* should be obtained in patients with suspected deep vein thrombosis. Thrombi are commonly located in the sinuses of the muscle veins or in their valve pockets. Optimum transparency of the contrast column is important for their detection.

A varicose small saphenous trunk, too, may not be plainly seen until the end of the examination. When the patient performs a Valsalva maneuver, only *that* quantity of opacified blood momentarily present between two valves of the popliteal vein can reflux into the small saphenous vein, and it may be no more than a few millimeters. Gradually, as the examination proceeds, the varicose saphenous vein is brought out more clearly by retrograde contrast sedimentation and blood flow.

With severe extrafascial varicosity, especially when accompanied by decompensated recirculating flow with marked perforating vein incompe-

Common technical errors in ascending pressure phlebography
Injection of contrast medium directly into the great saphenous vein
Tourniquet too loose, too tight, or too high on the leg
Inadequate or intermittent straining
Active contraction of leg muscles
Inadequate volume of contrast medium
Inadequate manual injection pressure
Omission of final fluoroscopic assessment

tence, it may not be possible to obtain clear views of the deep veins due to multiple superimposed vascular convolutions. One solution is to repeat the examination after tightly bandaging the lower leg.

Hemodynamic Aspects

A knowledge of the dynamics of venous blood flow in the lower extremity is of fundamental importance in understanding the technique of ascending pressure phlebography. Arnoldi (1964) describes the *hemodynamic cycle* as consisting of three phases: systole, diastole I, and diastole II.

In ascending pressure phlebography where the injected leg is relaxed and dependent, the hemodynamic conditions of *diastole II* prevail, characterized by a slow "-steady flow" in the deep veins. The flow rate in a supine position is 1–2 cm/s and falls as the patient is moved to a semiupright position due to the rising hydrostatic pressure. All valves are open, and venous outflow is driven entirely by pressure from the arteriolar side.
96 The *overflow effect* (higher-specific-gravity contrast medium spilling over into formerly unopacified veins at sites of venous confluence) is operative in this phase and permits proximal-to-distal filling of competent peripheral venous segments.

The pressure during diastole II is probably somewhat higher in the deep veins than in the superficial system. Accordingly, the valves in the perforating veins are closed, and only incompetent vessels can be opacified by a retrograde, outward-directed flow.

With rhythmic contractions of the calf muscles, producing a state of *systole*, the pressure rises sharply in the muscle veins and slightly in the popliteal vein, while it progressively falls in the great saphenous vein. Hence the perforating veins remain closed. A maximal muscular contraction can propel 50–75 ml of blood from the deep venous system to the pelvic level (Ludbrook 1972). Fluoroscopy will demonstrate how active stance or voluntary leg motion will abruptly expel the contrast medium from the lower limb, requiring another contrast injection in order to continue the examination.

During *diastole I*, the pressure in the calf muscles falls sharply, causing the blood to flow centrally through the perforating veins from the extrafascial vessels. With the influx from superficial and nutrient veins into the calf muscle sinuses, the venous pressure slowly rises. Once the pressure within the popliteal vein is exceeded, the "steady flow" condition of diastole II is restored.

Diastole I does not play a role in ascending phlebography with a Valsalva maneuver, because the tourniquet compression keeps the contrast medium from entering the superficial venous system. In this situation only unopacified blood could enter the intrafascial space, interfering with the examination.

The differentiated hemodynamics of the calf muscle pump explains why routine examination of the extrafascial venous system and important transfascial communications is best performed during diastole II. In this phase the main stem veins are well opacified by the slow, steady outflow of contrast medium. Competent perforating veins and saphenous trunks may be partially filled by the sedimentation effect; contrast may descend as far as the proximal sluice valve, producing a stump-like appearance. The muscle veins are routinely filled by retrograde overflow in the semiupright position.

May and Nissl Technique of Ascending Phlebography with Fluoroscopy

Suitable for evaluation of the deep leg veins, muscle veins and pelvic veins, ascending phlebography is an important method for the diagnosis of phlebothrombosis. May and Nissl (1973) developed the technique in a large clinical population and standardized it to the form practiced today.

Patient preparation and venepuncture are the same as for ascending pressure phlebography. A 30-ml dose of 60 % contrast medium is manually injected into a dorsal foot vein. If a staged procedure is dispensed with in favor of a global examination of the venous system, the recommended dose is 100 ml or more of a 40 %–45 % contrast solution, which may be administered by high-pressure injector (Schmitt 1977).

The patient stands on a raised platform at the foot of the tilted X-ray table, bearing no weight on the injected leg. Outflow of the contrast medium is achieved by manual calf compression or by active toe exercise. A distal-to-proximal filming sequence is used, following the centripedal progression of venous flow. Guided by television monitoring, six views of the leg veins are recorded on 24/30-cm film divided into two or 35/35-cm film divided into three: (1) a 30° internal rotation view of the lower leg veins, (2) a lateral view of the lower leg veins, (3) a lateral view of the popliteal vein, (4) a 30° internal rotation view of the popliteal vein, (5) a posteroanterior view of the superficial femoral vein, (6) and a posteroanterior view of the common femoral vein and iliac veins.

Ascending phlebography with a high dose of contrast medium in low concentration gives good delineation of the intrafascial stem veins and muscle veins, so it is useful in patients with clinical suspicion of deep vein thrombosis. The technique also gives good definition of the venous valves when combined with a Valsalva maneuver or deep inhalation. If a thrombus is detected, Valsalva maneuvers and compression tests are contraindicated due to the risk of embolism.
In the interest of radiation safety, time-consuming phleboscopy can generally be dispensed with during examinations for venous thrombosis. The experienced radiologist can draw his diagnostic conclusions from a dynamic observation of contrast outflow and incorporate them into his overall evaluation.

Ascending Phlebography with Phleboscopy in Severely Sick Patients in a Relaxed Oblique Position (Hach and Hach-Wunderle 1994)

Patients with deep leg vein and pelvic vein thromboses may be in poor general condition due to the primary disease or in poor condition due to the thromboembolic event and have to be transported in a laying position. They may not be able to stand up or actively hold on to side handles when in a vertical position. They may be immobile and have infusion needles in their arms because of injuries or surgery. In such situations, of course, special care must be taken during the examination. Two or three staff members should *passively* position the patients flat on the X-ray table, making them as comfortable as possible with a pillow. The leg muscles must be completely relaxed. Insofar as possible, it is advisable to remove compression bandages; they should at least be cut above the foot. Then a lukewarm wash cloth is placed on the forefoot, which is also kept warm a prewarmed towel. After 5 min the skin is warmed and X-ray examination can be performed under local anesthesia.
For phlebography the examination table should be slightly tilted – about 10°–15°; this should be sufficient to induce a sedimentation effect of the contrast agent. Normally a higher dose of contrast agent (80–100 ml) is required; a concentration of 45% is sufficient. The deep veins are sometimes not visible until a later phase of the examination via the overflow effect. Therefore, a second look is necessary. If the leg is very swollen, compression at the ankle has no effect. However, additional tourniquets should not be applied on the lower and upper thigh because of the risk of inducing lung embolus and of misdiagnosis.

Blind Technique of Ascending Pressure Phlebography (Almen and Nylander 1962; Haeger and Nylander 1967)

When image intensification video monitoring is not available, phlebograms can be taken with an overcouch tube on a Bucky table using a "blind" technique. The increased focus-film distance enhances image sharpness and eliminates dimensional distortion. The major *disadvantage* of this technique is that the visualization of specific vascular regions is left largely to chance due to the difficulty of estimating the rate of contrast outflow under normal and pathologic conditions. For this reason the blind technique is rarely used today.

Preparation of the patient is the same as for standard ascending phlebography. Views are best recorded on 96/20-cm film. A wedge filter can be used to correct the tube voltage for soft-tissue thickness. The first *exposure* is taken immediately after the injection of 20–60 ml of contrast medium, and three more exposures are taken at 15-s intervals following active plantar flexion of the foot or manual calf compression. It is unclear what filming mode is best in patients with severe varicose veins, acute deep vein thrombosis, malformations of the vascular system, or post-thrombotic syndrome.
The supine position gives rise to peculiar outflow conditions in the intrafascial venous system associated with layering of contrast material and flow-induced artifacts. The venous valves are poorly defined due to the unfavorable sedimentation effect. All this can lead to errors in interpretation of the phlebograms.
The technique can be improved by performing the examination on a tilt table and by using long cassettes,

which can be changed manually or with a Gärtner-Reisser changer. Even this technique is currently obsolete, however.

Noncompression Ascending Phlebography

Noncompression phlebography (superficial phlebography, "runoff" phlebography; Schneider and Fischer 1979) is best suited for the evaluation of the extrafascial venous system. The technique of contrast injection is similar to that for ascending pressure phlebography, using a connecting tube to inject the medium into the vein of the great toe or a dorsal foot vein. For selective visualization of the great or small saphenous vein, the needle is placed in the appropriate marginal foot vein. The table is tilted 20°–40°. Without tourniquet compression, most of the injectate flows through the saphenous veins, some also entering the deep veins by way of perforators in the foot and lower leg. This technique is not very satisfactory for defining the intrafascial vessels and the terminal valves of the saphenous veins. In selected cases, repeated contrast injections may be administered with and without compression to permit a comprehensive assessment. Today there are few recognized indications for the nontourniquet technique.

Varicography (May and Nissl 1973)

Varicography is used for the precise localization of incompetent perforating veins and to assess the drainage conditions about large varices prior to operative treatment. In special cases the procedure may be done as an adjunct to ascending phlebography, e.g., to demonstrate varicosity of Hach's profunda perforating vein or atypical connections related to congenital malformations of the venous system.

After the needle has been inserted into the vari-
104 cose vein and secured with adhesive tape, the X-ray table is brought to the horizontal position or tilted to a 20° head-down position. Then 5 ml of contrast medium is injected through a connecting tube and directed to the desired site by manual palpation under television control.

Due to the risk of local thrombophlebitis from prolonged contact of the contrast medium with the vein wall, it is best to perform the examination

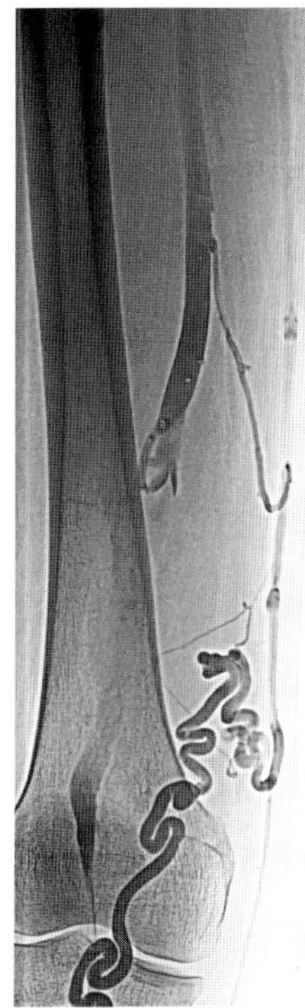

104. Varicography. Reticular varices and a competent Dodds perforating vein are demonstrated. Phlebography with electronic peripheral intensification

on the day before surgery. Varicography is not ideal for deep venous assessment due to the potential for misinterpretation.

Retrograde Pressure Phlebography (Gullmo 1956)

Retrograde pressure phlebography today is more often used in the diagnosis of primary and secondary femoral vein incompetence, especially before reconstruction or transplantation of values in the femoral vein. (Kistner and Ferris 1982; Raju and Fredericks 1988; Perrin et al. 1992.) It should be performed in conjunction with pelvic phlebography to detect pathologic changes. For the diagnosis of long saphenous varicosity ascending pressure phlebography appears better suited.

For *local anesthesia*, a skin wheal is raised with a vaccination gun in the supine patient 6 cm below the inguinal fold and 1.5 cm medial to the common femoral artery, and then about a 2-cm-wide area over the femoral vein is infiltrated as far as the inguinal ligament with approximately 8 ml of 0.5% mepivacaine. A larger dose might cause extrinsic compression of the vein, making the venepuncture difficult.

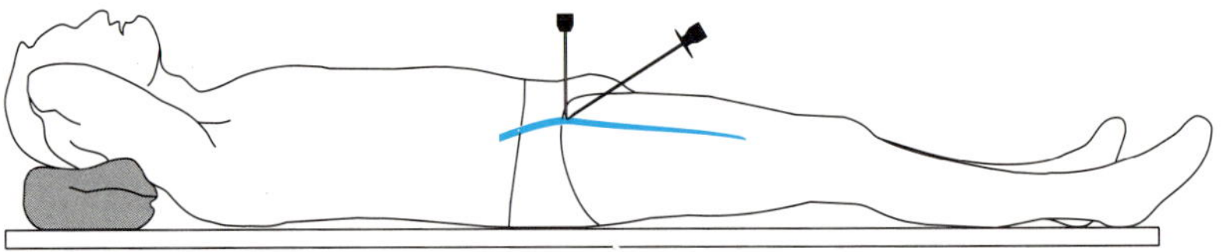

105. Vertical trial puncture and oblique venepuncture for retrograde pressure phlebography and pelvic phlebography

Epinephrine should not be added to the anesthetic solution due to the danger of severe circulatory impairment from an inadvertent arterial injection. The solution is not injected in a fanlike pattern but on a straight path over the course of the vessel. This safeguards against transient *paralysis of the femoral nerve*, which runs lateral to the femoral artery and supplies the extensor muscles of the thigh. Paralysis is manifested by inability to raise the leg and buckling of the leg during walking. The symptoms regress spontaneously in 3 h, and no special treatment is required.

The Seldinger system appears to be suitable for performing the *venepuncture*. The needle is introduced at a very oblique angle to the limb surface.
105 While this technique is relatively difficult and requires some practice, there is virtually no danger of needle displacement or paravenous injection during a Valsalva maneuver as there is with a perpendicular puncture. The examiner can determine the precise location of the vein by making vertical trial punctures with a no. 1-gauge disposable needle.

The vein can be successfully cannulated only when the hip joint is extended. Flexion at the hip makes the venepuncture impossible. Occasionally the insertion can be made easier by hyperextending the hip over a flat cushion placed beneath the buttock.

Pulsatile blood spurting from the hub signals the *inadvertent puncture of an artery*. The needle is withdrawn at once and the site manually compressed for 3–4 min. Then the examination may resume. For safety, we conclude the examination by covering the site with a pressure bandage secured with elastic tape and rest the limb for 2–4 h.

High-grade occlusion of the pelvic veins leads to a high-pressure *reflux of venous blood* from the needle that can simulate a punctured artery. Under normal conditions blood drains from the common femoral vein so slowly that, on making a trial puncture, the examiner must wait a moment or apply suction with a small syringe to confirm that the needle is within the vein.

The injection of 20 ml contrast medium is sufficient for *retrograde filling of the thigh veins*. The 106
patient should perform a Valsalva maneuver and continue straining during the injection. Under normal circumstances the contrast medium can reflux into the superficial and deep leg veins until it encounters a closed valve. With valvular incompetence, the retrograde flow may extend past the 107
knee. Generally the findings can be documented by one or two 24/30-cm films taken with a spot 108
film device. The digital subtraction technique also can be used.

In uncomplicated cases a simple adhesive bandage is placed over the venepuncture site at the end of the examination. An encircling bandage should not be used due to the danger of peripheral stasis. The patient is observed for 10–15 min before leaving the facility.

References

Almen T, Nylander G (1962) Serial phlebography of the normal lower leg during muscular contraction and relaxation. Acta Radiol (Stockholm) 57: 264

Arnoldi CC (1964) The venous return from the lower leg in health and chronic venous insufficiency. Acta Orthop Scand Suppl 64: 7

Arnoldi CC, Bauer G (1960) Interosseous phlebography. Angiology 11: 44

Chambraud R (1951) La phlebographie pelvienne par voie transosseuse. Gynéc Obstét 50: 477

Grollmann JH, Straede PD (1977) Rotating platform for ascending phlebography. Am J Roentgenol Radium Ther Nucl Med 129: 941

Gullmo AL (1956) On the technique of phlebography of the lower limb. Acta Radiol (Stockholm) 46: 603

Hach W (1974) Die aszendierende Preßphlebographie, eine Routinemethode zur Beurteilung der oberflächlichen Stammvenen. In: Friedrich HC, Hamelmann H (Hrsg) Ergebnisse der Angiologie, Bd 8. Schattauer, Stuttgart New York

Hach W (1976) Die schmerzlose Phlebographie. Fortschr Röntgenstr Nuklearmed 125: 98

Hach W (1981) Spezielle Diagnostik der primären Varikose. Demeter, Gräfelfing

Haeger K, Nylander G (1967) Die Phlebographie im akuten Stadium der Thrombose. Triangel 8: 18

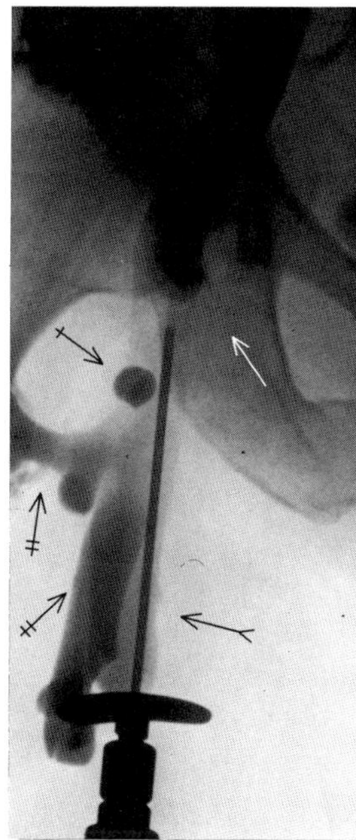

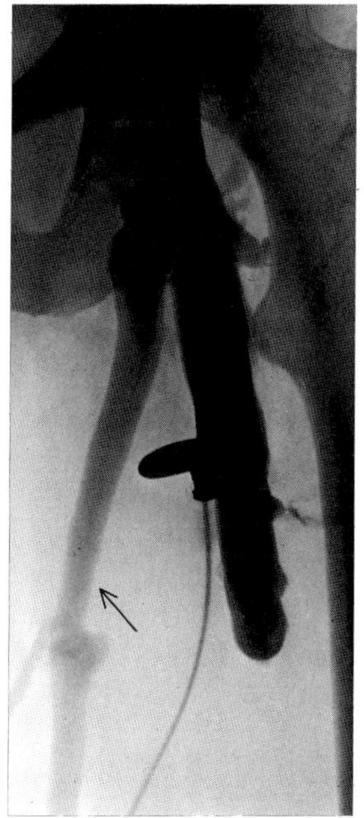

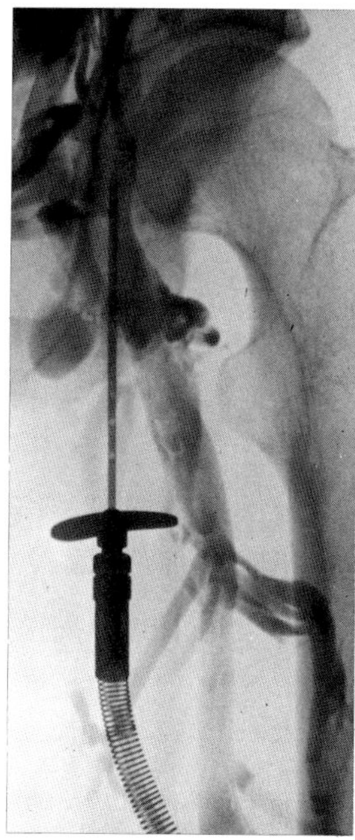

106 *(left).* A competent common femoral vein and its branches are demonstrated by retrograde phlebography with a Valsalva maneuver. → Terminal valve of the great saphenous vein, +→ terminal valve of the superficial circumflex iliac vein, ++→ muscle veins and profunda femoris, ↣ superficial femoral vein

107 *(middle).* Varicose great saphenous trunk (→) demonstrated by retrograde pressure phlebography

108 *(right).* Post-thrombotic syndrome of the leg and pelvic veins, demonstrated by retrograde phlebography. When the patient performs a Valsalva maneuver, contrast medium refluxes into the deep veins of the thigh. Note the septation of the vessel lumina

Höjensgard IC (1949) Phlebography in chronic venous insufficiency. Acta Radiol (Stockholm) 32: 375

Kistner RL, Ferris EB (1982) Femoral vein reconstruction in the management of chronic venous insufficiency Arch Surg 117: 1571

Lea Thomas M (1972) Phlebography. Arch Surg 104: 145

Ludbrook J (1972) The analysis of the venous system. Huber, Bern

May R, Nissl R (1973) Phlebographie der unteren Extremität. Thieme, Stuttgart

Perrin M, Bayon JM, Castells-Ferrer P, Hiltbrand B (1992) Résultats de la chirurgic restauratrice dans les reflux veineux profonds. In: Raymond-Martimbeau P, Prescott R, Zummo M (Eds) Phlebologie 92. J Libbey Eurotext, Paris

Rabinov K, Paulin S (1972) Roentgendiagnosis of venous thrombosis in the leg. Arch Surg 104: 134

Raju S, Fredericks R (1988) Valve reconstruction procedures of nonobstrutive venous insufficiency. Rationale techniqués and results in 107 procedures with 2 to 8 years follow-up. J Vasc Surg 7: 301

Schmitt HE (1977) Aszendierende Phlebographie bei tiefer Venenthrombose. Huber, Bern

Schneider H, Fischer H (1979) Die chronisch-venöse Insuffizienz. Enke, Stuttgart

Weber G (1978) Phlebographie und Venendruckmessung im Abdomen und Becken. Witzstrock, Baden Baden

Zeitler E (1973) Phlebographie. In: Haid-Fischer F, Haid H (Hrsg) Venenerkrankungen. Thieme, Stuttgart

Phlebography of the Pelvic Veins and Inferior Vena Cava

Radiographic examination of the pelvic veins differs from lower limb phlebography in that it may involve not just diagnostic problems in the vessels themselves but also *therapeutic aspects* of interventional radiology. These include the implantation of vena caval shields and stents, the removal of foreign materials with special instruments, and selective catheterization of the visceral veins to obtain blood samples for differentiated biochemical studies. In the investigation of organ diseases, phlebography has been completely superseded in recent times by more modern radiographic and sonographic techniques. The radiologist must know the precise nature of the inquiry so that he can select the most appropriate diagnostic procedure.

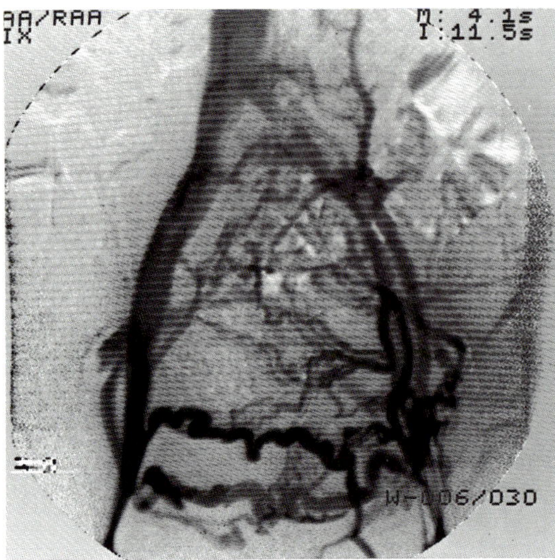

109. Digital subtraction pelvic phlebogram in a patient with post-thrombotic syndrome, obtained by simultaneous bilateral injection of 20 ml of 60 % contrast medium per side into foot veins

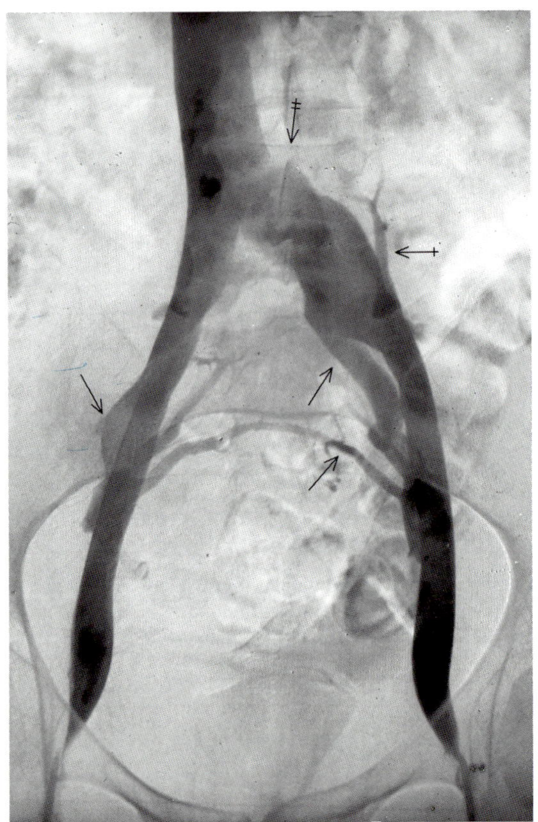

110. Pelvic veins demonstrated by the Seldinger technique. Photographic subtraction. → Internal iliac vein and presacral veins, ↔ ascending lumbar vein, ⇹ slight compression effect from the crossing right common iliac artery

Pelvic Phlebography

Phlebography of the pelvic veins and inferior vena cava (Helander and Lindbom 1959 a) has assumed considerable importance since the advent of thrombolytic therapy and the development of reconstructive venous surgery. *Digital subtraction
phlebography should be used if possible. 109
An alternative is to use a *cut film changer* and pho- 110
tographic subtraction. The iliac veins and vena cava are opacified by the simultaneous bilateral injection of 40 ml of contrast medium per side, injected manually into the common femoral vein through a connecting tube. Automated injection with a high-pressure pump infuses the medium at a rate of 8 ml/s. The exposures are made with a film plate changer. Usually four films are taken at intervals of 1.5 s, commencing after the injection of the first 15 ml of contrast. The patient is instructed to hold his breath without straining during the injection. Shallow breaths are taken during the examination.

The Valsalva maneuver has not proven helpful for evaluations of the visceral veins or internal iliac vein. Occasionally an oblique projection is useful for diagnosing extrinsic pressure syndromes in the region of the iliocaval junction.

When the common femoral vein is affected by acute
thrombosis or post-thrombotic occlusion, the iliac 111
veins can sometimes be opacified through superficial collateral pathways (uncircle technique). Trans- 112
osseous phlebography no longer has practical significance today, even in studies of the pelvic vessels.

Selective Techniques

The indications for selective phlebography have changed radically during recent years. While the

Technical errors in retrograde pressure phlebography and pelvic phlebography
Flexion at the hip
Unfavorable placement of the puncture site
Misdirection of the needle
Compression of the vein by local anesthetic depot
Addition of epinephrine to the local anesthetic solution
Puncture of the artery
Inadequate Valsalva maneuver

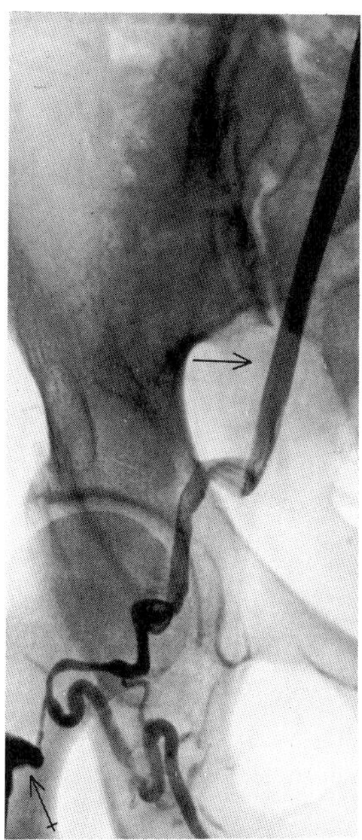

111. External iliac vein (→) demonstrated by injecting contrast medium into a collateral vein at the hip (↦) in a patient with post-thrombotic femoral vein occlusion

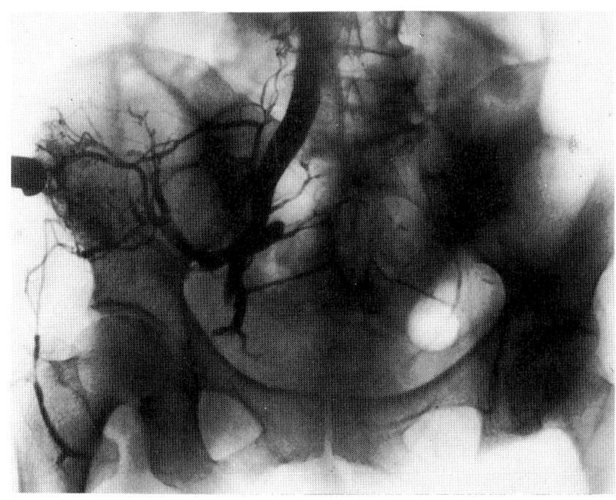

112. Historic transosseous phlebogram of the right internal and common iliac veins, obtained by injecting contrast medium at the iliac crest (Prof. Dr. Süsse, Frankfurt, 1972)

procedure has been superseded by computed tomography, magnetic resonance imaging and ultrasound for diagnostic applications, it has gained an established place in certain interventional radiologic procedures. Detailed information may be found in the textbooks by Günther and Thelen (1989) and Weber and May (1990).

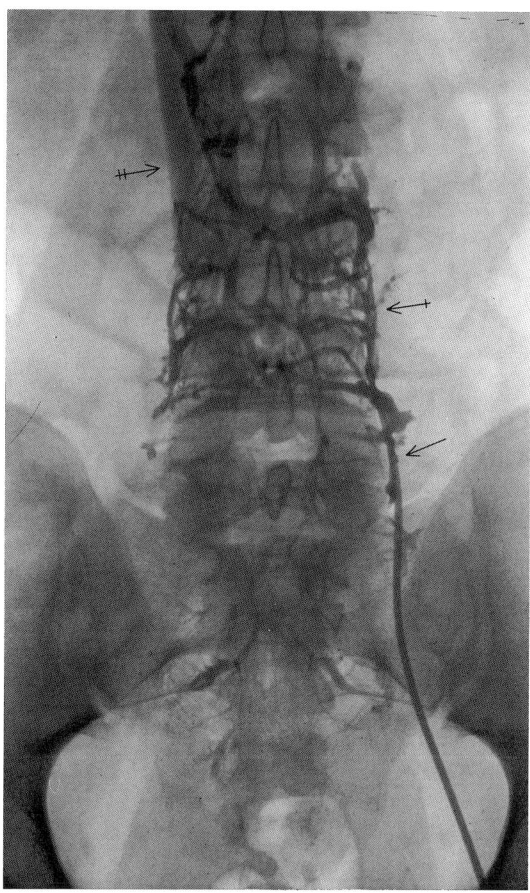

113. Lumbar veins (↦) and vertebral plexus. ⇸ Inferior vena cava. Demonstrated by selective phlebography of the ascending lumbar vein (→)

Selective Ascending Lumbar Phlebography

Selective ascending lumbar phlebography (Bücheler 1971; Bücheler et al. 1968) was formerly used for the investigation of retroperitoneal and especially vertebrospinal disease processes. It has few indications today.

The left ascending vertebral artery is relatively easy to catheterize from the common femoral vein. Contrast injection through the catheter opacifies the vertebral and paravertebral venous plexuses.

The origin of the left ascending lumbar vein is on the 113
lateral side of the common iliac vein, just past the termination of the internal iliac vein and approximately level with the inferolateral border of the fifth lumbar vertebra. The left vein ascends on a course that is a direct continuation of the external iliac vein; the right vein arises at a more acute angle.

Selective phlebography of the ascending lumbar vein is performed according to the Hettler principle using a

Phlebography of the vertebral and paravertebral venous systems by selective injection of the ascending lumbar vein
Puncture of the femoral vein
Catheterization of the ascending lumbar vein
Manual injection of 30 ml contrast medium
Serial angiography
Photographic (or digital) subtraction

sluice and conventional disposable catheters. The examiner should proceed gently and carefully; the delicate walls of the proximal veins are easily perforated, and endothelial damage can predispose to thrombosis. For this reason we flush the vessel intermittently with heparinized saline solution during the examination.
Following the manual injection of 30 ml of 60% contrast medium into the ascending lumbar vein, four serial films are taken at a rate of 1/s using a cut film changer. If facilities are available, the digital subtraction technique is used. Owing to the numerous interconnections and absence of venous valves, generally the entire vertebral and paravertebral vascular tree can be opacified from the left ascending lumbar vein as far as the azygos-hemiazygos system with very good contrast resolution (Bücheler 1971; Weber 1978).

Selective Internal Iliac Phlebography (Helander and Lindbom 1959 b)

Thromboembolitic disease occasionally arises within the internal iliac system, but the diagnosis of internal iliac vein thrombosis still poses major difficulties (Lea Thomas et al. 1972). Retrograde phlebography by the femoral route gives unsatisfactory results due to the contrast washout effect from the countercurrent blood flow and the extensive presacral collaterals to the opposite side. In some cases the internal iliac vein can be selectively
114 visualized by the occlusive technique using a bilumen Swan-Ganz or Dotter-Lukas catheter (Gillot 1974; Weber 1978). By using sonography, the venous system can be visualized.

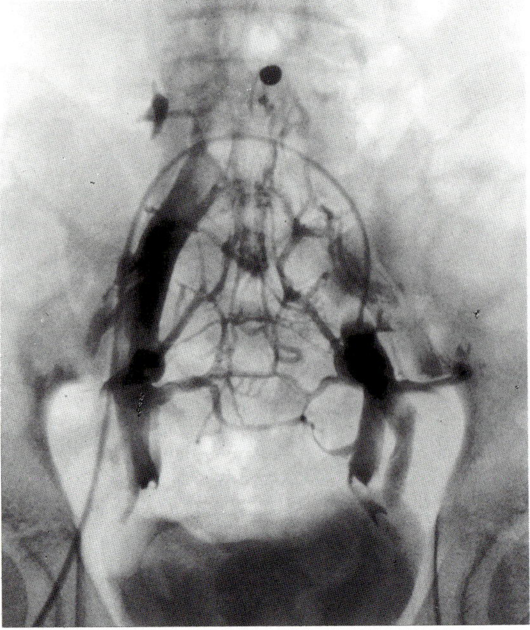

114. Occlusive phlebography of the left internal iliac vein with a Swan-Ganz catheter. (Phlebogram courtesy of Dr. J. Weber, General Hospital Altona)

Selective Phlebography of the Kidneys, Adrenals, and Liver

Retrograde phlebography of the major visceral
115 veins (Gillot et al. 1965; Gillot and Stuhl 1966; Weber 1978) has been largely supplanted by magnetic resonance imaging and advanced ultrasound techniques. Rarely, varices in the region of the renal pelvis and ureters can cause a compression syndrome with hematuria, necessitating direct visualization. Phlebography continues to be useful in special laboratory studies that require selective blood sampling from the visceral veins.

The examination is performed according to the Hettler technique, making the venepuncture at the common femoral vein. The use of occlusive catheters is favorable. The delicate walls of the visceral veins call for a meticulous working technique.

Selective Phlebography of the Spermatic Vein

Since *varicocele* has been recognized as a cause of impotence, radiographic visualization of the spermatic veins has assumed practical importance. Se- 116
lective catheterization may be done as part of a preoperative diagnostic workup or as a prelude to sclerotherapy (Seyfarth et al. 1980). Spermatic phlebography is also useful for the differential diagnosis of testicular agenesis and undescended testes.

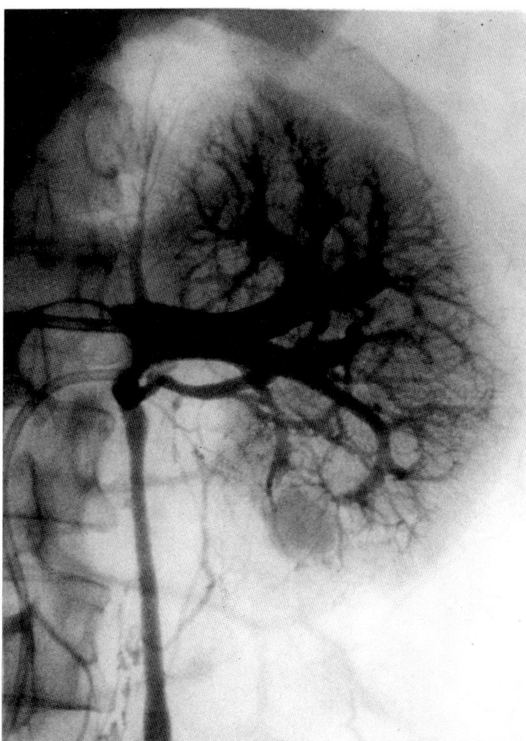

115. Occlusive phlebography of the left kidney with a Dotter-Lucas balloon-tipped catheter in a 45-year-old woman with chronic pyelonephritis. (Phlebogram courtesy of Dr. J. Weber, General Hospital Altona)

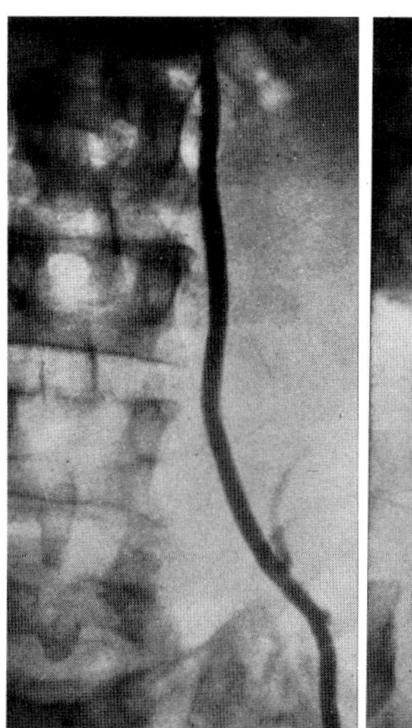

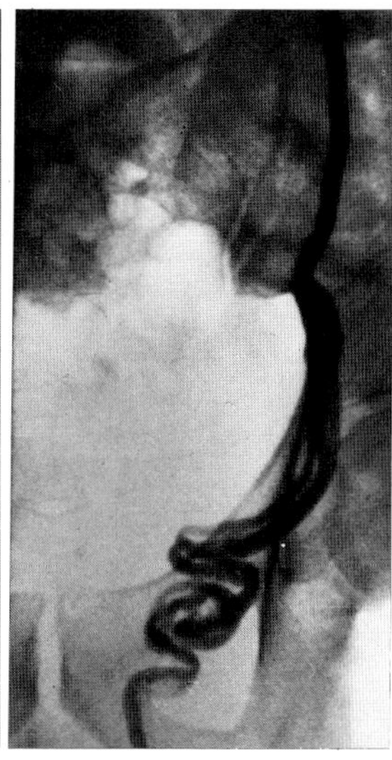

116. Selective phlebography of the left spermatic vein. *Left,* cranial segment; *right,* caudal segment. (Phlebograms courtesy of Prof. Dr. med. E. Zeitler, Nuremberg Municipal Clinics)

Generally the right spermatic vein drains into the inferior vena cava and the left spermatic vein into the renal vein. The catheter is inserted into the right common femoral vein through an introducer system (Hettler principle) under television control. Catheters with various curvatures may have to be tried. A dose of 10–20 ml of 60% contrast solution is injected by hand within 7 s. One or two spot films are taken at the end of the injection to encompass the central and peripheral portions of the vein. The semiupright position and use of the Valsalva maneuver during filming are beneficial. A varocele is sclerosed by injecting 2 ml of 3% polidocanol.

References

Ahlberg NE, Bartley O, Chidekel N, Frijesson A (1966) Phlebography in varicocele scroti. Acta Radiol [Diagn] 4: 517

Bücheler E (1971) Die direkte Angiographie der Vertebralplexus, der lumbalen Venen und des Azygosvenensystems. Röntgenanatomie und klinische Anwendung. Ergebn Med Radiol 3: 1

Bücheler E, Düx A, Venbrocks HP (1968) Die direkte vertebrale Venographie bei lumbalen Bandscheibenhernien. Fortschr Röntgenstr 109: 593

Chermet J, Bigot JM (1980) Venography of the inferior vena cava and its branches. Springer, Berlin Heidelberg New York

Gillot C, Stuhl H, Ecoiffier J (1965) La phlébographie rénale occlusive; technique et résultats normaux. Presse Med 73: 2215

Gillot C, Stuhl L (1966) La phlébographie rénale occlusive; documents pathologiques obtenu en sériographie. Presse Med 74: 1041

Gillot C (1974) Die Beckenvenenphlebographie mit Okklusion. Vasa 3: 126

Günther RW, Thelen M (1988) Interventionelle Radiologie. Thieme, Stuttgart

Helander CG, Lindbom A (1959a) Venography of the inferior vena cava. Acta Radiol (Stockholm) 52: 257

Helander CG, Lindbom A (1959b) Retrograde pelvic venography. Acta Radiol (Stockholm) 51: 401

Lea Thomas M, Browse NL (1972) Internal iliac thrombosis. Acta Radiol (Stockholm) 2: 660

Seyfarth W, Richter EI, Grosse-Vorholt R (1980) Phlebographie der Vena spermatica interna. Radiologe 20: 440

Weber J (1978) Phlebographie und Venendruckmessung im Abdomen und Becken. Witzstrock, Baden-Baden

Weber G, May R (Hrsg) (1990) Funktionelle Phlebographie. Thieme, Stuttgart

Other Techniques in Venous Diagnosis

The diagnostic protocol for the investigation of venous disorders has changed fundamentally in recent years. Ascending pressure phlebography can provide a *reference standard* (Hach 1973) for assessing the specificity and sensitivity of other clinical and instrumental diagnostic techniques. Comparisions of this kind have shown that apparently proven methods yield high incidences of false-negative and false-positive results. This applies to deep vein and pelvic vein thrombosis as well as primary varicose disease.

Despite all limitations, the clinical status and a
117 noninvasive examination score will continue to form the basis for a *staged diagnostic workup* of venous disease.

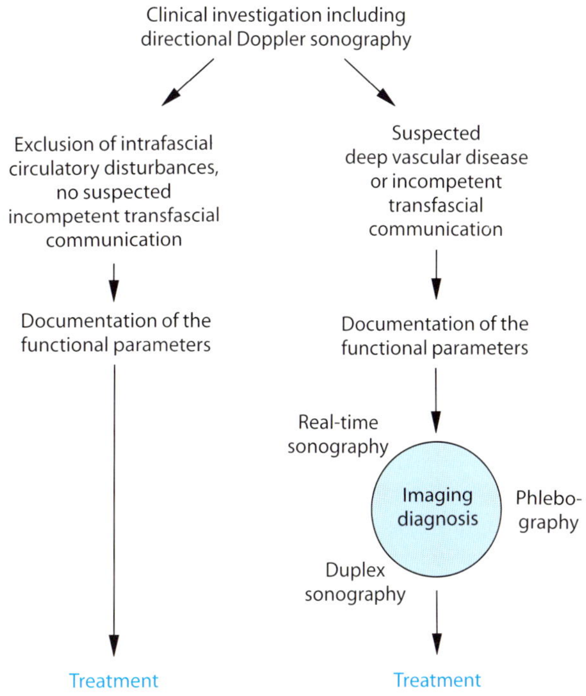

Clinical investigation including directional Doppler sonography

Exclusion of intrafascial circulatory disturbances, no suspected incompetent transfascial communication

Documentation of the functional parameters

Treatment

Suspected deep vascular disease or incompetent transfascial communication

Documentation of the functional parameters

Real-time sonography

Imaging diagnosis

Phlebo-graphy

Duplex sonography

Treatment

117. Staged investigation score for peripheral vascular disease

Clinical Examination

A carefully elicited history is a crucial source of information in *acute venous diseases*. The physician has the often difficult task of evaluating the symptoms described by the patient and fitting them into a nosologic scheme. Most laypeople's understanding of lower limb symptomatology does not go beyond *varicose veins* and *leg pain*, and they do not usually appreciate the important distinctions between phlebothrombosis and thrombophlebitis.

The history is also an important guide in *chronic venous diseases*. Previous therapeutic measures commonly affect the current clinical presentation. For example, even severe varicosity of the great saphenous trunk may be completely missed in cases where smaller side-branch tributaries have been repeatedly sclerosed. A temporal connection between the onset of venous flow impairment and a severe trauma should raise suspicion of post-thrombotic syndrome.

The *clinical examination* begins with visual inspection. Occasionally this is diagnostic, as with typical forms of primary varicosity, severe leg and pelvic vein thrombosis, or post-thrombotic disease with arthrogenic venous insufficiency. Attention is given to the arrangement and location of varices, subtle color differences between the lower legs, and retromalleolar edema in Bisgaard's region. Changes in the skin and subcutaneous tissue in the supramelleolar region with sites of pigmentation, induration, scars, and atrophy with pallor are typical features of chronic venous insufficiency. They are seen exclusively in association with outflow disturbances in the deep leg veins.

Palpation of the extremity in the supine and erect positions is an important part of the examination. The different forms of peripheral edema can be distinguished from one another by their typical tissue turgor. For the experienced examiner, palpable tension in the deep compartments of the leg will provide a very high index of suspicion for phlebothrombosis. Varicosity of the great and small saphenous trunks can often be diagnosed by its typical palpable features. Cockett's veins are best evaluated by sliding the index finger along their projected course. The extent of a thrombophlebitis or subcutaneous induration can be determined by palpation.

In the case of unusually severe venous disease with extensive varicosity, *auscultation* of the large stem veins in the popliteal fossa, thigh, and groin is also recommended. A loud, continuous vascular murmur is diagnostic for arteriovenous fistula.

A careful clinical examination should take note of *surrounding structures* such as the arterial and lymphatic systems. Myostatic insufficiency, neurologic deficits, and dermatologic conditions frequently provide an indication for a phlebographic workup.

Instrumental Diagnostic Studies

The past two decades have brought significant progress in the instrumental diagnosis of venous disease. Some of these methods, such as B-mode sonography and Doppler ultrasound, provide information on the functional and morphologic status of a *particular vessel* or *venous system*. Others, such as peripheral phlebodynamometry, light-reflection rheography, and venous occlusion plethysmography, assess the *global venous circulation* in terms of the parameters of *pressure*, *volume*, and *flow pattern*. Other modalities such as thermography and radionuclide imaging are reserved for special inquiries.

The results of these studies *add* information to that furnished by contrast phlebography. Modern ultrasound techniques, moreover, can *replace* phlebography in certain areas.

Ultrasonography

Basically two sonographic techniques are available for the examination of blood vessels: real-time B-mode sonographic imaging and Doppler flow sampling. Duplex scanning refers to the combination of B-mode and Doppler ultrasound. In color-coded duplex scanning, the acoustic Doppler signal is converted into colors representing different Doppler frequency shifts (p. 80).

B-Mode or Real-Time Sonography

Real-time sonography is based on the pulse-echo principle. When pulsed ultrasound waves transmitted into the body encounter an interface between tissues of different acoustic impedances, part of the energy is reflected back to the ultrasound receiver. Each reflected pulse is transformed into an electrical signal and displayed as a bright spot on the monitor. The sum of the bright spots constitutes a B-mode ultrasound image (B=brightness). Instead of using different shades of gray, various color schemes are now available; these enable the examiner to make a detailed, individual assessment and constitute a color codifi- 118
cation of the intensity of the impulse echo.

By using real-time sonography, intravasal structures are easy to see in thrombosis. The vessel wall and perivascular tissues can be assessed, as can the caliber of the vessel, any abnormalities of flow and aneurysms. Real-time sonography forms an important part of sonographic thrombosis workup.

Nondirectional and Directional Doppler Sonography

In the *continuous wave mode,* continuous ultrasound waves are transmitted by the source and picked up by a receiver. If they encounter a stationary interface, they are reflected back at the same wavelength. However, if the reflector is moving toward or away from the source, the frequency of the reflected waves will be higher or lower, respectively, than the source frequency. The difference is called the *Doppler shift* and happens to lie within the audible range.

The acoustic reflectors in flowing blood are the red cells. The frequency of the Doppler shift depends upon the *source frequency* and the *blood flow velocity,* in accordance with the Doppler formula. Velocites slower than 3 cm/s cannot be detected with conventional 4- to 8-MHz Doppler probes.

Two basic types of Doppler instrument are available. The simple *unidirectional pocket-sized unit* converts the Doppler shift to an audible signal; the direction of flow can be determined only from theoretical deductions. The more complex *directional Doppler instruments,* on the other hand, can assess both the direction and pattern of blood flow and display them as an analog waveform.

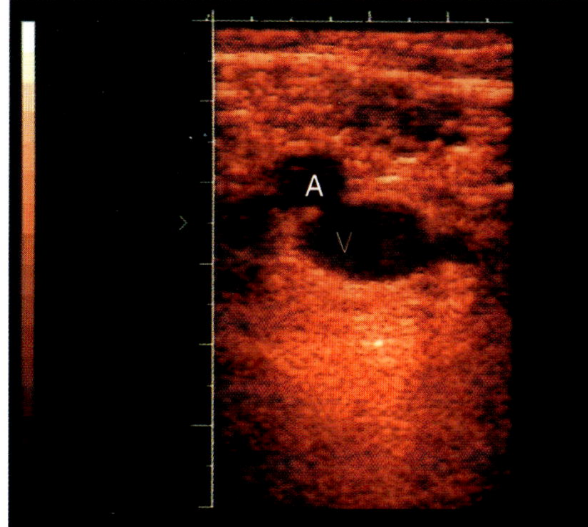

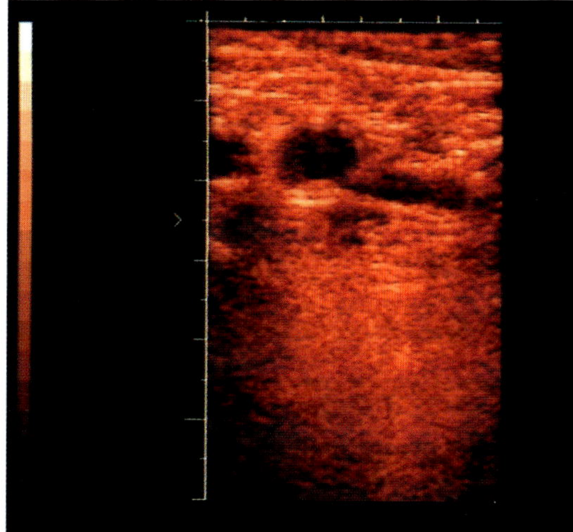

118. Real-time sonogram with color coding. Acuson 128 XP/10, color imaging sepia. Demonstration of the right groin. *Top*, cross-section of the common femoral artery and vein. The vascular wall is easy to assess. *Bottom*, compressibility of the vein. Normal perivascular tissue structures

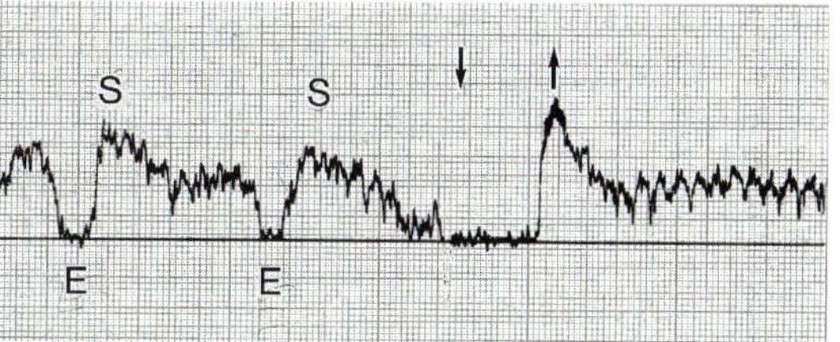

119. Directional Doppler sonography. Normal breathing modulations (S sounds) over the common femoral vein (*S*). Brief interruption of flow during expiration (*E*). Valsalva maneuver with persisting flow interruption (↓). Overshoot phenomenon (↑)

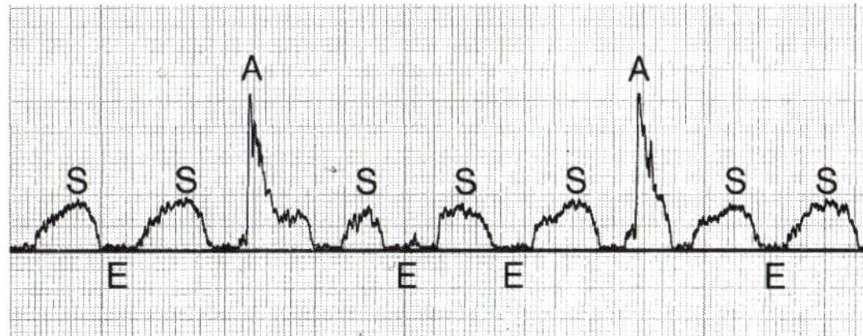

120. Directional Doppler sonography. Normal breathing modulations (S sounds) over the common femoral vein. Brief interruption of flow during expiration (*E*). Augmented sounds (A sounds) during the calf compression test (*A*)

The Doppler examination serves to determine whether blood is *flowing* or whether the vessel is occluded. It can also establish flow direction. Additionally, provocative tests can be used during the Doppler examination to assess valvular competency.

Blood flow in the large stem veins of the leg is normally respiration dependent. Absence of flow is recorded at the end of inspiration due to the elevated intra-abdominal pressure, and loud flow signals reappear during expiration. These are called the "S sounds" (spontaneous sounds). The presence of phasic respiration variations confirms
free blood flow in the proximal venous segments. 119
Manual compression of the calf or thigh muscles
produces an augmented flow wave that can be
heard and recorded as an "A sound" (augmenta- 120
tion sound). The A sound, too, is characteristic of
unimpeded venous flow. In the case of vessel occlusion, pathologic Doppler signals are found (see p. 162).

A quite different procedure involves the use of directional Doppler sonography to assess *valvular
function*. The Valsalva maneuver or calf *de*com-
pression test is used to provoke retrograde flow as 121
proof of valvular incompetence. The *Valsalva maneuver* is performed in the supine patient to detect great saphenous varicosity or test valvular competency in the deep veins of the inguinal region. For the *calf decompression test*, the patient stands upright with the leg as relaxed as possible. On calf compression the blood flows proximally, and on release of compression, i.e., calf *de*compression,
there is normally only a brief return flow until the
valve closes; if the venous valves are incompetent, 164
the blood flows back distally.

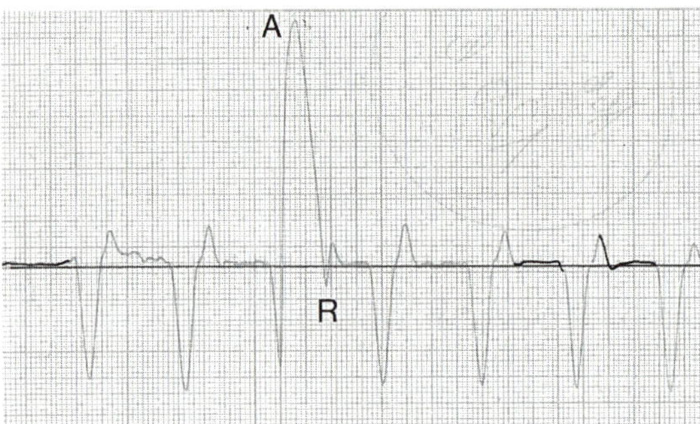

121. Directional Doppler sonography using the analog technique. Calf compression test with normal A sounds (*A*). Brief return until the valve closes. Calf *de*compression test (*R*). Drainage via the superficial femoral artery and vein. Arterial pulsations in the negative range

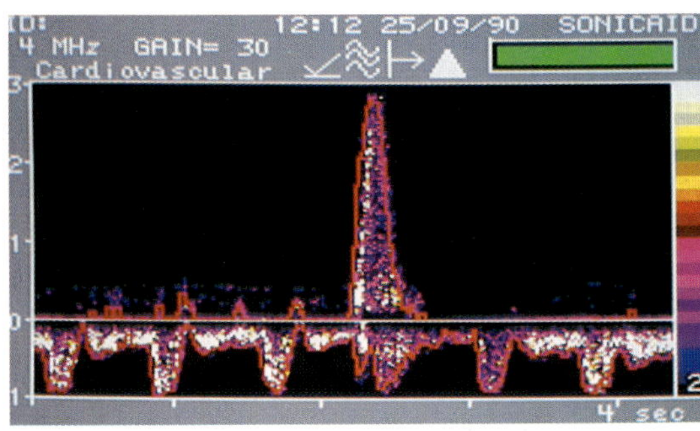

122. Color-coded spectrum analysis. Calf compression test with a high A sound; no negative vascular flow competents following complete valve closure. Arterial pulsations in the negative range. (Sonicaid, 8-MHz transducer)

The *nondirectional technique* of Doppler sonography is so simple and quick to perform that – like blood pressure measurement – it should be regarded as a *routine procedure* for a thorough investigation of the venous system. *Directional Doppler ultrasound* has a definite role as an adjunct to phlebography; for example, it allows conclusions to be drawn concerning the extent to which physiologic phlebectasis of the great saphenous vein in post-thrombotic syndrome already shows signs of reverse flow components in the sense of secondary saphenous varicosity (see p. 182).

Frequency Spectrum Analysis

The analog waveform represents the sum of all the frequencies in the Doppler spectrum (corresponding to the speed components of the flow) over time; in contrast, in spectrum analysis the Doppler shift signal is divided up into its individu-
122 al frequencies. This is done technically by means of rapid Fourier transformation. The values of the individual flow components that the ultrasound beam encounters can be read off the curve. Although this procedure is very important in the diagnostic workup of the arteries, it is of only limited importance in phlebology. The instruments needed for spectrum analysis are also considerably more expensive that those needed for the analog technique.

Duplex Sonography and Color-Coded Duplex Sonography

Duplex sonography is a combination of real-time sonography and directional Doppler sonography. By means of a technical variation, the pulsed ultrasound beam can be accurately positioned on a particular part of the vessels lumen and the Doppler signals derived at this point (*sample volume*). 123
In the arterial diagnostic workup, this enables vessel stenoses to be analyzed; in phlebology, however, the main concern is to provide evidence of the bloodflow per se and to rule out the possibility of a fresh thrombosis.

A more recent development is that of *color-coded duplex sonography*. Here, too, pulsed ultrasound waves are transmitted, and these are evaluated in terms of both real time and the Doppler shift; the Doppler shift is color coded, often using red for the waves that are approaching the transducer and 124
blue for those moving away from the transducer. Combining real-time sonography and color-coded Doppler shift forms the color-coded image of duplex sonography.

The fact that duplex sonography is noninvasive and does not require the use of contrast media is a considerable *advantage* compared to phlebography. However, it has the disadvantage that a detailed diagnosis of smaller veins and the venous valves is not possible with duplex sonography. Evaluation of the vessels of the abdominal and pelvic cavity is sometimes difficult in obese patients or if an excessive amount of gas is present. Furthermore, possible incidences of bypass circu-

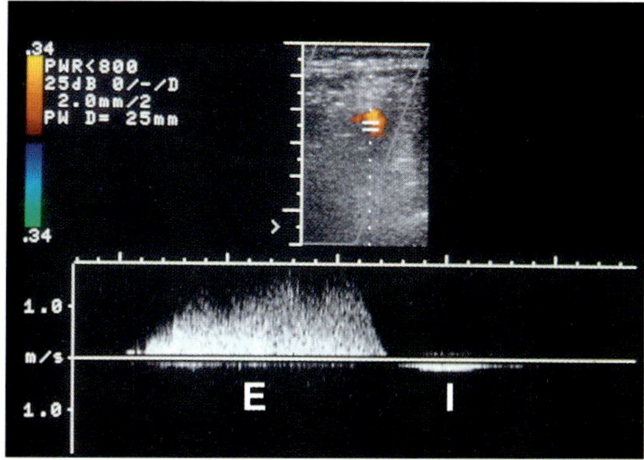

123. Color-coded duplex sonography. The sample volume drains away via the common femoral vein. Antegrade flow profile during expiration in the positive range, hence the veins are coded *red*. Brief, minimal retrograde flow at the beginning of inspiration. (Acuson, 128 XP 10.7-MHz linear transducer)

lation are not revealed. However, duplex sonography allows an optimal evaluation of the vessel wall and perivascular structures using the real-time technique. In many cases in which a detailed phlebologic diagnosis is required, the best results are obtained by *combining* phlebography and real-time sonography or color-coded duplex sonography.

Venous Pressure Measurements

The peripheral venous pressure consists of various components. The filling pressure, vascular tonus, and flow pressure play a role in recumbency, and the hydrostatic pressure is added in the erect posture. Venous pressure measurements are of interest in practical phlebology for two reasons: They aid in assessing pelvic vein hemodynamics prior to reconstructive surgery (*femoral pressure measurement*), and they help to determine global circulatory conditions in the leg veins (*peripheral phlebodynamometry*). Both studies can be performed immediately following phlebography.

Femoral Pressure Measurement

The common femoral venous pressure in the supine patient is 10–15 mmHg during the expiratory phase. If there is an outflow obstruction in the pelvic venous system with inadequate collateraliza-

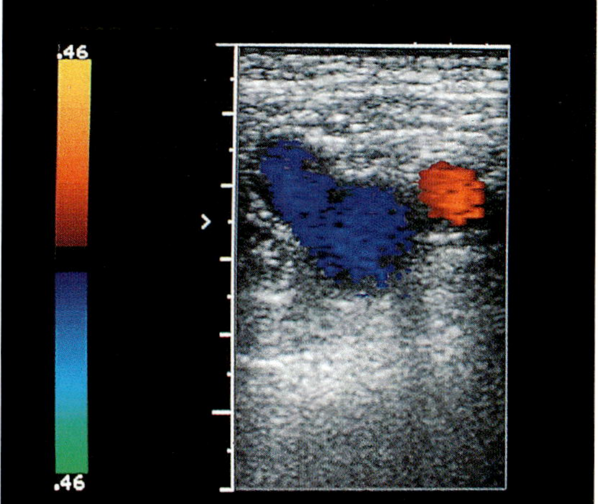

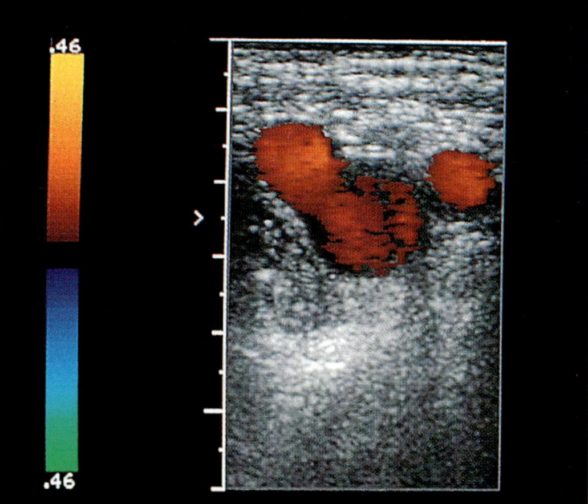

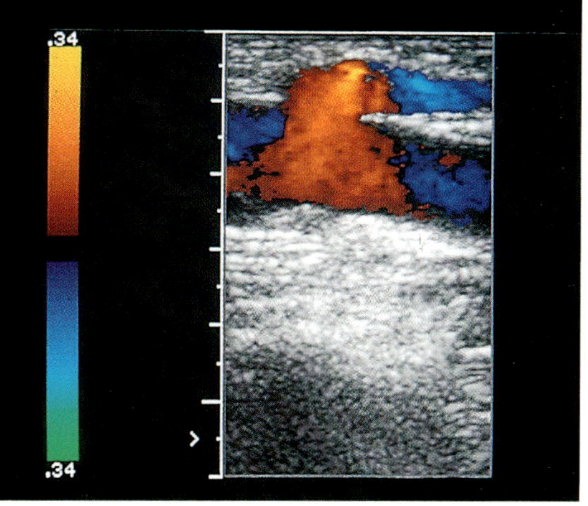

124. Terminal section of the great saphenous vein in saphenous varicosity. Demonstrated using color-coded duplex sonography with a 7-MHz linear transducer. Cross-section of the left groin. *Top*, veins during expiration with centripetal flow direction (*blue*). Common femoral artery with centrifugal flow direction (*red*). *Middle*, complete reversal of flow in the veins during a Valsalva maneuver (coded *red*). *Bottom*, turbulent flow profile in the proximal superficial femoral vein during a Valsalva maneuver and return flow in the enlarged great saphenous vein

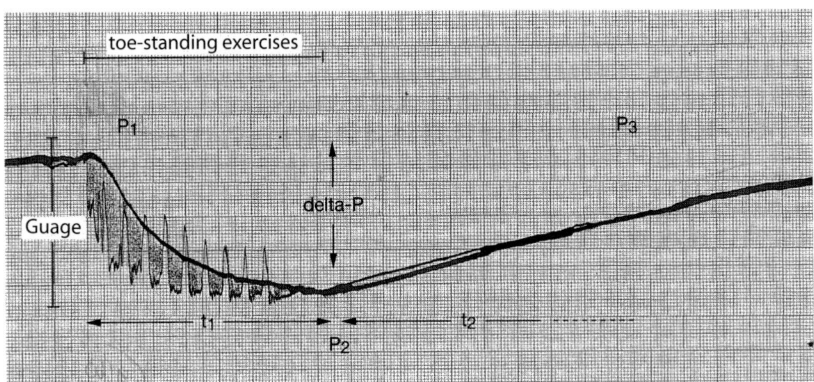

125. Normal peripheral vein pression curve. Fall in pressure delta-P caused by exercises involving standing on the tips of the toes, long period of pressure compensation *t2*. *P1*, resting pressure during standing; *P2*, maximal pressure decrease after weight-bearing; *P3*, resting pressure after weight-bearing; *t1*, period of pressure decrease; *t2*, period of pressure compensation

tion, the pressure rises. A pressure elevation at least three times the normal level should be present before bypass surgery is considered.

The examination is performed in the supine patient. A needle is inserted into the common femoral vein, and the intravenous pressure is measured with a Statham element and plotted on a calibrated recording system.

Peripheral Phlebodynamometry

Peripheral invasive venous pressure measurement during exercise is considered the most accurate physical method for evaluating global venous circulatory function. The response of the blood pressure and volume in the leg veins to dynamic exercise provides useful information on the transport capacity of the vessels (Weber 1978; Hach 1981a).

A dorsal foot vein is punctured with a butterfly needle and connected to the Statham element by polyethylene tubing; pressure pulses are transmitted electromechanically to a multiple-pen recorder. After the resting pressure is recorded, the patient performs ten toe-standing exercises timed by a metronome.

Activation of the calf muscle pump causes a *pressure drop* represented by the *delta-P* value in the tracing. The lower the delta-P, the more severe the impairment of ve-
125 nous hemodynamics. A shortening of the *filling time t1*
(due to retrograde flow components) has a similar interpretation. The delta-P and *t1* values are highly reproducible parameters of the global transport capacity of the leg veins. This gives peripheral phlebodynamometry a significant role in medical disability assessment and scientific research. It cannot identify the nature of the underlying disease, however.

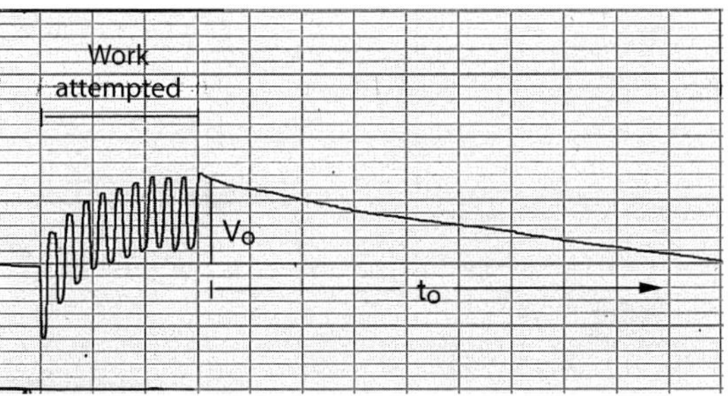

126. Normal photoplethysmographic curve. Work attempted during exercises involving lifting the foot, with increasing drainage of the vascular plexus (rising curve). *Vo*, minal volume; *to*, period of volume compensation (>30 s)

Light-Reflection Rheography (Photoplethysmography)

Light-reflection rheography provides information on peripheral venous hemodynamics that corresponds roughly to the *t2* value in peripheral phlebodynamometry. A different principle is employed, however. Light waves of a certain wavelength are partially absorbed and reflected in the tissue. The physical reactions depend on the blood content of the large subdermal venous plexuses, which are emptied by activation of the calf muscle pump during exercise and subsequently refill during rest. The rheography tracing, then, represents 126
a mirror image of the venous pressure curve.

Light-reflection rheography is a simple, noninvasive study that can be repeated as often as desired.

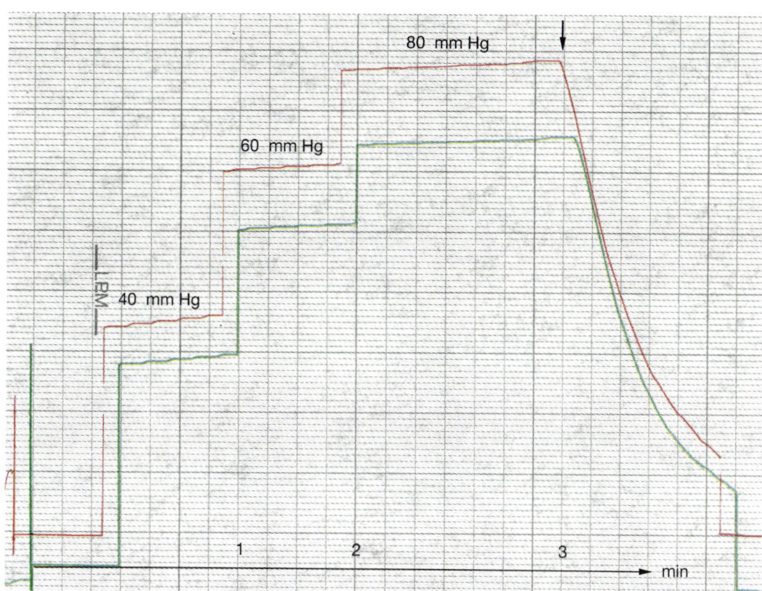

127. Normal curves of vascular occlusion plethysmography in both legs. Staged congestion by application of a tourniquet on the thigh up to 80 mmHg to determine the vascular capacity: right 6.6 ml, left 4.3 ml blood/100 ml tissue. Drainage determined by decreasing the pressure (↓): right 83.7 ml, left 72.9 ml blood/100 ml tissue/min

The determination of venous refill time is sufficient for a gross assessment of the transport capacity of the venous system. As a global method, however, light-reflection rheography cannot furnish a specific diagnose of venous disease. Its greatest value lies in the long-term follow-up of post-thrombotic syndrome and of secondary popliteal and femoral vein incompetence. Peripheral phlebodynamometry is preferred in disability assessment cases owing to its excellent reproducibility.

Venous Occlusion Phlethysmography

Venous occlusion phlethysmography is based on the principle that both the arterial inflow of blood into an extremity and the venous outflow produce transient volume fluctuations that can be measured by the mercury strain-gauge method or by other systems. A pneumatic cuff is placed on the thigh and inflated in stages to a pressure of 80 mmHg; this still permits arterial inflow while occluding venous outflow. The continuous tracing of the calf circumference moves to a new plateau that is a measure of venous capacity. On sudden release of the cuff, the tracing falls sharply indicat-
127 ing the rate of venous outflow.

Venous occlusion plethysmography is considered a sensitive screening test for occlusive ileofemoral vein thrombosis and post-thrombotic syndrome, in which venous capacity and outflow are diminished. Increased values are seen in severe saphenous varicosity with secondary popliteal and femoral vein incompetence. The procedure offers a quantitative supplement to phlebographic findings and is utilized for disability assessment.

References

Habscheid W (1991) Die bildgebende Sonographie in der Diagnostik der tiefen Beinvenenthrombose. Schattauer Stuttgart

Hach W (1974) Die aszendierende Preßphlebographie, eine Routinemethode zur Beurteilung der oberflächlichen Stammvenen. In: Friedrich HC, Hamelmann H (Hrsg) Ergebnisse der Angiologie, Bd 8. Schattauer, Stuttgart New York

Hach W (1981a) Spezielle Diagnostik der primären Varikose. Demeter, Gräfelfing

Hach W (1981b) Nicht-invasive instrumentelle Diagnostik venöser Thrombosen. In: Vinazza H (Hrsg) Thrombose und Embolie. Springer, Berlin Heidelberg New York

Hach-Wunderle V (1995) Venöser Gefäßstatus. Internist 36: 525

Hennerici M, Neuerburg-Heusler D (1988) Gefäßdiagnostik mit Ultraschall. Thieme, Stuttgart New York

May R, Kriessmann A (Hrsg) (1978) Periphere Venendruckmessung. Thieme, Stuttgart

May R, Stemmer R (Hrsg) (1984) Die Licht-Reflexions-Rheographie. Perimed, Erlangen

Rabe E (Hrsg) (1994) Grundlagen der Phlebologie. Kargerer, Bonn

Weber J (1978) Phlebographie und Venendruckmessung im Abdomen und Becken. Witzstrock, Baden Baden Köln New York

Wienert V (1991) Anwendungsfehler und Fehlinterpretationen bei der Lichtreflexionsrheographie. Phlebologie 20: 126

Wuppermann Th, Wille B (1983) Was leistet die Venenverschlußplethysmographie bei Venenkrankheiten und wie wird sie durchgeführt. Phlebol Proktol 12: 105

Wolf KJ, Fobbe F (1993) Farbcodierte Duplexsonographie. Thieme, Stuttgart New York

Clinical Aspects of Phlebography

Phlebology has undergone fundamental changes in its diagnostic and therapeutic concepts during the past 20 years. Until the middle of this century, the treatment of venous disorders was overwhelmingly conservative and delivered in outpatient settings. However, the development of a differentiated surgical approach to primary varicose veins, the introduction of fibrinolysis, and the surgical reconstruction of venous channels in patients with thrombosis or post-thrombotic syndrome have established an active role for the surgical clinic in the management of selected severe venous disorders.

The prognostic assessment of different therapeutic options is based on the results of functional *and* morphologic studies. In this sense the importance of phlebography has increased steadily up to the present day. The radiographic examination of the veins of the lower extremity permits a *comprehensive assessment* of anatomic relationships and pathologic structures. No other diagnostic study can equal or surpass phlebography in information content, although ultrasound can provide a useful adjunct in some situations.

Primary Varicose Veins

In *primary varicose veins*, the superficial extrafascial vessels undergo a varicose degeneration of multifactoral etiology. By definition, the etiology of primary varicose veins is unrelated to changes in the deep venous system, although deep vein pathology can seriously complicate the subsequent course of the disease. *Secondary varicose veins* are caused by an organic or severe functional outflow impairment in the intrafascial venous system. There is no strict dividing line between the two types of disease.

It has proven useful to classify primary varicosities into specific disease entities according to clinical criteria. The classification is based on the anatomy of the extrafascial venous system, in which the saphenous trunks and their main tributaries, the "side branches," are distinguished from the reticular veins and perforating veins. It should be noted, however, that today a more *synoptic view* is taken which forms the basis for the current theory of recirculating flow patterns in varicose disease.

Characteristics of primary varicose veins
Primary involvement of the extrafascial veins and perforators
No prior damage to the deep veins
Multifactorial etiology
Favorable prognosis with appropriate treatment
High complication rate in certain forms that are allowed to progress

Radiography can help to differentiate among the disease states and recirculation patterns in cases where clinical findings are equivocal. The different phlebographic techniques offer different capabilities in this regard, but only ascending pressure phlebography can furnish *comprehensive* information.

Saphenous varicosity, perforator incompetence, and the transfascial forms of side-branch varicosity differ in their pathogenesis from other varices in that they are based on an acquired or congenital valvular dysfunction in these vessels before their entry into the deep venous system. This results in a retrograde blood flow from the deep trunks to the superficial veins when the patient performs a Valsalva maneuver. Diagnosis centers on the detection and localization of these *incompetent transfascial connections*, and the only method that appears suitable for this task, besides Doppler flow detection, is ascending pressure phlebography. Treatment consists in surgical division of the incompetent connections at their junction with the deep venous system.

The extrafascial type of side-branch varicosity and reticular varices are mainly caused by pri-

Veins of the extrafascial system	
Important vessels	**Characterization**
Great saphenous vein Small saphenous vein	Saphenous trunks
Lateral accessory saphenous vein Medial accessory saphenous vein Anterior arcuate crural vein Posterior arcuate crural vein	Side branches of the great saphenous trunk
Femoropopliteal vein	Side branch of the small saphenous trunk
Unnamed	Reticular veins
Kuster's veins Cockett's veins Sherman's vein Boyd's vein Hunter's vein Dodd's veins May's vein Popliteal perforator (of Dodd) Profunda perforator (of Hach)	Perforating veins

Classification of primary varicose veins
Saphenous varicosity with compensated/ decompensated reflux circuit
Complete forms
Incomplete forms
Side-branch varicosity with/without reflux circuit
Transfascial forms
Extrafascial forms
Reticular varicosity
Varicose perforators

Preferred modes of treatment for primary varicose veins	
Varicose saphenous trunk	Operation
Side-branch varices	
Transfascial	Operation
Extrafascial	Sclerotherapy
Varicose reticular veins	Sclerotherapy
Varicose perforators	Operation

Differential diagnosis of primary varicosity by different phlebographic methods							
Method	Saphenous varicosity			Transfascial side-branch varicosity	Reticular varicosity	Perforating varicosity	Secondary popliteal and femoral vein insufficiency
	Terminal valve	Vascular stem	Incomplete form				
Ascending pressure phlebography	+	+	+	+	–	(+)	+
Ascending phlebography	–	–	–	–	–	(+)	+
Noncompression runoff phlebography	–	+	(+)	(+)	+	(+)	–
Varicography	–	(+)	–	+	+	+	–
Retrograde pressure phlebography	+	+	–	–	–	–	+

mary vessel wall damage due to the action of various exogenous and endogenous factors. These lesions are best managed by sclerotherapy, so they do not require a comprehensive diagnostic work-up.

Long Saphenous Varicosity

(Complete) varicosity of the great saphenous trunk progresses distally from the incompetent terminal valve of the saphenous vein to an anatomically predetermined site called the *distal point of incompetence*. The rare tubular form of great saphenous varicosity (stage IV disease) is probably based largely on congenital structural abnormalities in the vessel wall itself.

Clinical symptoms of great saphenous varicosity
Primary symptoms
Palpable dilatation of the vessel in the inguinal fold
Positive cough test
Positive percussion test
Secondary symptoms (with decompensated reflux circuit)
Spider webs at the supramalleolar level
Chronic venous insufficiency
Arthrogenic stasis syndrome

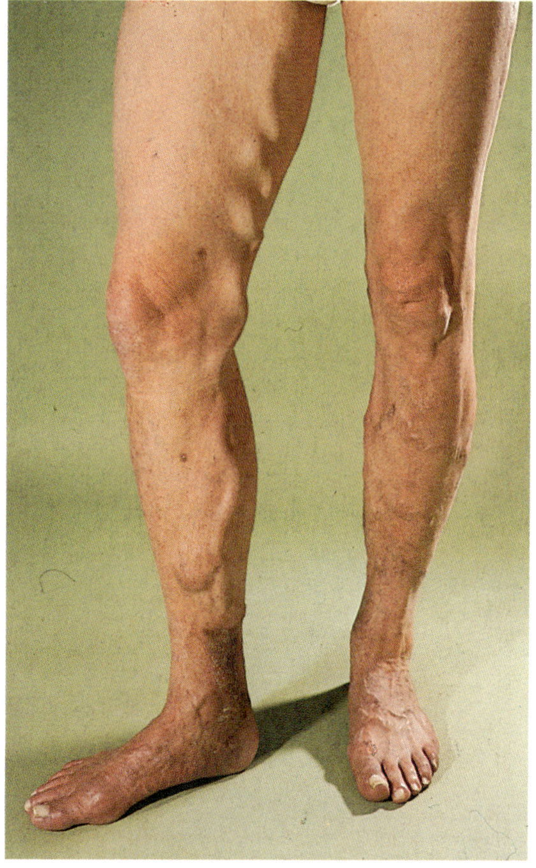

128. Great saphenous varicosity in a 64-year-old man with a more than 40-year history of disease. The patient had chronic venous insufficiency with a decompensated type IV reflux circuit

Clinical Aspects

In thin patients and patients with pronounced signs and symptoms, the diagnosis is usually made clinically. In the standing patient, the varicose great saphenous vein appears as a dilated, sometimes slightly tortuous vessel that can be traced from the groin to its junction with a branch varix at the distal point of incompetence, or rarely
128 as far as the medial malleolus.

The ectatic vein is easiest to palpate in the inguinal fold. A pressure wave is plainly felt within the vessel during coughing. The percussion of a peripheral segment can be felt at the groin and proves the continuity of the vessel (*percussion test*). The Trendelenburg test no longer has clinical importance today.

Besides direct signs of disease in the vessel itself, there are a number of indirect signs involving the skin and subcutaneous cellular tissue of the distal lower leg that reflect the volume and pressure overload of the deep venous trunks in the setting of *chronic venous stasis syndrome* (chronic venous insufficiency). The total incidence of these findings in our patients, drawn from a metropolitan population, was 27.7%. The indirect signs include areas of brawny induration, pigmentation, stasis dermatitis, and ulceration. The frequency and extent of these changes relate directly to the prevailing pattern of recirculating flow.

Spread of the inflammatory process to the ligaments of the ankle and subtalar joints sets the
129 stage for *arthrogenic stasis syndrome*, the most serious local complication (Hach et al. 1983). To relieve pain, the patient holds the foot in equinus until ankylosis eventually supervenes. At that point the patient must recurvate the knee to bear weight on the sole of the foot. There is failure of the major peripheral venous muscle pumps in the ankle and calf. The peripheral venous pressure can no longer fall during exercise, and intractable crural ulcers develop.

In the great majority of cases, a varicose saphenous trunk becomes clinically apparent early in the third decade of life. It is probably based on a congenital defect in the terminal valve that gradually, over a period of years or decades, leads to overt disease. Saphenous varicosity, then, has its
onset *in youth*, and the associated retrograde flow 130
circuit increasingly decompensates with aging. This fact is incorrectly interpreted in most epidemiologic studies. Our statistical studies indicate that there is only a small age peak of the onset of disease in the seventh decade (Hach 1981b).

Factors that affect the *manifestation* of saphenous varicosity include hormonal influences due to pregnancy or contraceptive use, prolonged standing, very strenuous physical and athletic exertion, or inactivity. Morphologic and hemodynamic factors also play a crucial primary

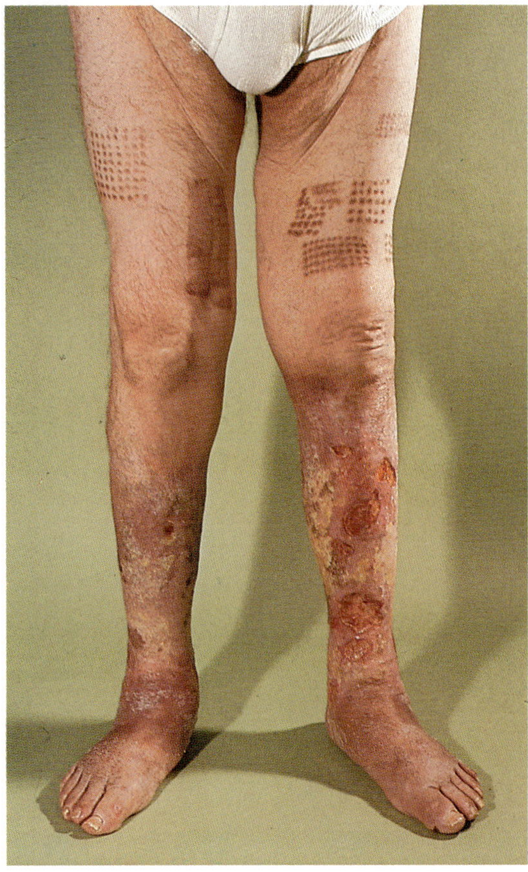

129. Arthrogenic stasis syndrome due to untreated great saphenous varicosity with a decompensated type III reflux circuit in a 67-year-old man with a 42-year history of varicose veins and 40-year history of ulceration (he had repeated, prolonged hospital stays for intractable crural ulcers). Scars are visible from numerous meshed skin grafts. Patient has bilateral equinus deformity and difficulty walking, with marked recurvatum at the knees when standing on level ground. Peripheral phlebodynamometry shows no venous pressure fall during exercise

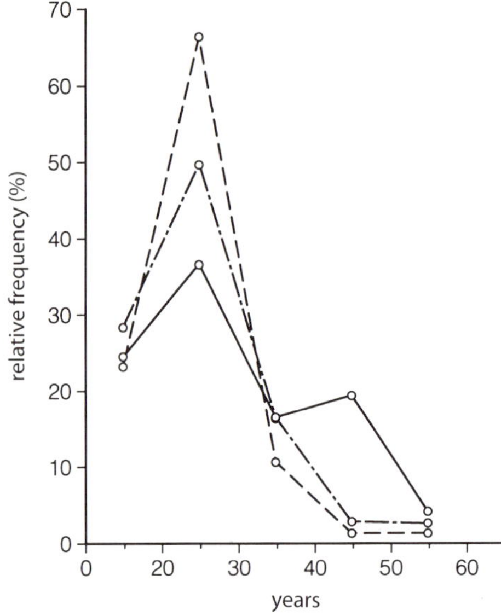

130. Average age at clinical manifestation of great saphenous varicosity according to stages. Total of 385 limbs. *Unbroken line*, stage II; *dotted/dashed line*, stage III; *dashed line*, stage IV. (From Hach 1981)

Symptoms of chronic venous insufficiency with a decompensated reflux circuit in saphenous varicosity
Supramalleolar region
Edema
Spider webs
Siderosis
Dermatoliposclerosis
White atrophy
Crural ulcer
Ulcerous scars
Foot
Corona phlebectatica paraplantaris
Stasis track
Pedal ulcer

role. Once established, the recirculating flow pattern that is linked to the saphenous varicosity does not change spontaneously with passage of time, although decompensation can occur.

The pathoanatomy of great saphenous varicosity may involve primary damage to the elastic fibers in the vessel wall, to the muscular fibers, or to the polyvalent cells located between the intima and media. Electron microscopic findings point to a transformation of the muscle cells, which in turn leads to the formation of inferior-grade connective tissue fibers by way of extracellular lysosomes. Endogenous and exogenous factors as well as hormonal influences or unfavorable static conditions can predispose to these changes (Staubesand 1977).

Characteristics of arthrogenic stasis syndrome
Chronic venous congestion
Intractable crural ulcers
Scars from failed skin grafts
Limitation of ankle motion
Difficulty walking and standing due to equinus deformity
Diminished venous pressure fall during exercise

Biochemical wall changes also have been implicated in several studies (Niebes and Laszt 1971; Svejar et al. 1964).

Radiographic Signs of a Competent Saphenous Terminal Valve

Ascending pressure phlebography is used routinely to evaluate saphenous dysfunction. The ankle tourniquet initially directs all of the contrast medium into the deep veins. As the medium enters the common femoral vein, the functional competence of the saphenous terminal valve is tested by having the patient perform a *Valsalva maneuver*. In the normal great saphenous vein, contrast medium will fill only a short segment of the vein as far as its highest valve. Intermittent straining will sometimes propel the medium down through
131 competent preterminal valves, however, so contrast reflux alone does not signify valvular incompetence.

Normally the venous valves are open. On straining, a small amount of blood refluxes until the commissures have closed. This reflux can be observed fluoroscopically. It can also be detected by Doppler ultrasound as an initial reflux with stop (Hach 1981b).

Earlier (see p. 6) we referred to the anatomic peculiarities in the proximal portion of the great saphenous vein. The highest (terminal) valve establishes a broad, funnel-shaped connection with the common femoral vein. The saphenous vein caliber is progressively reduced below each of the two lower, preterminal valves, creating a *sluice effect*. These abrupt caliber changes at the sluice valves are manifested on phlebograms by the *telescope sign*, which affords proof of the functional compe-
44 tence of the whole preterminal region.

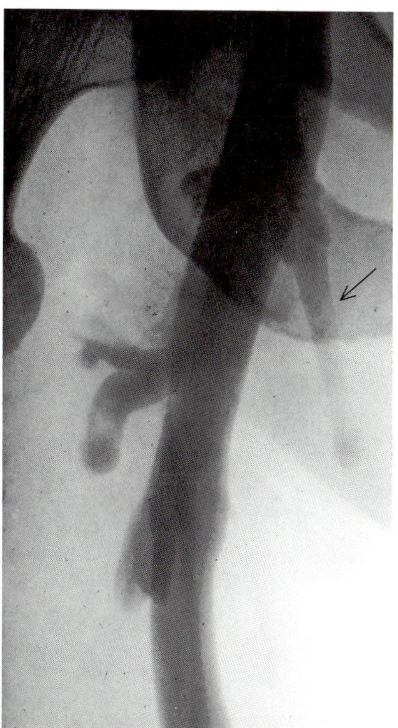

131. Competent sluice valves of the great saphenous veins with telescope sign (→), demonstrated by ascending pressure phlebography

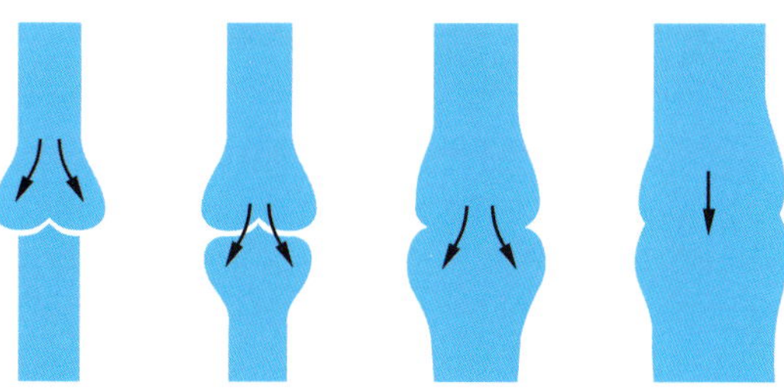

132. Progressive development of saphenous varicosity due to terminal valve incompetence

Radiographic Signs of Proximal Valvular Incompetence

A knowledge of the pathogenesis of saphenous varicosity is necessary in order to assess radiographically the functional competence of the great
132 saphenous vein. This knowledge will permit a consistent interpretation of borderline findings.

In cases where the terminal valve cusps can no longer close completely, a pressure surge in the common femoral system will cause blood to reflux into the great saphenous vein. The pressure of the downthrusts against the vessel wall, shear forces, and turbulent phenomena cause an ampullary distention of the vessel just below the valvular plane. This process, called *infravalvular dilata-* 133
tion, is analogous to poststenotic dilatation in the arterial system.

When reflux occurs through a venous valve, the valve ring, which is more rigid than the vein adjacent to the valve, forms a relative constriction within which, according to Bernoulli's law, flow velocity increases and wall pressure declines. The opposite conditions prevail past the constriction, where the flow velocity slows and there is increased pressure on the vessel wall. The reflux

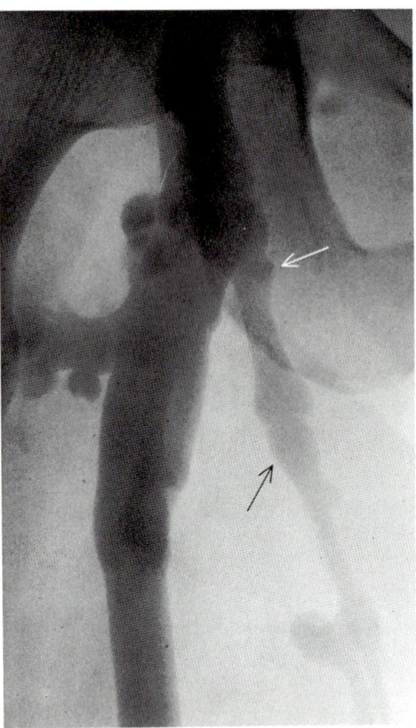

133. Stage II great saphenous varicosity with ampullary dilatation just below the plane of the proximal sluice valves (→). The valve cusps are intact. Demonstrated by ascending pressure phlebography

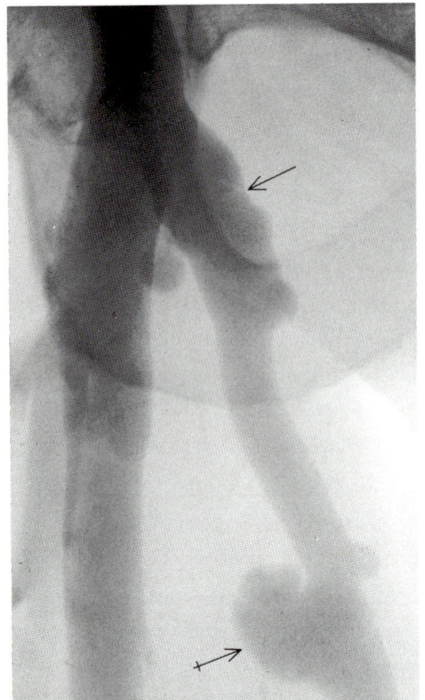

135. Stage III great saphenous varicosity with loss of the telescope sign. There is irregular dilatation of the vessel lumen in the preterminal region. The valve attachment is still faintly visible (→). Farther distally is an infravalvular aneurysm (↔)

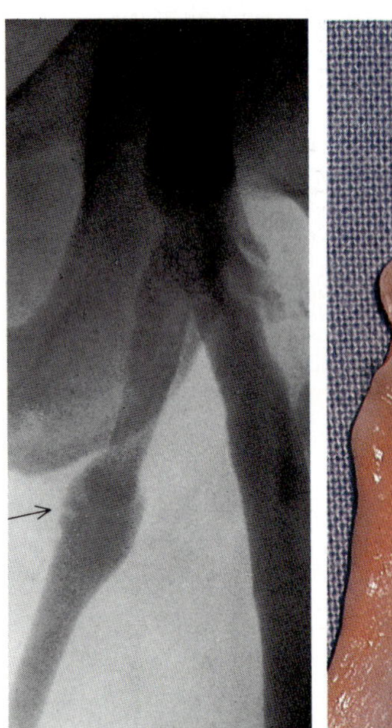

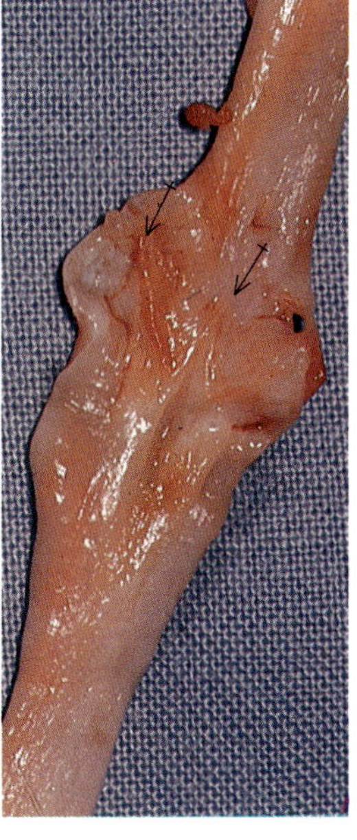

134. Stage III great saphenous varicosity. *Left,* ampullary dilatation distal to the plane of the middle sluice valve (→). The valve cusps are still intact. Demonstrated by ascending pressure phlebography. *Right,* surgical specimen. ↔ Valve attachment

is not continuous, but is intermittent and of varying intensity. This gives rise to turbulent flow, with an associated vibration of the vein wall that can lead to mechanical injury.

As dilatation progresses, the normal caliber reductions at the sluice valves are effaced so that the characteristic "telescope" shape of the vessel is replaced by the tubular shape of *global dilatation.* 134
The valve cusps at this stage may still be well defined on radiographs. Later they degenerate and appear only as vestigial elevations on the vessel 135
wall.

With progression of disease the flow waves and pressure waves impinge upon the next lower valve, which becomes stretched and incompetent, again leading to infravalvular dilatation. In this way the varicosity progresses distally to an anatomically predetermined site, the distal point of incompetence.

When the valvular incompetence is asymmetrical, the retrograde pressure jet is not directed toward the center of the lumen, but impinges on one part of the vessel wall below the valvular plane, causing a localized dilatation that becomes expanded 136–139
through hemodynamic forces into a *saphenous vein aneurysm.* 321–325

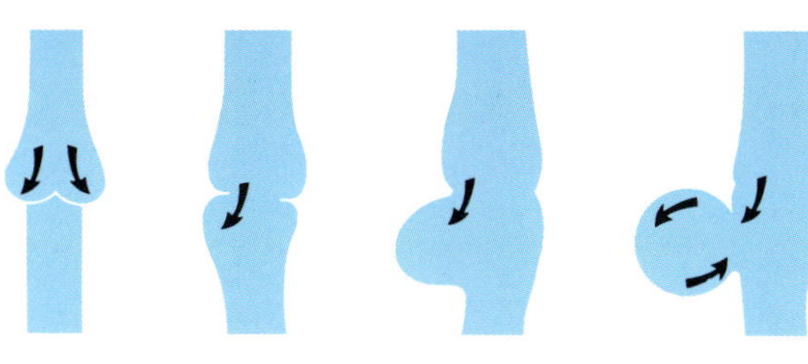

136. Progressive development of a venous aneurysm in a varicose saphenous vein with an incompetent sluice valve

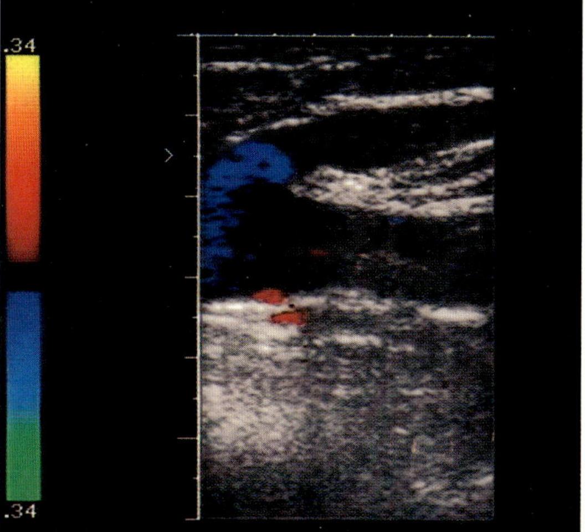

138. Great saphenous varicosity with infravalvular dilatation. Demonstrated by color-coded duplex sonography. (Acuson, 7-MHz transducer)

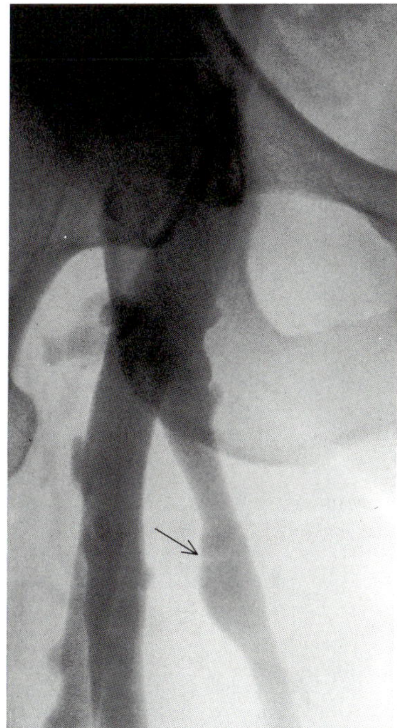

137. Stage II great saphenous varicosity, with asymmetric dilatation of the vessel lumen below the middle sluice valve; the valve cusps are still well defined (→). Demonstrated by ascending pressure phlebography

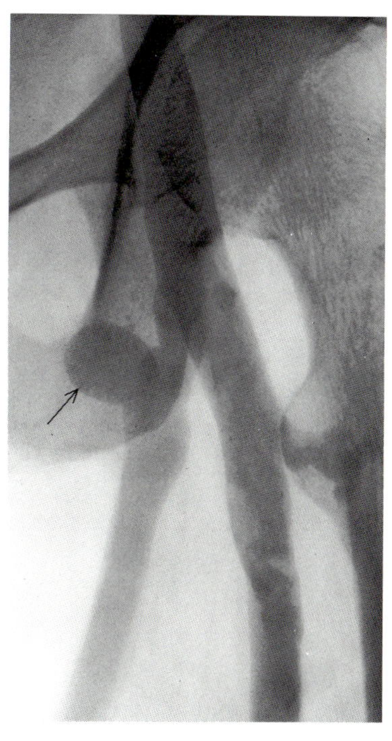

139. Stage IV great saphenous varicosity. Ascending pressure phlebography demonstrates a cherry-size aneurysm (→) with a narrow pedicle below the terminal valve ▷

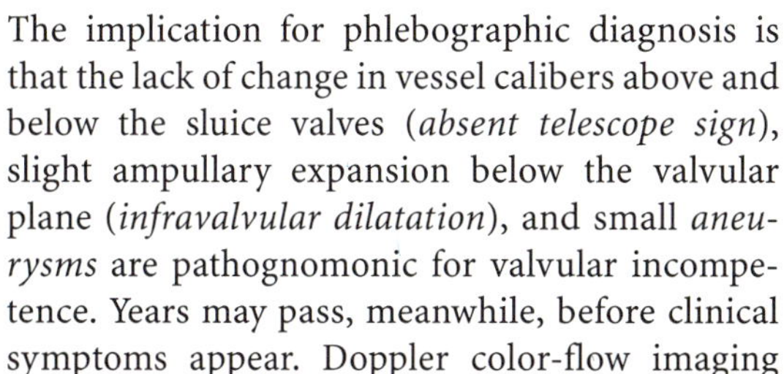

The implication for phlebographic diagnosis is that the lack of change in vessel calibers above and below the sluice valves (*absent telescope sign*), slight ampullary expansion below the valvular plane (*infravalvular dilatation*), and small *aneurysms* are pathognomonic for valvular incompetence. Years may pass, meanwhile, before clinical
138 symptoms appear. Doppler color-flow imaging can demonstrate the blood flow reversal during a Valsalva maneuver.

Stages of Great Saphenous Varicosity

The valvular dysfunction leads to an increasing
dilatation of the great saphenous trunk. Loops 139

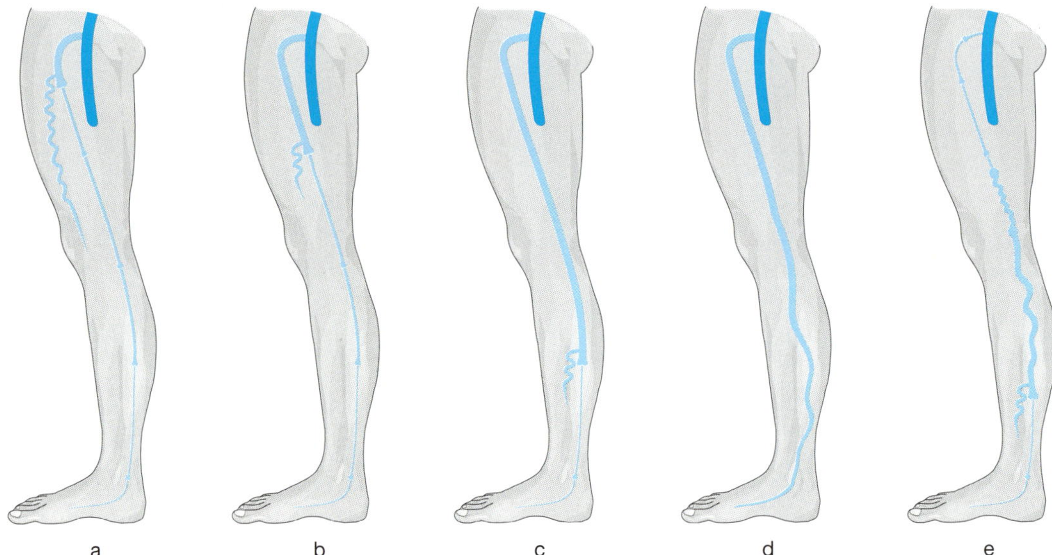

140 a–e. Definition of the proximal and distal points of incompetence in great saphenous varicosities (deep vein system not shown). **a** Distal point of incompetence in the groin, with a varicose main tributary branching from the dilated saphenous sinus ("side branch" varicosity of the lateral accessory saphenous vein). **b** Distal point of incompetence above the knee in stage II disease. **c** Distal point of incompetence below the knee in stage III disease. **d** Distal point of incompetence below the malleolus in stage IV disease. The exact distal site of incompetence often cannot be ascertained. **e** Incomplete great saphenous varicosity, with a proximal point of incompetence in the thigh

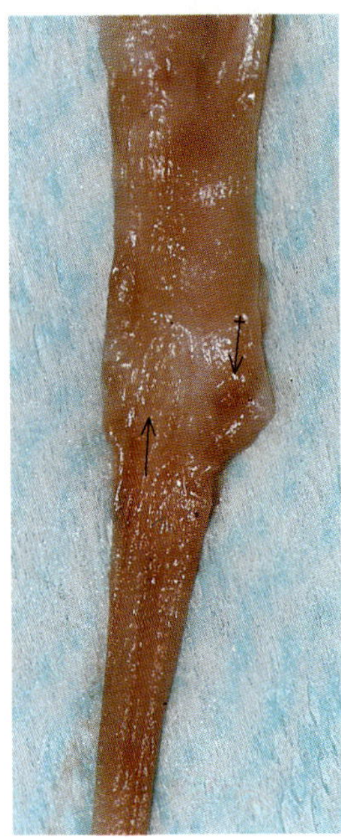

141. Distal point of incompetence in a resected specimen. Competent venous valves are clearly visible (→). A large varicose tributary branches from the valve sinus (↔)

and tortuosities develop, and valves are no longer visible. Finally the vessel degenerates into a varix about the diameter of the thumb. In most cases the varicose degeneration does not affect the entire great saphenous trunk. Close radiographic scrutiny will reveal a point at which a major varicose tributary branches off distally and where the incompetent portion of the great saphenous vein 146
terminates at a competent valve. The location of
this site, called the *distal point of incompetence*, 140
forms a basis for classification of the saphenous 141
varicosity that takes into account not just the morphology of the disease but also its clinical course and severity. The distal point of incompetence in stage II varicosity is located in the distal thigh; it is a handswidth below the knee in stage III disease, and at or below the malleolus in stage IV disease. The *proximal point of incompetence* is located at the site of the incompetent transfascial communication (see p. 108) and characterizes the complete and incomplete forms.

Stage I saphenous varicosity has been redefined in the light of the theory of recirculating flow patterns (reflux circuits). The distal point of incompetence in stage I cases is located in the groin at the base of an abnormally dilated and elongated

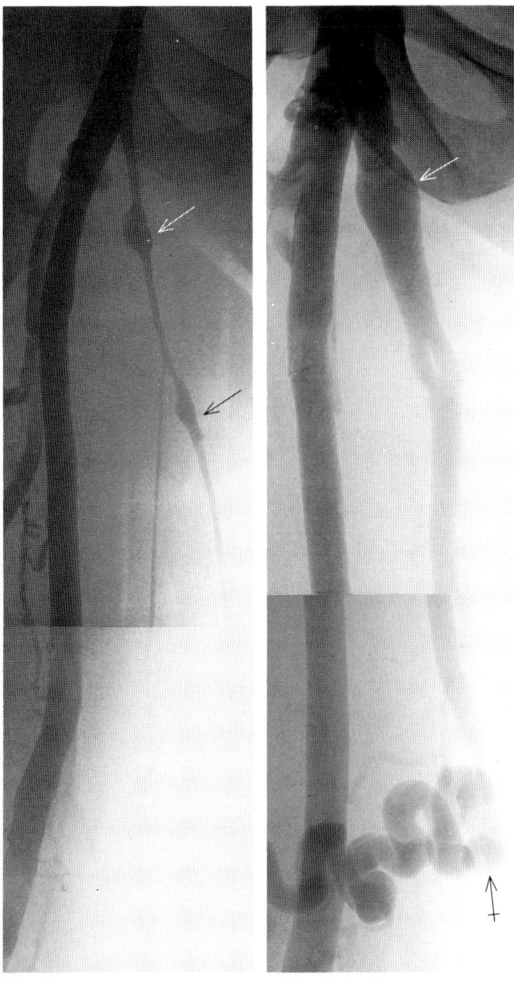

142 *(left)*. Stage II great saphenous varicosity. A slight telescope sign is still present. There are infravalvular dilatations (→) below the proximal venous valves, but the trunk itself is not dilated. Demonstrated by ascending pressure phlebography

143 *(right)*. Stage II great saphenous varicosity. The saphenous trunk is dilated to finger thickness, and there is infravalvular dilatation in the preterminal region (→). The distal point of incompetence, marked by a conspicuous branch varix, is located at the junction of the middle and lower thirds of the thigh (↔). Decompensated type II reflux circuit with dilatation and valve destruction in the superficial femoral vein signifying secondary popliteal and femoral vein insufficiency

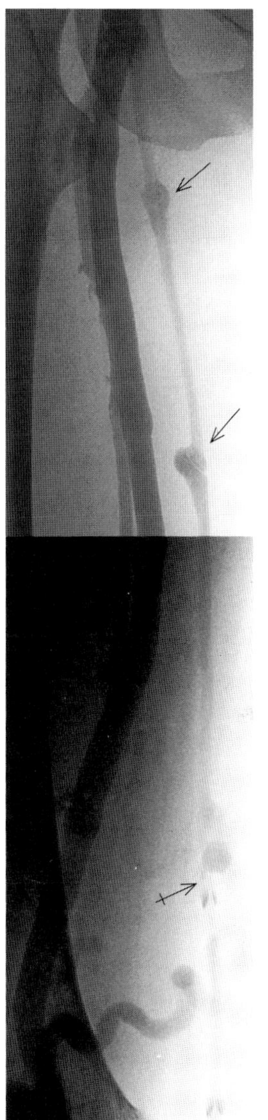

144. Stage II great saphenous varicosity. The trunk is distended to pencil thickness and shows multiple infravalvular dilatations (→). The distal point of incompetence, marked by a branch varix, is a hands width above the knee (↔). Compensated type II reflux circuit

saphenous sinus. As in the other stages, a branch varix passes distally from that site. We commonly refer to this as a "side-branch varicosity" of the lateral accessory saphenous vein.

142–144 In *stage II* cases, varicose degeneration of the great saphenous vein extends from the terminal region to a fairly constant valve located a handswidth above the knee. The distal point of incompetence is marked by a large branch varix, which permits the reflux of blood to the periphery. A distal point 145–146
of incompetence could not exist without this varicose tributary. The varicose segment of the great

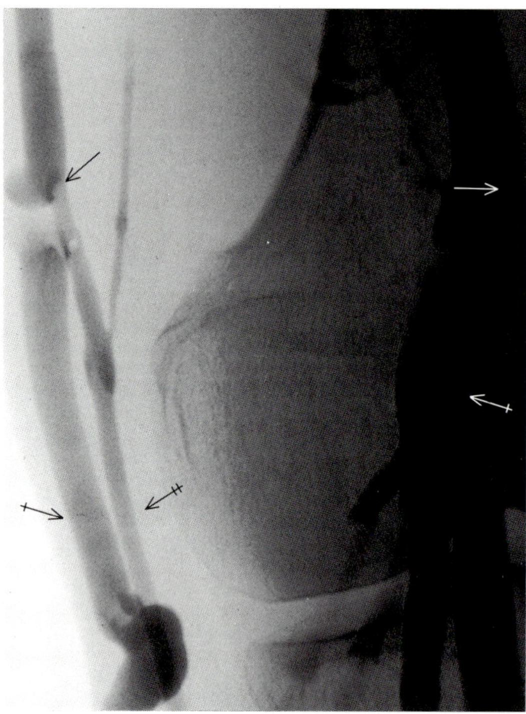

145. Distal point of incompetence (→) in a stage II great saphenous varicosity, with a branch varix (↛) and competent saphenous trunk distal to the point of incompetence (⇸)

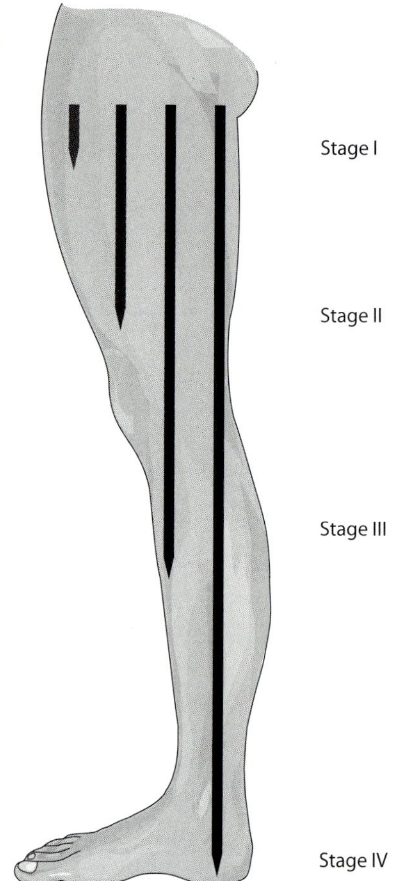

147. Stages of great saphenous varicosity

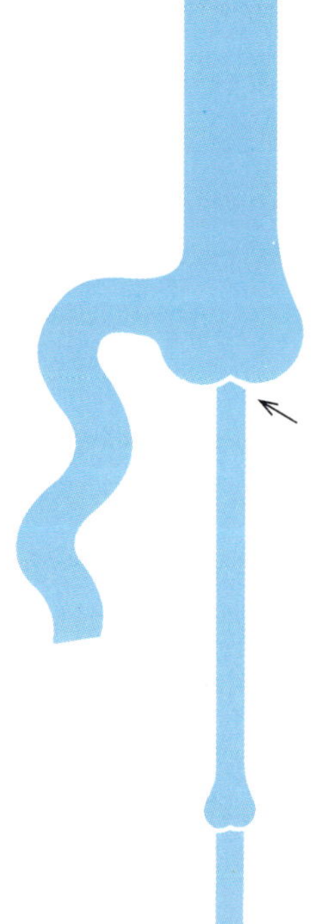

◁ **146.** Distal point of incompetence in a varicose great saphenous vein, marked by a branch varix directly above the highest competent valve in the venous trunk (→)

saphenous trunk is markedly dilated to the diameter of a pencil or small finger. Clinical symptoms are mild at this stage, although a small varicose knot can be felt on the medial side of the thigh.

In *stage III* the great saphenous incompetence extends from the groin to a venous valve located a handwidth below the knee. Again, the distal point of incompetence is marked by the termination of a prominent branch varix. Often the saphenous trunk is already dilated to finger thickness when the patient presents for treatment, and many patients have symptoms of chronic venous insufficiency due to decompensation of the reflux circuit. 147, 148

Stage IV varicosity can produce severe symptomatology, even in young patients. In the tubular form the great saphenous trunk is only moderately di- 149, 150

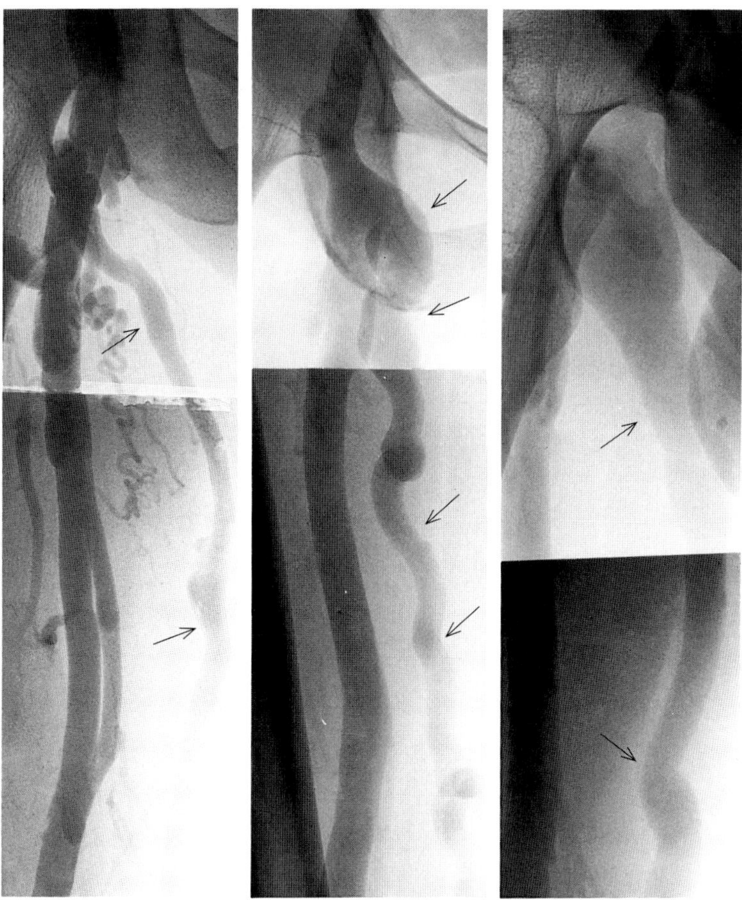

148 *(left)*. Stage III great saphenous varicosity. The inguinal portion of the vessel is dilated to small-finger thickness (→). The distal point of incompetence is below the knee. Compensated reflux circuit

149 *(middle)*. Stage IV great saphenous varicosity. The vein is dilated to the thickness of the thumb (→) and shows marked tortuosity. Reflux extends distally past the level III point of incompetence. Decompensated reflux circuit

150 *(right)*. Stage IV great saphenous varicosity. The vein is massively dilated (→) and very tortuous. Reflux extends past the level III point of incompetence. The vessel is weakly opacified due to severe circulatory impairment caused by secondary popliteal and femoral vein insufficiency in the decompensated reflux circuit

lated but passes in a straight line from the groin to the foot, permitting a rapid reflux of blood to the
128 periphery. This contrasts with the "circoid" form in which the vein is dilated to the thickness of the thumb and shows marked tortuosity. Though it develops more gradually, this form also leads to early cutaneous changes (see p. 102).

The reflux circuit appears to decompensate at an early age, with secondary popliteal and femoral vein insufficiency making the condition difficult to distinguish from congenital aplasia of the venous valves. Without phlebography, the severe chronic venous insufficiency is clinically indistinguishable from post-thrombotic syndrome.

The coexistence of saphenous varicosity with an *incompetent Cockett's perforator* is particularly 151
detrimental and is commonly associated with severe chronic venous insufficiency. The distal lower leg shows areas of brawny induration, pigmentation, and statis dermatitis. Ulcers, scars, and white atrophy are present about the ankle, indicating a microcirculatory disturbance.

The inflammatory response may spread to involve the capsule of the ankle joint. Initially the patient favors the limb by holding the foot in equinus, and

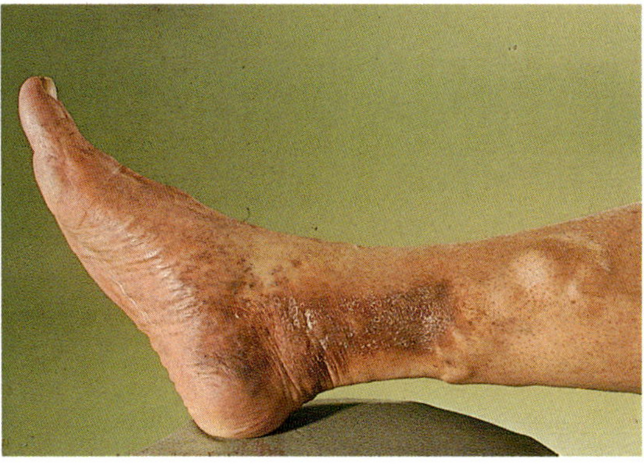

151. Chronic venous insufficiency in stage IV great saphenous varicosity with an incompetent upper Cockett perforator. Pigmentation, dermatoliposclerosis, small ulcer scars, white atrophy, mild contact dermatitis. (Close-up of the limb in Fig. 128)

Radiographic criteria of saphenous varicosity
Retrograde saphenous flow
Absence of telescope sign
Infravalvular dilatations
Venous aneurysms
Dilatation and tortuosity of the saphenous vein

129 an *arthrogenic stasis syndrome* ensues. Failure of the peripheral venous pumps leads to a severe impairment of venous hemodynamics. The ankle ulcers either do not heal, or they quickly recur under hydrostatic loading after prolonged hospitalization with immobilization and skin grafting. The supramalleolar region is extensively involved by dermatolipofasciosclerosis with chronic stasis eczema, hypodermitis, and recurrent bouts of contact dermatitis. Computed tomography (CT) and magnetic resonance imaging (MRI) show an increasing fibrosis of the retromalleolar space and the gliding tissues about the Achilles tendon, the latter showing a diffuse decrease in density that correlates with the severity of the chronic venous insufficiency (Schmeller 1990). The only curative treatment is surgical ablation of the affected extrafascial vessels, paratibial fasciotomy, and remobilization of the ankle.

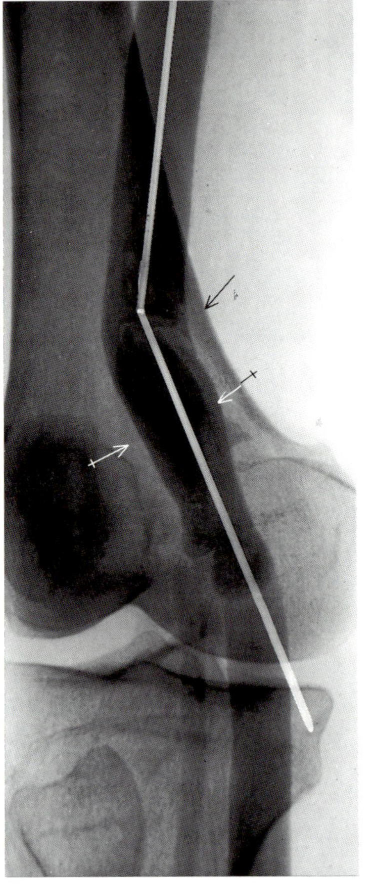

152. Radiographic signs of incipient popliteal and femoral vein insufficiency secondary to great saphenous varicosity: increasing popliteofemoral angulation (→) and dilatation of the vessel lumen (↔). The valves in the popliteal vein are still functionally competent

Secondary Popliteal and Femoral Vein Insufficiency

With passage of time, the recirculating blood volume associated with the great saphenous varicosity produces marked structural changes in the deep venous system, which we refer to as secondary popliteal and femoral vein insufficiency (Hach et al. 1980). The phlebographic picture is
characteristic: The deep veins of the lower leg ap- 152
pear slightly dilated, but their valves are compe- 153
tent. Regressive changes are usually seen in the muscle veins, which contain fewer valves than normal. The popliteal vein and superficial femoral vein are *dilated*. The popliteofemoral junction forms a bend at the level of Hunter's canal that becomes sharper with the severity of the disease; ul- 156
timately the angle may fall below 135°. In ad-

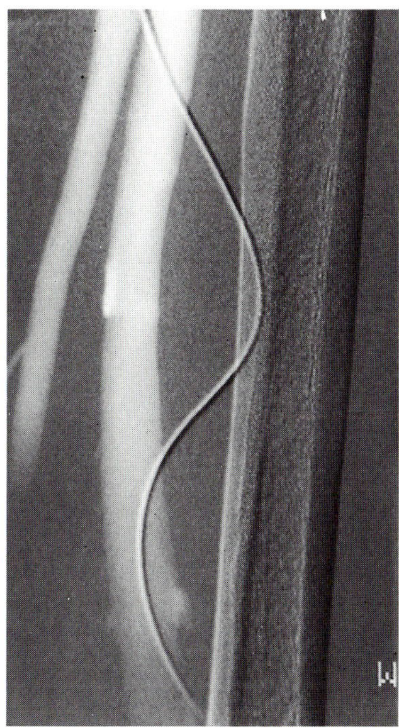

153. Great saphenous varicosity with secondary popliteal and femoral vein insufficiency. Demonstrated by retrograde pressure phlebography. Distally decreasing retrograde flow in the superficial femoral vein. Digital image

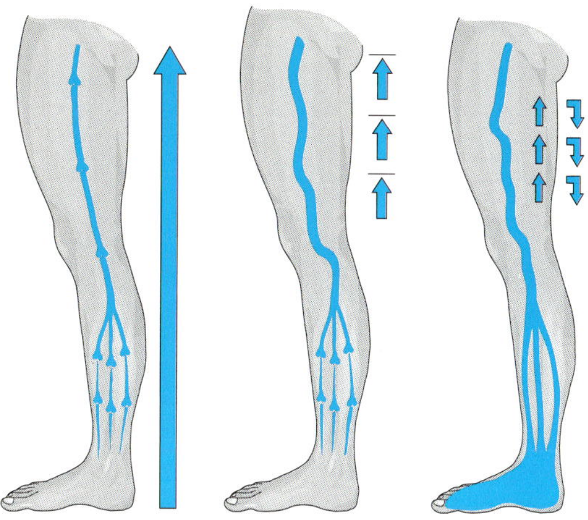

154. Antegrade flow components in the deep veins during ascending phlebography with manual calf compression. *Left,* normal situation; *middle,* secondary popliteal and femoral vein insufficiency; *right,* post-thrombotic syndrome

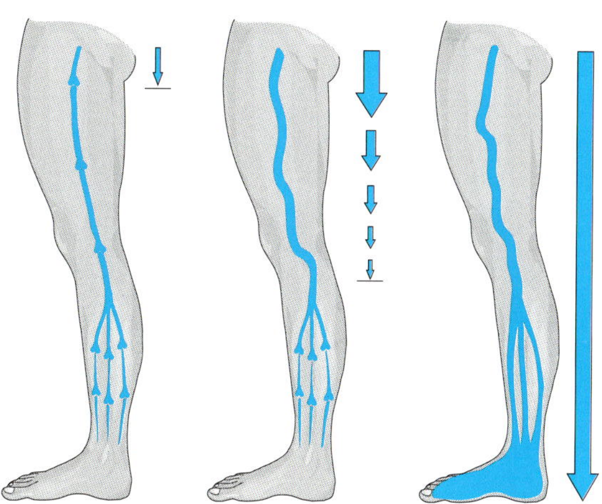

155. Retrograde flow components in the deep veins during retrograde pressure phlebography. *Left,* normal flow conditions; *middle,* secondary popliteal and femoral vein insufficiency; *right,* post-thrombotic syndrome

vanced cases the junction may become *kinked* and functionally occluded. The superficial femoral vein is slightly tortuous, and its valves are no longer visible. The changes are best appreciated by comparison with the opposite side.

Another radiographic sign of secondary popliteal
and femoral vein insufficiency is a generally faded
158 or *washed-out appearance* of the phlebogram. Es-
159 pecially in the thigh region, the axial veins are not
portrayed with the usual sharpness and density,
even when a larger contrast dose is used. The
154 cause is apparent during fluoroscopy: Manual calf
compression in the relaxed, dependent limb no longer produces an outrush of blood into the pelvic region; instead, the bolus is merely propelled a few centimeters and then stops. The contrast medium becomes increasingly mixed and diluted with blood, producing the typical washed-out phlebographic signature.

The special hemodynamics of secondary popliteal and femoral vein insufficiency represents an *antegrade* form of deep venous insufficiency. This contrasts with the *retrograde* insufficiency of post-thrombotic syndrome, in which all the venous valves are destroyed, and blood can reflux into the peripheral venous pools on quiet standing or Valsalva straining. The flow reversal
in post-thrombotic syndrome is easily document-
ed by retrograde pressure phlebography follow- 155
ing contrast injection into the common femoral 156
vein.

With *antegrade insufficiency* due to secondary 157
popliteal and femoral vein damage, the valves in
the lower leg veins are functionally competent.

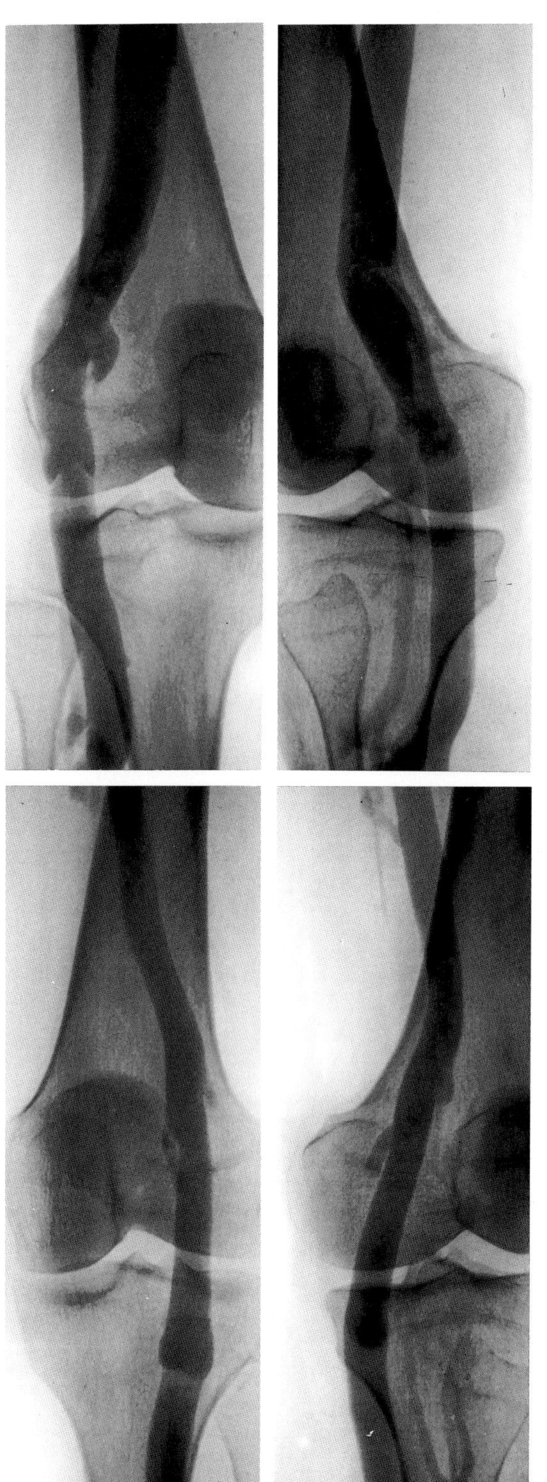

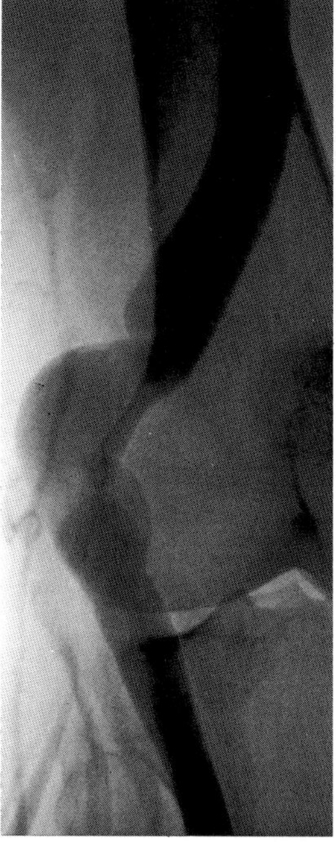

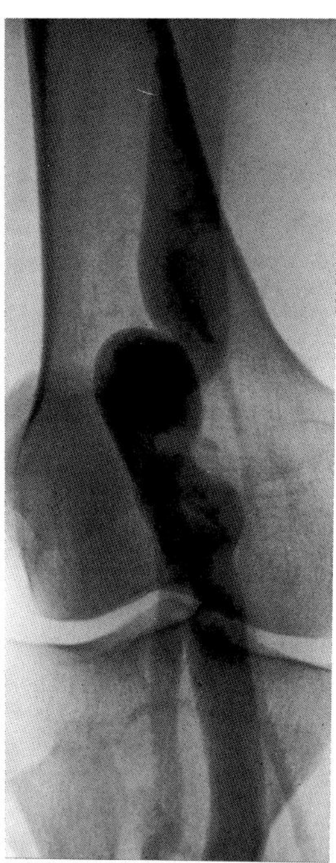

157. Very severe secondary popliteal and femoral vein insufficiency with kinking and loss of valvular function in a 67-year-old woman with a long history of inadequately treated stage IV great saphenous varicosity and a decompensated reflux circuit. Chronic venous insufficiency with frequent swelling. No post-thrombotic syndrome. Ascending phlebography, internal rotation (*left*) and lateral view (*right*)

◁

156. Incipient secondary femoral and popliteal vein insufficiency on the right side (*top*), with normal left phlebograms for comparison (*bottom*). The popliteofemoral angle is 142° on the right and 153° on the left, with respective vessel diameters of 23 mm and 13 mm. Ascending pressure phlebography, internal rotation (*upper left*) and lateral view (*upper right*), in a 44-year-old woman with severe stage III great saphenous varicosity and a decompensated reflux circuit. Chronic venous insufficiency on the right side, persistent edema after surgery

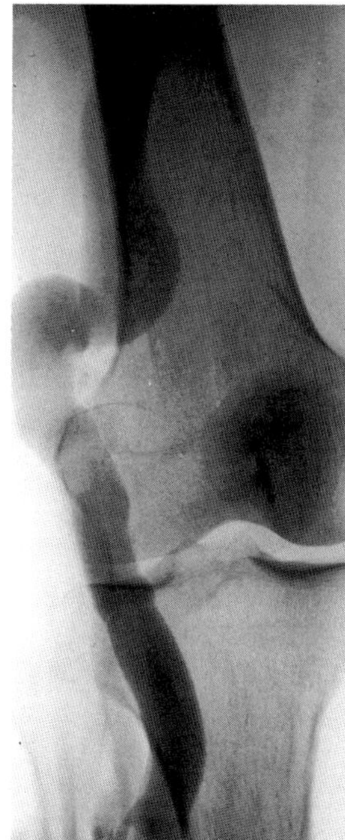
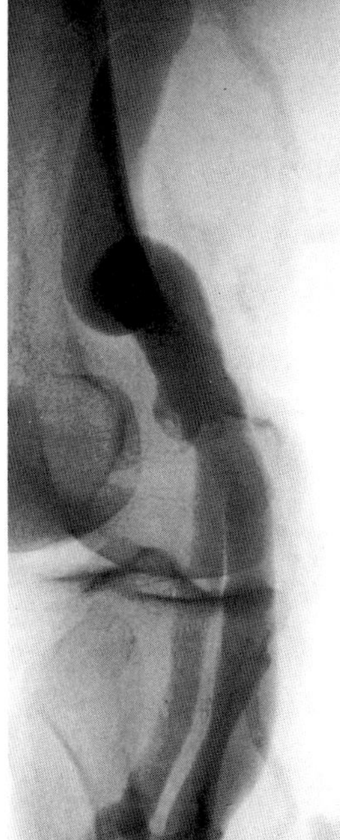
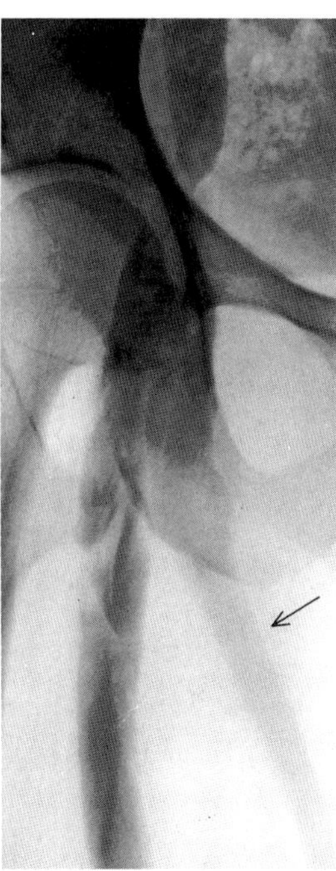

158. Secondary popliteal and femoral vein insufficiency with 90° kinking in a 59-year-old woman with stage IV great saphenous varicosity (→; *right*) and a decompensated reflux circuit. Weak opacification of the vessels due to greatly imparied hemodynamics. Ascending pressure phlebography, internal rotation (*left*) and lateral views (*right*)

Antegrade and retrograde venous insufficiency		
	Phlebographic diagnosis	Disease
Antegrade	Ascending pressure phlebography (with stem vein test)	Secondary popliteal and femoral vein insufficiency
		Post-thrombotic syndrome without recanalization
		Regressive vascular changes
		Arteriovenous fistula
		Functional pump incompetence
Retrograde	Retrograde pressure phlebography	Post-thrombotic syndrome of the lower extremity
		Avalvulia
		Vascular dysplasia

Thus, reflux can occur in the proximal part of the thigh during a Valsalva maneuver only until the capacity of the dilated stem veins is exhausted. Retrograde phlebography down the femoral vein
with a Valsalva maneuver plainly shows that the 99
velocity and quantity of the reflux decrease rapidly in the distal direction. The popliteal vein is not opacified by the retrograde study.

The pathophysiologic conditions of antegrade and retrograde deep venous insufficiency are easily assessed by Doppler ultrasound. Both directional Doppler and duplex scanning indicate very short reverse flow signals during retrograde flowmetry. There is a typical constellation of physical parameters, marked initially by an increase of venous capacity and drainage. Phlebodynamometry or photoplethysmography additionally demonstrates a severe impairment of the pump function in the leg. Clinically the limb is swollen and exhibits the more or less pronounced features of chronic venous insufficiency due to venous hypertension.

As the term implies, *secondary popliteal and femo-* 158
ral insufficiency chiefly affects the popliteal vein 159
and the superficial femoral vein. The vessels of the

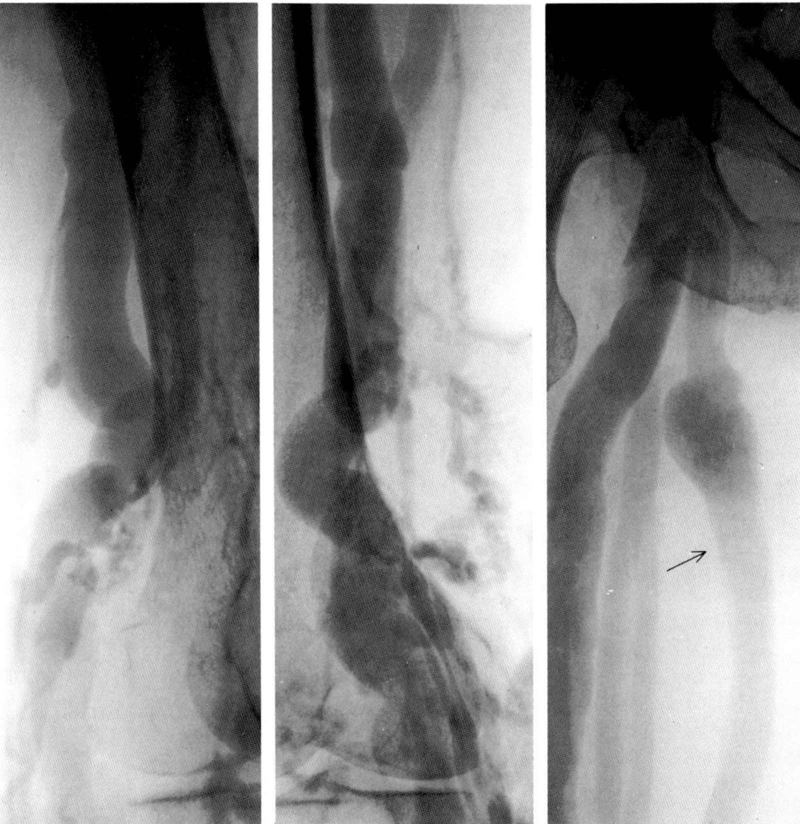

159. Secondary popliteal and femoral vein insufficiency with multiple kinks and severe venous dilatation (*left, middle*). The vessels are weakly opacified due to impaired hemodynamics. Woman 72 years of age with neglected stage IV great saphenous varicosity (*right*, →) and a decompensated reflux circuit; chronic venous insufficiency

lower leg appear slightly dilated, but their valves are still competent. The explanation is clear: The recirculating blood volume in the lower leg is distributed among six vessels that contain abundant valves and are each supported by a vascular sheath and surrounding muscles. The distribution of a volume load in a multitube system is much less susceptible to disturbances than in a single-tube system. In view of this, the term deep vein insufficiency also seems justified.

When there is severe varicosity of a Cockett perforator, a *secondary tibial vein insufficiency* can develop that is fully analogous to the flow changes occurring in the thigh. The heavy volume load leads to dilatation and tortuosity of the deep vein with regional incompetence of its venous valves.

Primary Reflux Circuits

The concept of primary recirculating flow patterns (Hach 1989) permits us to take a synergistic view of the various manifestations of varicose disease. This in turn enables us to draw appropriate diagnostic and therapeutic inferences for a given case and make an individual prognostic assessment.

Every reflux circuit hinges on a varicose saphenous trunk. That is why we touch upon the subject of recirculating flow in the present chapter, although a knowledge of details given in subsequent chapters is needed to have a thorough understanding.

The notion of a blood volume recirculating in a limb with severe varicose veins is a century old. The Bonn surgeon Fritz Trendelenburg first described this as a "private circulation" in 1891 in his famous paper on proximal saphenous vein ligation as a treatment for lower leg varices: "The blood present in the reservoir of the saphenous vein must drain into the deeper veins and then be replaced by blood from the femoral vein. In this way a 'private circulation' is established in the lower extremity as blood is pumped up the deep veins of the leg and then partly spills down again into the saphenous system."

We have adopted Trendelenburg's principle of the "private circulation" in saphenous varicosity and modified it in the light of recent scientific discoveries. In accordance with the four stages of great saphenous varicosity described earlier, we recognize four types of associated reflux circuits, which initially are compensated with respect to the deep venous system but can decompensate under certain conditions. Phlebography is considered the basic diagnostic modality for defining the morphologic substrate of the recirculating flow; additional information can be derived from the results of physical measurements.

The *reflux circuit III* associated with great saphenous varicosity begins with retrograde blood flow into the saphenous trunk at the groin and continues into the varicose side branch located at the
160 distal point of incompetence. The blood then reenters the deep venous system through competent perforators. The four types of reflux circuit (I–IV) are easily conceptualized by referring to the corresponding stages of saphenous varicosity.

Over time the recirculating blood volume overloads the deep venous channels. These dilate until their valve cusps can no longer coapt, and secondary popliteal and femoral vein insufficiency ensues. With this *decompensation* of the reflux circuit, the dynamic venous pressure rises, leading to *Cockett's perforator varicosity* with the complications of chronic venous insufficiency.

The time at which decompensation occurs in a given case depends on various factors. A key factor is the location of the distal point of incompetence and the associated branch varix. The saphenous trunk is a straight vessel with a high transport volume. The varicose side branch, by contrast, always has a very tortuous course that reduces the flow velocity and limits retrograde flow. The peripheral divisions into small reticular vessels produce a similar effect. Thus, the long varicose branch in a type I reflux circuit is far more efficient in protecting the limb from hemodynamic stresses than the shorter branch varix in a type III circuit. The absence of a branch varix in the type IV circuit has a particularly devastating effect.

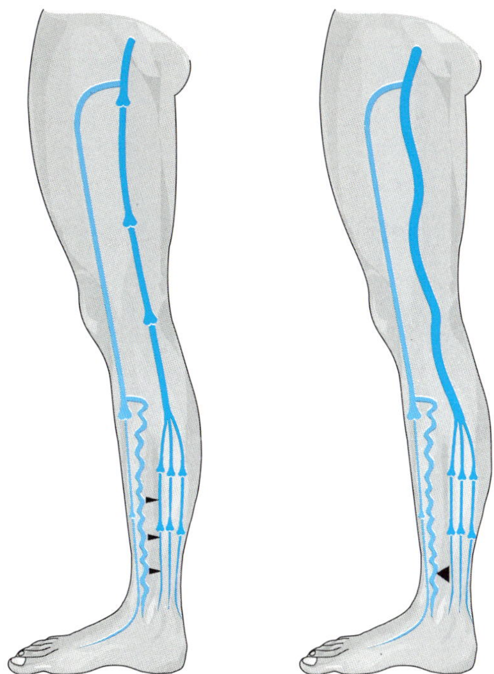

160. Reflux circuit III. Return blood flow from the groin into the great saphenous vein, at the distal point of incompetence into the side-branch varicosity and from there via the perforating veins into the deep venous system. Compensated stage (*left*) and decompensation with secondary popliteal and femoral vein insufficiency (*right*)

Drawing an analogy with landscape ecology, we note that a meandering brook has a very slow rate of flow. It can transport only a limited volume of water, so it provides for efficient hydration of adjacent fields. If the stream bed were straightened, the flow rate would be greatly increased, and neighboring meadows and marshes would dry up. The size of the waterway is of minor importance. The river into which the straight channels run is in flood.

In a ***type I reflux circuit,*** the varicose lateral accessory saphenous vein arises from an abnormally 161
enlarged sinus of the great saphenous vein. The varicose side branch is so long that there is virtually no danger of deep venous decompensation, 196
regardless of the development of the branch varix. 197
The disease is hardly ever associated with chronic venous insufficiency.

The branch varix is also relatively long in a ***type II reflux circuit,*** extending from the thigh to the malleolar region. This type of circuit takes several decades to decompensate, if at all.

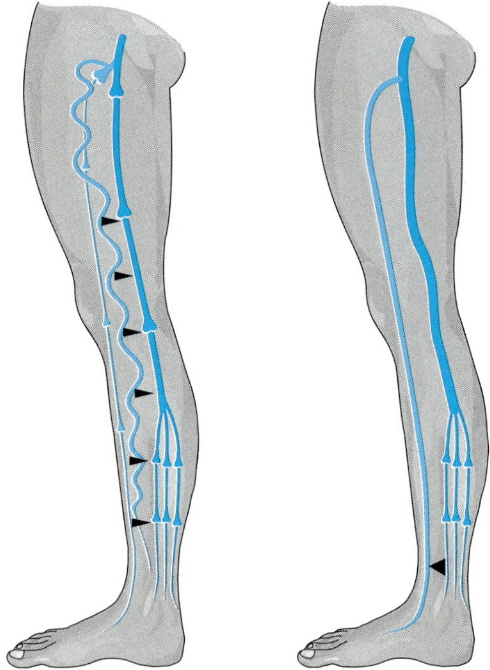

161. Extreme reflux circuits. In circuit I, there is maximal development of the side-branch varicosity and thus hemodynamic protection of the deep venous system (*left*). In circuit IV, there is no conjugated side-branch varicosity and thus early decompensation (*right*)

Factors that promote the decompensation of a reflux circuit
Location of the points of incompetence
Hereditary factors
Hormonal influences
Physical training
Orthostatic load
Thermal effects
Body weight

Characteristics of the reflux circuits associated with great saphenous varicosity		
Type of circuit	Compensated/ decompensated	Chronic venous insufficiency
I	Always/Never	Absent
II	Long/very late	Rare
III	Moderate/one to two decades	Mild to severe
IV	Short/immediate	Very severe

160 In a ***type III reflux circuit*** – the pattern most common in great saphenous varicosity – the branch varix develops below the knee. Decompensation occurs after an average of one to two decades, or sooner under unfavorable conditions.

The ***type IV reflex circuit*** carries the worst prognosis. The regurgitant blood volume is so large from the outset that secondary popliteal and femoral vein insufficiency develops rapidly. Most patients become symptomatic in adolescence, and venous ulcers form early. Usually the saphenous varicosity is of the tubular form, especially in tall, thin patients with an asthetic constitution. But the circoid type also progresses swiftly to decompensation with an unusually severe course.

161 The reflux circuits associated with stage IV saphenous varicosity are relatively rare in a surgical population, with an incidence of about 1 in 500. Accordingly, this condition is overdiagnosed in radiologic practice. One reason for this is that the distal portion of the great saphenous vein is poorly filled by retrograde flow during ascending pressure phlebography. More precise information could be obtained by superficial phlebography and varicography, but the experienced surgeon can usually dispense with these studies and rely on a clinical assessment.

The proximal point of incompetence also affects the timing of decompensation in the deep venous system. Incomplete forms of saphenous varicosity generally take a favorable course with no danger of secondary popliteal and femoral vein insufficiency, although this might result with Dodd's perforator type of incomplete varicosity. The side-branch type, posterior type, or the rare perforator types of incomplete saphenous varicosity rarely cause dermatologic complications.

We do not yet fully understand the laws that govern the *timing of the decompensation* of reflux circuits, and we cannot make a definitive prediction in a given case. We know only that the timing is affected by hereditary and hormonal influences in addition to morphologic factors, and that daily living habits are important. Minimal athletic conditioning in an individual whose work involves prolonged standing, heavy lifting, and possibly heat exposure promotes the development of secondary popliteal and femoral vein insufficiency.

This accounts for the frequency and severity of cases in bartenders, bakers, and butchers. Clinical experience indicates that chronic venous insufficiency develops more rapidly in obese individuals.

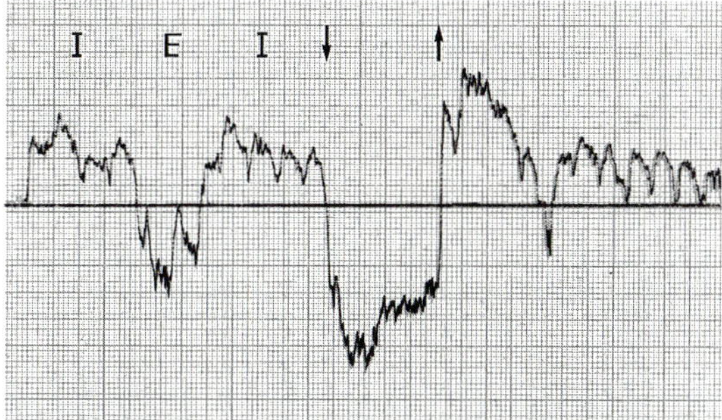

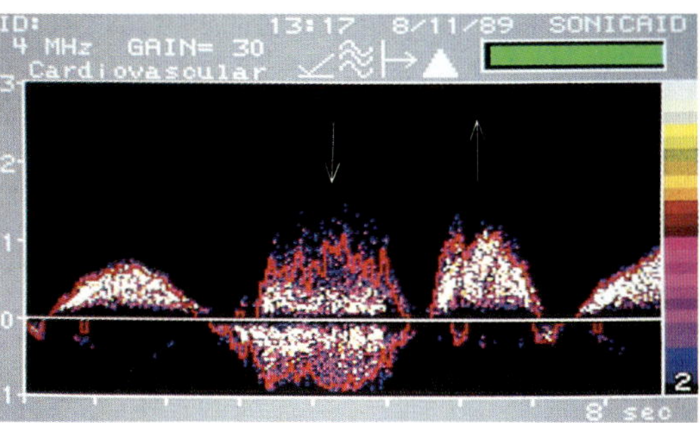

162. *Top*, directional analog curve in severe saphenous varicosity. During expiration (*E*), the retrograde flow component can already be clearly seen. Valsalva test with considerable retrograde flow. Overshoot phenomenen after the Valsalva test (↑). Drainage via the terminal region of the great saphenous vein. *Bottom*, frequency analysis. Considerable flow turbulence during the Valsalva test (↓). Overshoot phenomenen (↑). Centripetal flow in the positive and centrifugal in the negative range. (Sonicaid, 8-MHz transducer)

Comparison of Phlebography with Other Diagnostic Methods

As an invasive procedure, ascending pressure phlebography requires a strict medical indication in cases where the procedure will have therapeutic implications. The varicose saphenous trunk is the most important component of a primary reflux circuit; hence its diagnosis should not be considered in isolation but as part of the overall assessment of the peripheral circulation of the extremity. Moreover, the surgical treatment concept should not be limited to the varicosity itself but should encompass the recirculation pattern as a whole.

The surgeon requires specific information on the proximal point of incompetence, in part to establish the upper limit of an incomplete saphenous varicosity. He must also know the location of the distal point of incompetence so that he can plan the stripping procedure.

Ascending pressure phlebography has the value of a reference standard for identifying the points of incompetence. The most important clinical examination, *venous palpation in the groin*, has a sensitivity of only 41.5 %, 56.1 % and, 75.7 % in stages II, III, and IV, respectively, although its specificity, at 92.7 %, is high (Hach 1981).

Doppler ultrasound can detect (complete) great saphenous varicosity with a specificity of 93.6 % and a sensitivity of 91.2 % (Hach 1981 b), the directional and nondirectional techniques providing equivalent diagnostic information. The examination starts at the groin in the recumbent patient, with a Valsalva maneuver eliciting inexhaustible retrograde saphenous flow in positive cases. When the patient stops straining, there is an
162 audible overshoot phenomenon caused by an antegrade surge of venous blood pooled in the leg.

The calf *de*compression test during Doppler examination in the standing position relies on patient cooperation and demonstrates saphenous varicosity by the detection of retrograde blood flow during quiet orthostasis. The probing is carried out directly above the vessel with an 8-MHz transducer. Again, a *continuous, inexhaustible reflux* must be present to establish a positive diagno- 163
sis. An initial retrograde flow followed by zero flow signifies delayed but complete closure of the venous valves. The distal point of incompetence can be difficult to locate, because the Doppler signal from the origin of the varicose side branch is identical to that from the incompetent varicose trunk. Clinical findings, however, can generally help clarify the situation.

Diagnostic imaging by *real-time sonography* and in particular *color-coded duplex scanning* has proven valuable, especially for evaluations of the crosse region. Sonographic imaging offers a sensitivity of 96 % and specificity of 75 % (Wuppermann 1991). The latest generation of high-resolution instruments can document fine morphologic features in the terminal portion of the saphenous vein as well as infravalvular dilatations and aneurysms. Color flow imaging provides impressive views of venous flow patterns under various con-

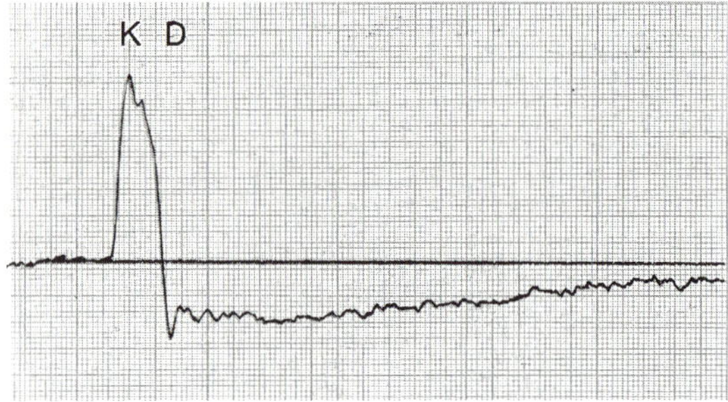

163. Directional Doppler sonography. Inexhaustible return flow via the great saphenous vein in severe saphenous varicosity. Calf compression test (*K*) and decompression test (*D*)

164 ditions. As in the analog techniques, significant
165 diagnostic problems are encountered only with
the incomplete forms of saphenous varicosity.

Thus, agreement between clinical and sonographic findings provides a high level of diagnostic confidence. If a discrepancy exists, phlebography should definitely be included in the preoperative workup.

Physical measuring techniques that supply information on global parameters of venous function have adjunctive importance for the investigation of saphenous varicosity. They are useful for making a general evaluation of the recirculating flow.

Secondary popliteal and femoral vein insufficiency is a dynamically progressive disease process that must be held responsible for the rising complication rate in patients with primary varicose veins and especially for the development of chronic venous insufficiency. Decompensation of the reflux circuit is diagnosed mainly by detecting a reduction in the pump function of the leg. Accurate data are provided by *peripheral phlebodynamometry* which, combined with phlebography, allows for a comprehensive assessment of venous hemodynamics. *Photoplethysmography* furnishes a comparable impression by noninvasive means. It appears that fluoroscopy permits a semiquantitative assessment of the insufficiency when the femoral vein test is applied.

Venous occlusion plethysmography yields data on venous capacity and drainage. Both quantities increase with the severity of deep venous insufficiency due to progressive enlargement of the flow channel.

Secondary popliteal and femoral vein insufficiency is defined phlebographically. With precise technique, the diagnosis can also be established by *di-*

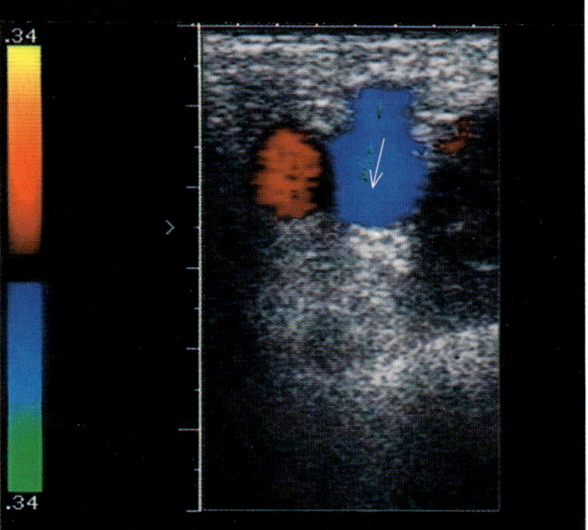

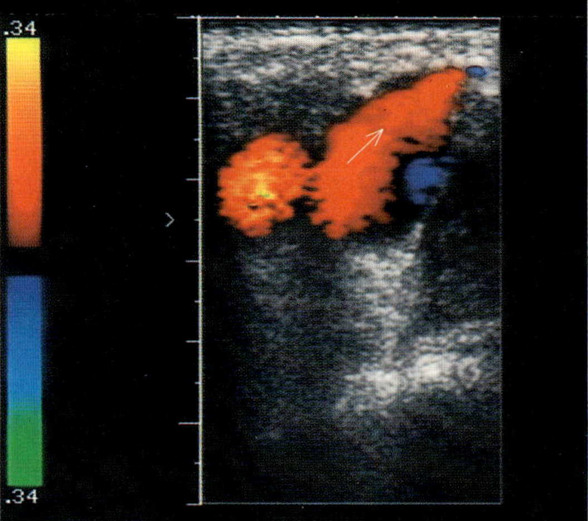

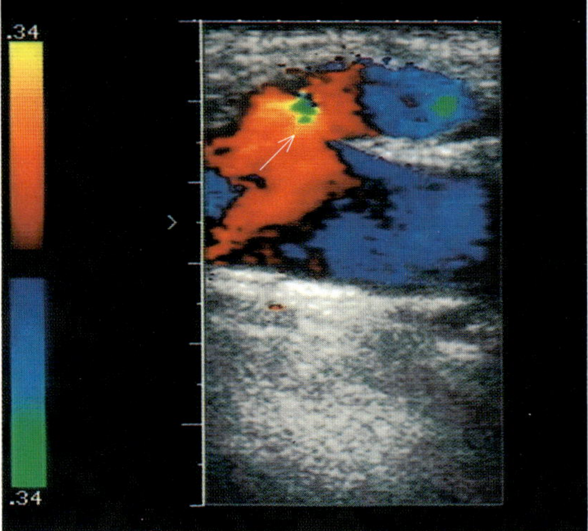

164. Great saphenous varicosity. Color-coded duplex sonography in the groin region. Cross-section with antegrade flow into the great saphenous vein (↓) during expiration (*top*). Retrograde flow into the great saphenous vein during the Valsalva test (↑); cross-section (*middle*) and longitudinal section (*bottom*). Flow turbulence. (Acuson, 7-MHz transducer)

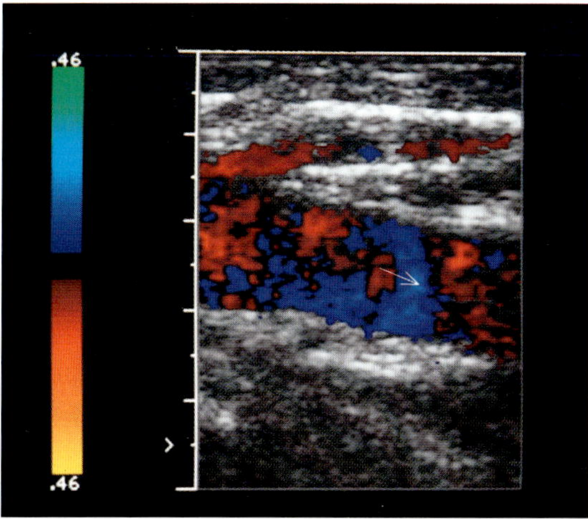

165. Secondary popliteal and femoral vein insufficiency in great saphenous varicosity. The superficial femoral vein is considerably enlarged, and there is retrograde flow turbulence during the Valsalva test. Color-coded duplex sonography. (Acuson, 7-MHz transducer)

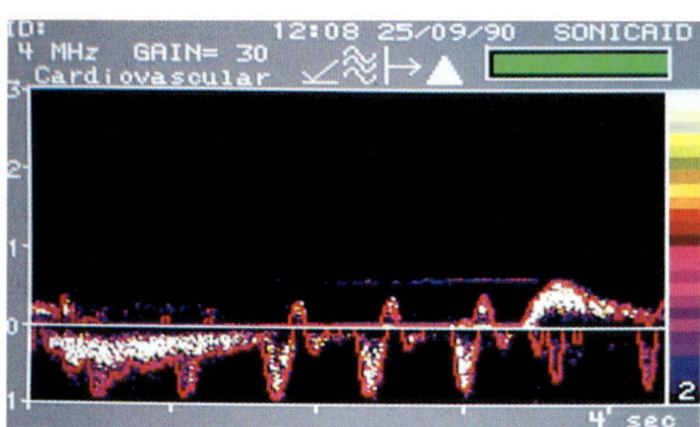

166. Evidence of secondary popliteal and femoral vein insufficiency provided by the calf *de*compression test via the superficial femoral vein in the proximal thigh. Return flow phenomenen in the negative range over two cardiac cycles (*left*). Greatly weakened A sound during the calf compression test (*right*). Centripetal flow in the positive and centrifugal in the negative range. Frequency analysis. (Sinocaid, 8-MHz transducer)

Comparative values of peripheral phlebodynamometry

Reflux circuit (RC)	Semiquantitative stem vein test	n	delta-P (mmHg)	t_2 (s)
Compensated				
Control group	0	24	64.0±7.4	28.4±4.1
RC II	0	14	62.5±5.1	5.9±7.7
Decompensated				
RC III	1–2	15	34.0±5.4	6.1±1.9
RC IV	>3	14	15.0±3.9	2.8±1.19

False-positive misdiagnoses of saphenous varicosity by Doppler ultrasound flowmetry

- Side-branch varicosity of lateral accessory saphenous vein
- State after crossectomy, inguinal varices
- Functional valvular incompetence
- Primary femoral vein insufficiency
- Post-thrombotic syndrome

Physical parameters associated with progressive secondary popliteal and femoral vein insufficiency

Severity of disease (phlebographic stem vein test)	Pump function: Venous pressure	Pump function: Refill time (t_2, t_0)	Venous capacity	Venous drainage
+	↓	↓	↑	↑
++	↓↓	↓↓	↑↑	↑↑
+++	↓↓↓	↓↓↓	↑↑↑	↑↑↑

False-positive diagnoses of saphenous varicosity by Doppler ultrasound flowmetry

- Anatomic variations
- Obesity
- Incomplete forms
- Inadequate compliance

rectional frequency analysis and duplex scanning.
166 On calf compression, only an attenuated A sound with a small flow wave is detected over the superficial femoral vein, with decompression producing a brief reflux effect. A reasonably confident diagnosis can be made only when findings are pronounced. Comparative quantitative evaluations are not yet available.

Formulating the Diagnosis

The phlebographic diagnosis supplied to the attending physician must cover the essential features of the saphenous varicosity, i. e., the stage of the disease and any complications that are present. It should convey information that is both concise and adequate for drawing therapeutic and prognostic conclusions.

Examples:

1. Stage II great saphenous varicosity with a compensated reflux circuit
2. Severe stage IV great saphenous varicosity with a decompensated reflux circuit; incompetent middle Cockett's perforator; varicose degeneration of the posterior arch vein; secondary popliteal and femoral vein insufficiency

Special Problems and Pitfalls

Long saphenous varicosity is best detected by the demonstration of retrograde blood flow from the groin. This is contingent upon several conditions. First there must be a *staged transport* of the contrast bolus during the examination to ensure that the concentration in the groin is still adequate for retrograde filling of the superficial vessels. Extra tourniquets above and below the knee alter the flow conditions and generally do not permit a differentiated diagnosis.

Another problem is the significant hemodynamic impairment caused by secondary popliteal and fe-
158 moral vein insufficiency. In pronounced cases the contrast medium is greatly diluted by blood due to the antegrade deep venous insufficiency, resulting in *poor opacification* of the extra- and intrafascial
159 veins above the knee. In this case the contrast dose must be doubled or tripled, and even then the radiographs present a washed-out appearance with deficient opacification of the vessels.

A major error is *incomplete performance of the*
103 *Valsalva maneuver.* Some patients strain ineffectively without actually bearing down through the abdomen. Others incorrectly tense their calf muscles, producing an outrush of contrast medium that is easily detected by fluoroscopy. Active leg movements by the patient also cause an accelerated outflow.

Weak or elderly patients often cannot sustain a Valsalva maneuver long enough for filming at the optimum phase, and the contrast injection must be repeated. Also, most patients cannot force the contrast medium down the great saphenous vein as far as the lower leg, and the opacification becomes increasingly faint as the bolus descends. Thus, a diagnosis of stage IV disease is made as soon as the bolus passes the level III point of incompetence a handswidth below the knee.

The Valsalva maneuver places a strain on the cardiovascular system, so it should either be omitted or performed only briefly in patients with *cardiovascular risk.* Patients with pulmonary emphysema, severe obesity, or dizzy spells also have difficulty straining for various reasons. However, these patients usually are not candidates for operation, so the indication for ascending pressure phlebography should be thought over again.

Therapeutic Implications

The treatment of choice for a complete great saphenous varicosity is crossectomy followed by saphenous stripping from the groin to the distal point of incompetence. This procedure, called a *partial saphenectomy* (Hach 1981 a), is preferred for various reasons over Babcock's operation in patients with stage II and stage III disease. It is a lesser operation, it does not damage the prefascial lymphatic bundle, and it avoids postoperative sensory disturbances in the lower leg and foot due to saphenous nerve injury. Partial saphenectomy preserves the distal, competent venous segment, which generally remains functional and can be
used at some future time for transfer into ob- 167
structed arterial systems. Even with stage IV saphenous varicosity, we do not carry the stripping procedure much past the knee in every case for the reasons cited above.

With a compensated reflux circuit, surgical treatment is essentially complete with the partial saphenectomy. The varicose side branch can be extracted through tiny skin incisions or obliterated with a sclerosing injection; frequently it regresses without treatment. The disease is regarded as cured.

In cases where the reflux circuit has decompensated, a *complete ablative procedure* is indicated (Hach 1991) that includes partial saphenectomy, removal of the branch varix, and selective dissection of incompetent Cockett's perforators. *Paratibial fasciotomy* has proven beneficial in patients with severe chronic venous insufficiency or arthro-

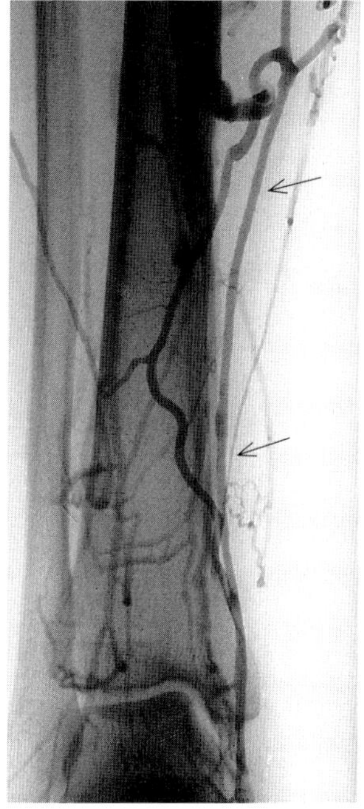

167. Phlebogram taken 5 years after partial saphenectomy in a 45-year-old woman demonstrates an intact, competent segment of the great saphenous vein in the lower leg (→)

Development of secondary popliteal and femoral vein insufficiency during the spontaneous progression of saphenous varicosity		
Diameter (mm)	Previous examination	Follow-up examination at 7.6 (2–10) years
Popliteal vein	15 (12–18)	17 (14–22)
Superficial femoral vein	15 (12–16)	17 (13–21)

Follow-up of secondary popliteal and femoral vein insufficiency after complete extrafascial ablative procedures		
Diameter (mm)	Before operation	After operation 6.6 (2–12) years
Popliteal vein	20 (15–35)	17 (12–23)
Superficial femoral vein	18 (14–22)	16 (10–18)

genic stasis syndrome. This procedure was developed by the authors in 1983 to replace the larger operations of Linton and Cockett. Through a small skin incision, the crural fascia is split at its tibial attachment from the malleolus to just below the knee, and the incompetent perforators are dissected. Special instruments are used for this procedure. With a broad communication thus established between the intra- and extrafascial tissue spaces, the increased pressure in the dorsal muscle compartments is disminished and the severe microcirculatory disturbances in the skin will resolve within a short time. The operation is simple and can be performed in any small hospital. It requires no special vascular surgical training and takes only a few minutes. The best way of performing it is now in combination with the *endoscopic technique* or at least during ischemia produced by using a Lövqvist tourniquet (Hach and Hach-Wunderle 1994). Even in very severe and longstanding cases, the cure rate is approximately 90 %.

In all cases great saphenous varicosity should be diagnosed as early as possible, preferably during adolescence. The main concern is to prevent decompensation of the reflux circuit and effect a permanent cure. Once secondary popliteal and femoral vein insufficiency has supervened, there will be a risk of recurrence even after a technically perfect and complete extrafascial ablative procedure. A regression of deep venous insufficiency can be documented by phlebography after only a few weeks. Under favorable conditions radiographic morphology will return to normal, dilatation will regress, and the valve cusps will coapt without leakage. There is an associated improvement in the measurable parameters of global function studies.

Phlebography has proven *the causal relationships* between saphenous varicosity, recirculating blood volume, and secondary popliteal-femoral vein insufficiency (Stranzenbach and Hach 1990). Long-term follow-ups in untreated cases have demonstrated luminal enlargement of the popliteal and superficial femoral veins from an average of 15 mm to 17 mm. By contrast, in patients with secondary popliteal and femoral vein insufficien- 168
cy who underwent the complete extrafascial ablation described above, the popliteal vein diameter decreased from 20 mm to 17 mm on average, and the superficial femoral vein diameter from 18 mm to 16 mm.

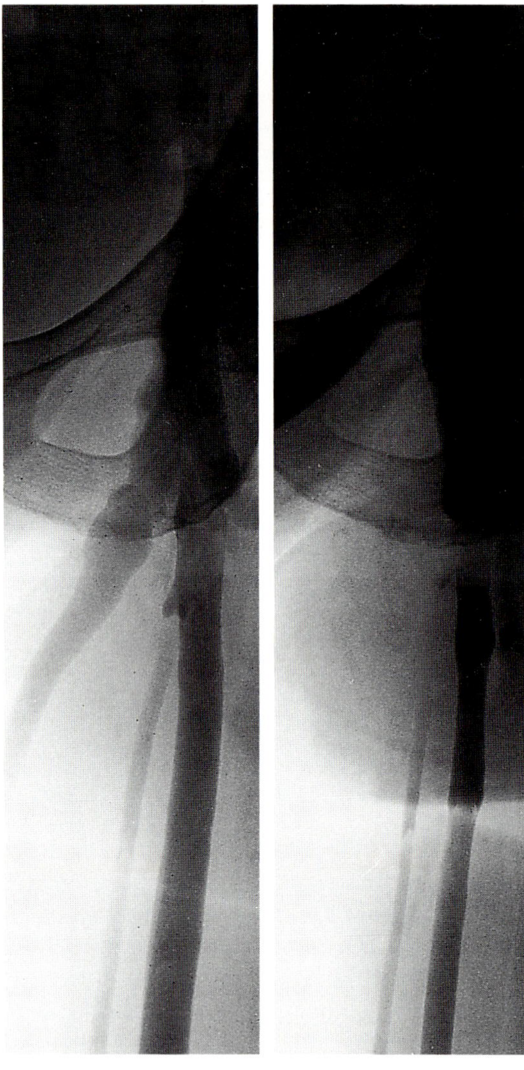

168. Secondary popliteal and femoral vein insufficiency in stage III varicosity of the left great saphenous vein (*left*). Complete involution after complete extrafascial operative treatment. Venous valves can be distinguished again (*right*). Demonstrated by ascending pressure phlebography

Incomplete Great Saphenous Varicosity

Ascending pressure phlebography has identified a new entity called incomplete saphenous varicosity (Hach 1981 b). Though clinically indistinguishable from complete saphenous varicosity in most cases, this condition has assumed considerable practical importance due to the availability of special procedures for its surgical treatment. Complete forms are more prevalent than the incomplete forms by a ratio of 12:1.

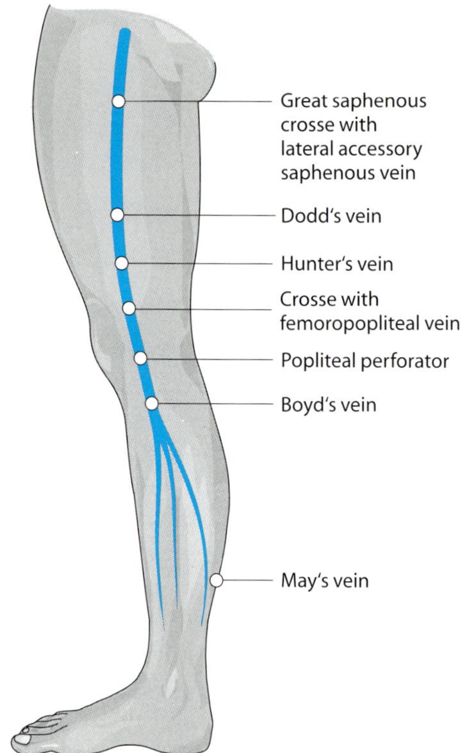

169. Potential sites where transfascial communicating veins can form the proximal point of incompetence for an incomplete great saphenous varicosity

Forms

Complete varicosity of the great saphenous vein is
defined as a varicose degeneration of the vessel
that results from incompetence of its terminal
valve and progresses in a proximal-to-distal direction. With *incomplete* varicosity, the terminal and
sluice valves are functionally sound. The saphenous trunk becomes incompetent at a lower level, 169
the *proximal point of incompetence*, where the 170
incompetent transfascial communicating vein
unites with the saphenous trunk. In 27.8% of cases this vein is an incompetent Dodd's perforator,
so the term *perforator type* is applied to this entity.
It is less common than the *side-branch type*, which
is present in 55.5% of cases. Here the proximal
point of incompetence is at the origin of the varicose lateral accessory saphenous vein, which arises from an enlarged saphenous sinus and enters
the great saphenous vein at the midthigh level
with the distal accessory anastomosis. The *poste-* 19
rior type denotes an incompetent communication 20
between the small saphenous vein and great sa-

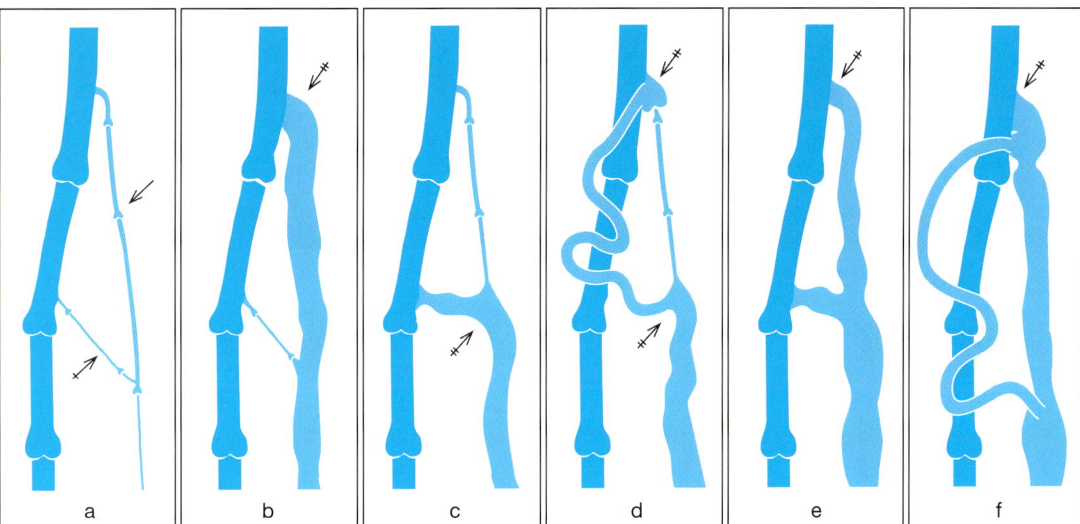

170 a–f. Various forms of incomplete great saphenous varicosity. **a** Normal situation. → Great saphenous vein; ⇸ Dodd's perforator. **b** Complete saphenous varicosity. ⇻ Proximal point of incompetence in the groin. **c** Dodd's perforator type of incomplete saphenous varicosity. ⇻ The proximal point of incompetence is at the midthigh. **d** Side-branch type of incomplete saphenous varicosity involving the lateral accessory saphenous vein. **e** Complete saphenous varicosity with an incompetent Dodd's perforator. **f** Complete saphenous varicosity with varicose degeneration of the lateral accessory saphenous vein

Forms of incomplete great saphenous varicosity	
Side-branch type- via lateral accessory saphenous vein	55.5 rel%
Perforator type- via Dodd's perforator	27.8 rel%
Posterior type- via femoropopliteal vein	16.7 rel%

phenous vein via the femoropopliteal vein and
21 medial accessory saphenous vein, the Giacomini
anastomosis. The disease is based on a congenitally enlarged ostial sinus of the small saphenous
vein. The posterior type of incomplete great saphenous varicosity accounts for 16.7% of cases
(Hach 1981 b).

Clinical Symptoms

Direct signs of disease are usually less prominent in incomplete saphenous varicosity than in the complete form, because the reflux circuit includes very tortuous vessels of the side-branch type, or valve-bearing segments are situated about the varicose portion of the great saphenous vein. These

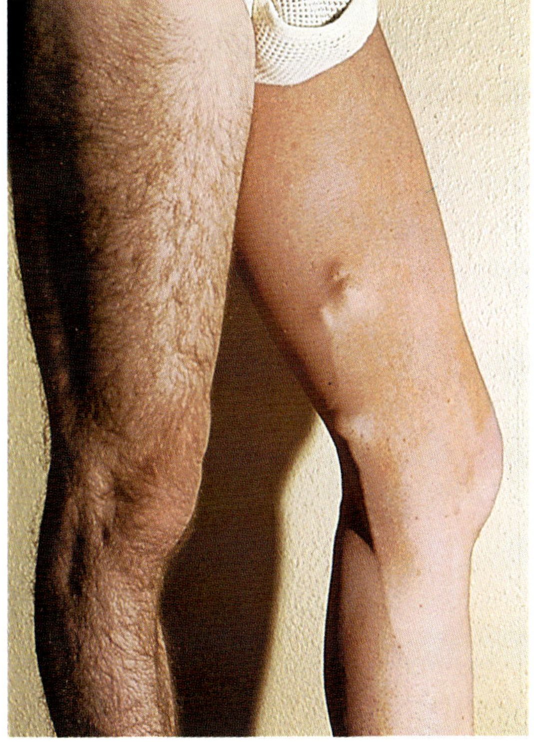

171. Dodd's perforator type of incomplete great saphenous varicosity in a 38-year-old man with a 10-year history of disease

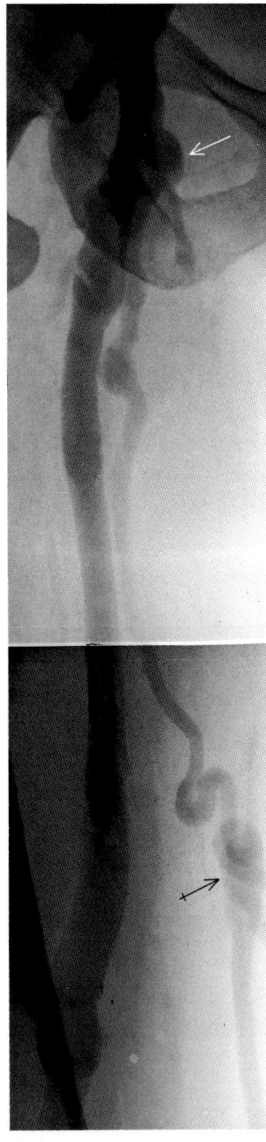

172. Side-branch type of incomplete great saphenous varicosity. The lateral accessory saphenous vein branches from an enlarged ostial sinus (→) above the competent saphenous terminal valve. ↔ Proximal point of incompetence. Demonstrated by ascending pressure phlebography

171 factors limit the retrograde blood flow. In the perforator type, palpable findings and function tests in the groin are negative. The side-branch type via the lateral accessory saphenous vein and the posterior type are extremely difficult to diagnose without phlebography.

Clinical manifestation of the disease has a later onset than in complete saphenous varicosity, occurring at 34 years of age on average. There is no clear statistical evidence of a general predilection for younger age groups, however.

Secondary clinical symptoms include broom straws at the supramalleolar level (61 %) and mild localized edema (38.9 %). The reflux circuit remains compensated for years, so chronic venous insufficiency is uncommon. Reticular and branch varicosities are frequent misdiagnoses.

Phlebographic Diagnosis

Ascending pressure phlebography is suitable for the radiographic evaluation of incomplete saphenous varicosity. The ***side-branch type*** is based on a
congenital anomaly of the saphenous sinus, which 197
is pathologically dilated and up to 4 cm in length. The *terminal valve* is located at the neck of the funnel-shaped sinus and appears to be competent. The anomalous entry of the lateral accessory
saphenous vein directly into the ostial sinus above 19
the terminal valve is a necessary factor in the pathogenesis of incomplete saphenous varicosity (*inguinal type*). On Valsalva straining, blood can freely enter the vessel from the pelvic level and reflux through the accessory anastomosis to the 20
proximal point of incompetence, where the retro- 172
grade pressure waves cause varicose degeneration of the great saphenous trunk. The terminal and sluice valves remain competent. Strictly speaking, the side-branch types of incomplete saphenous varicosity have two proximal and two distal points of incompetence.

The varicose saphenous trunk below the distal point of incompetence is opacified relatively late in the examination, so ascending pressure phlebography should always conclude with a final fluoroscopic check of the peripheral medial soft tissues of the thigh. This second look ensures that atypical, incompetent transfascial connections and an incomplete saphenous varicosity are not missed.

A femoral termination of the lateral accessory 20
saphenous vein (see p. 22) in itself cannot incite an incomplete saphenous varicosity, but it can exert a hemodynamic effect on the great saphenous vein if there is coexisting preterminal valvular incompetence (complete saphenous varicosity) and a 173
distal accessory anastomosis.

The perforator type is visualized in an earlier
phase of the examination, so usually it is more 170, 171
densely opacified than the side-branch type.

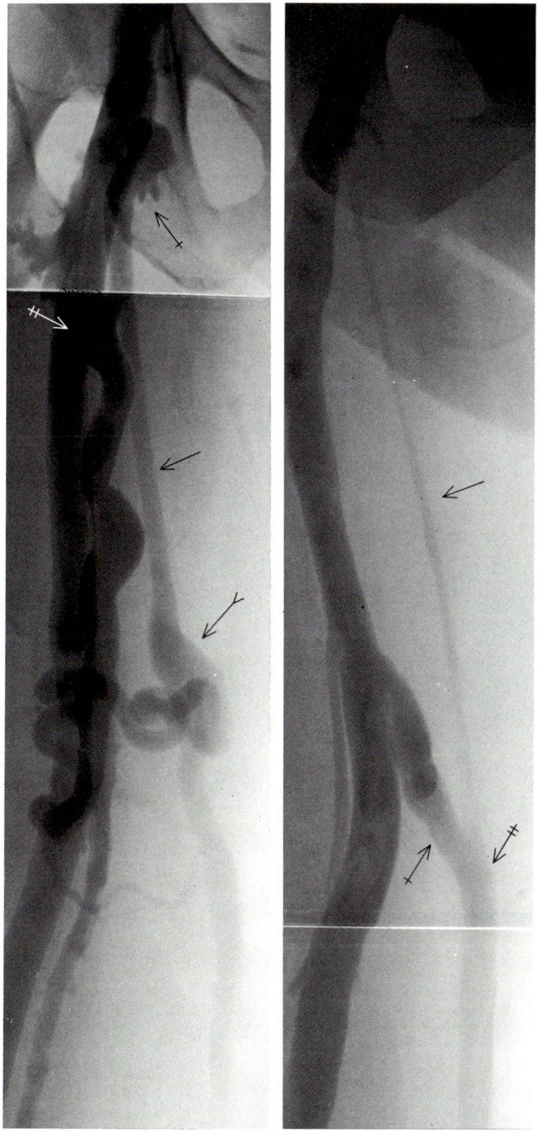

173 *(left).* Great saphenous varicosity (→). The second closed terminal valve (↔) indicates duplication of the vessel with nonvisualization of the second trunk. The varicose lateral accessory saphenous vein branches from the varicose saphenous trunk (⇸) (femoral mode of termination). The lumen of the great saphenous vein is dilated below the distal point of incompetence (↣). Demonstrated by ascending pressure phlebography

174 *(right).* Perforator type of incomplete great saphenous varicosity. → Competent portion of vessel; ↔ incompetent Dodd's perforator; ⇸ proximal point of incompetence

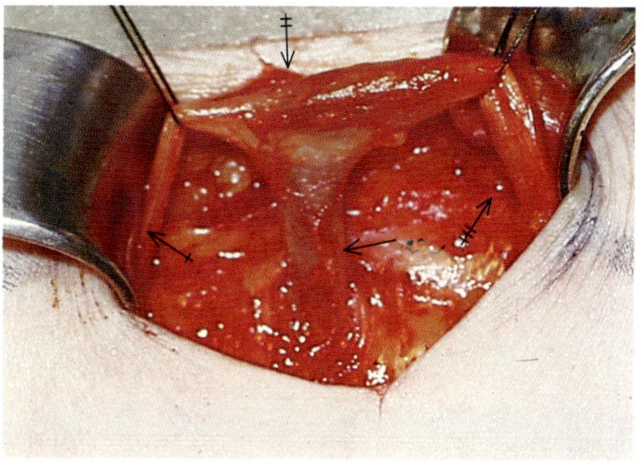

175. Perforator type of incomplete saphenous varicosity as viewed at operation. → Dodd's vein; ↔ competent segment of great saphenous vein; ⇸ proximal point of incompetence with Dow's sign; ⇻ incompetent distal portion of great saphenous vein

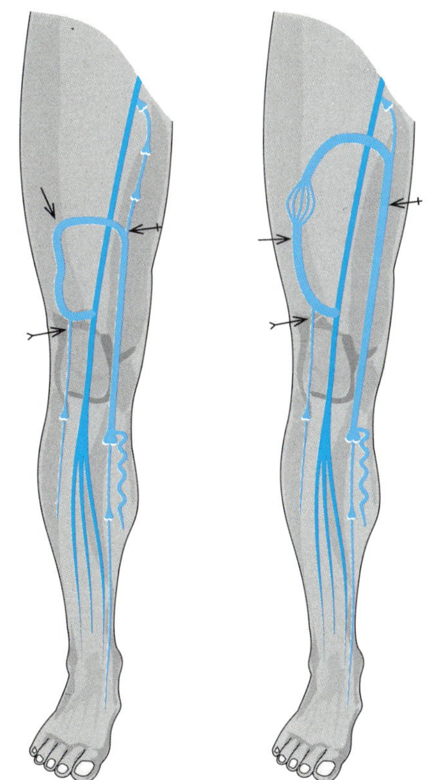

176. Posterior type of incomplete great saphenous varicosity with the femoropopliteal vein (→) functioning as a transfascial communicating vessel. There is circumscribed varicose degeneration of the great saphenous vein with proximal (↔) and distal (↣) points of incompetence. *Left,* junction of the femoropopliteal vein and the great saphenous vein. *Right,* insertion of the medial accessory saphenous vein via Giacomini's anastomosis

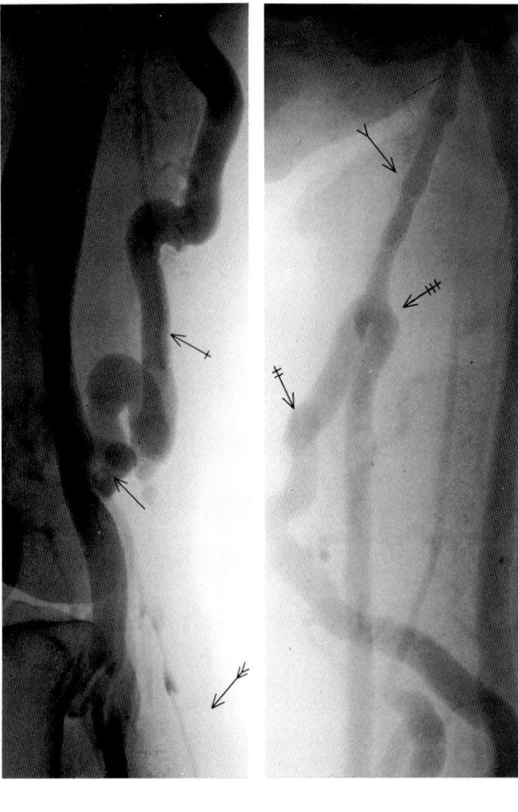

177. Posterior type of incomplete great saphenous varicosity in the left leg. Blood flows from the large incompetent sinus of the small saphenous vein (→) through the varicose femoropopliteal vein (+→) and Giacomini's anastomosis (not shown) to the medial accessory saphenous vein (++→), forming a proximal point of incompetence (+++→). Competent segment of the great saphenous vein (↣). Competent small saphenous vein (»→). Ascending pressure phlebography, internal rotation (*left*) and lateral view (*right*)

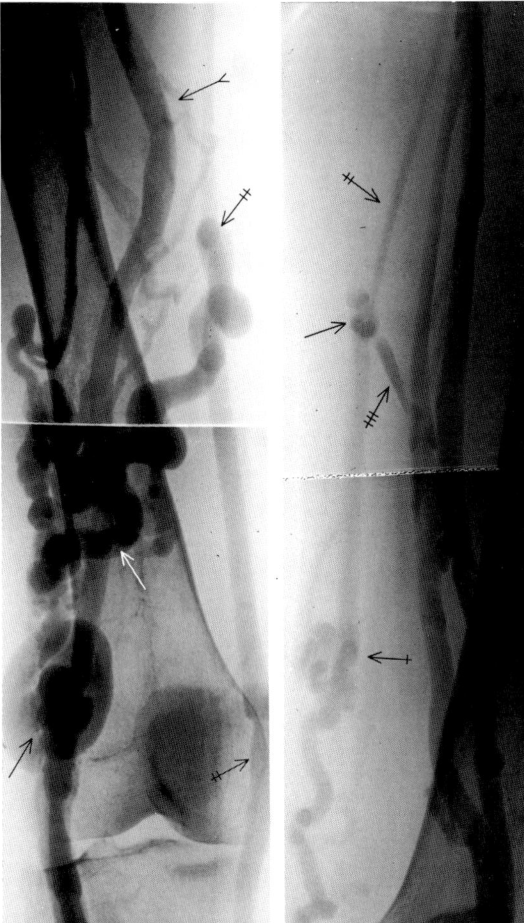

178 *(left).* Varicose popliteal perforator entering the great saphenous vein, which shows incomplete varicosity. → Perforating vein; ++→ incomplete great saphenous varicosity; ↣ superficial femoral vein

179 *(right).* Stage II incomplete great saphenous varicosity of the perforator type. The varicosity begins at the proximal point of incompetence at the junction of the upper and middle thirds of the thigh (→) and extends to the distal point of incompetence a handswidth above the knee (+→), marked by a branch varix. ++→ Competent segment of the great saphenous vein; +++→ incompetent Dodd's perforator with Dow's sign. The varicosity is weakly opacified due to the small caliber of the incompetent transfascial connection

Dodd's perforator may dilate to a greater than
174 thumb-size diameter and permit a rapid reflux of
contrast medium to the extrafascial vessels. The
proximal point of incompetence is easily recognized on the monitor by the abrupt caliber change
in the great saphenous trunk. Frequently there is a
175 localized outpouching of the vessel wall (Dow's
171 sign) opposite the site of entry of the incompetent
perforating vein.
176 Identification of the ***posterior type*** of varicosity
179 may present difficulties. Because of the relatively
21 long, small-caliber connection between the ostial
sinus of the small saphenous vein and the proximal 177
point of incompetence in the great saphenous vein, the incomplete saphenous varicosity is visualized at a relatively late stage in the examination, and the varicose segment of the great saphenous vein is more weakly opacified than usual. Often the diagnosis must wait until the final fluoroscopic

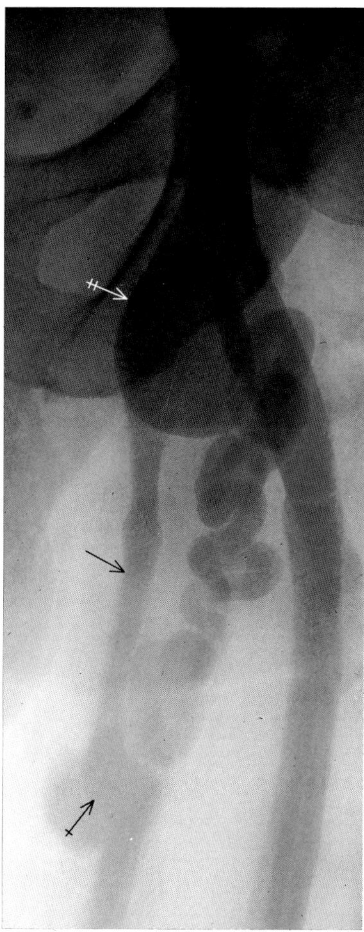

180. Great saphenous varicosity (complete form →) and varicose lateral accessory saphenous vein forming a distal point of incompetence (+→). The great saphenous vein caliber increases distally, and the saphenous sinus is greatly enlarged (++→). Demonstrated by ascending pressure phlebography

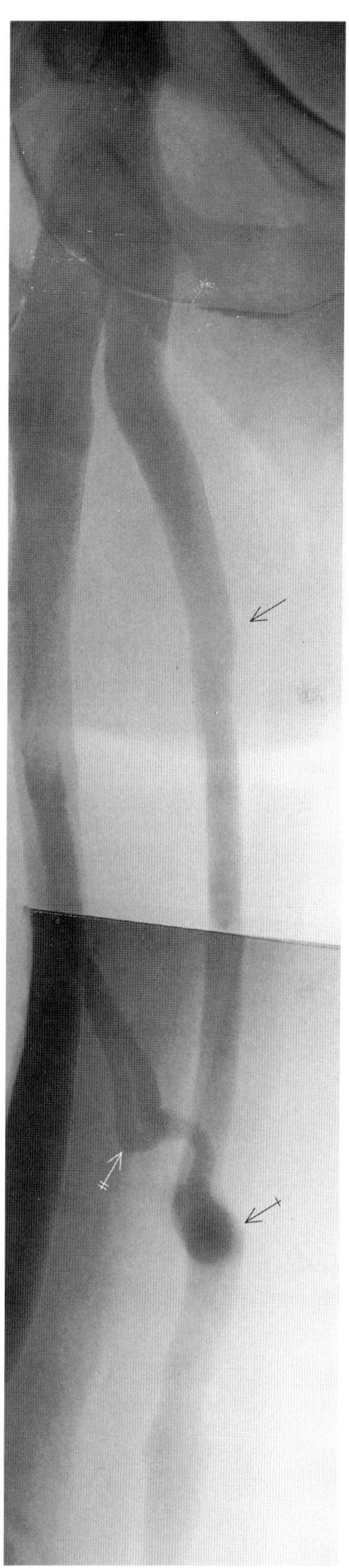

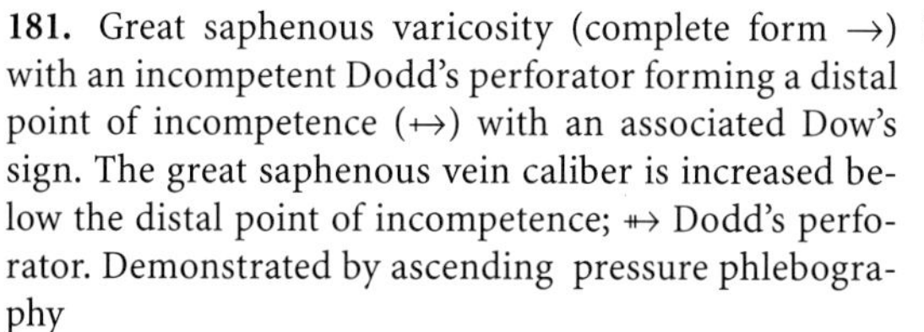

181. Great saphenous varicosity (complete form →) ▷ with an incompetent Dodd's perforator forming a distal point of incompetence (+→) with an associated Dow's sign. The great saphenous vein caliber is increased below the distal point of incompetence; ++→ Dodd's perforator. Demonstrated by ascending pressure phlebography

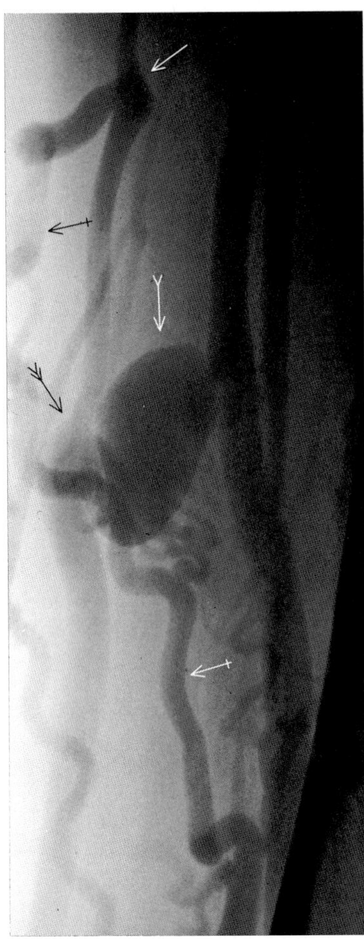

182. Incomplete great saphenous varicosity with two separate transfascial communications. One proximal point of incompetence is at the termination (→) of the varicose medial accessory saphenous vein (+→), which receives blood from the small saphenous sinus. An incompetent, massively dilated Dodd's perforator (≻→) forms a second proximal point of incompetence (≫→). Ascending pressure phlebography (left leg)

observation is made. The varicose femoropopliteal vein is either pulled directly towards the great
190 saphenous vein or it is connected further proximally via Giacomini's anastomosis with the medial accessory saphenous vein as the communicating vessel.

Peripheral types of incomplete saphenous varicosity are uncommon. They are always caused by
178 incompetent perforating veins. An incompetent popliteal perforator can still produce marked clinical symptoms, but the hemodynamic effects associated with incompetent perforators below the knee are mild.

The definitive diagnostic assessment of incomplete saphenous varicosity is like that for the com- 176
plete forms. The distal point of incompetence may be above or below the knee. Its location deter- 179
mines whether the disease is classified as stage II or stage III, so the varicose degeneration appears to be limited to a relatively short segment of the great saphenous vein. The varicose transformation may extend to the foot, but it does not cause pronounced clinical symptoms. Hemodynamic conditions are more favorable in the incomplete forms of saphenous varicosity than in the complete forms.

In some cases of incomplete great saphenous varicosity, the proximal segment of the saphenous trunk undergoes varicose degeneration. This condition is referred to as *complete saphenous vari-* 170
cosity with a branch varix or *varicose Dodd's per-* 180–182
forator. The saphenous trunk shows a characteristic abrupt caliber increase at the site of entry of the 203
incompetent transfascial vein.

Comparison of Phlebography with Other Diagnostic Methods

When the hemodynamic situation is known, certain transfascial communicating veins such as the lateral accessory saphenous vein or Dodd's perforating veins can be detected with Doppler ultrasound, while others such as the posterior or peripheral type of incomplete saphenous varicosity are far less accessible to Doppler investigation. Sometimes the blood flow velocities in the varices are so slow that equivocal signals are obtained. Even with real-time B-mode and duplex scanning, the sites of origin of the transfascial communicating vessels are very easily overlooked, especially since there are no fixed reference points due to the variability of the venous system. Thus, phlebography is the only consistently reliable study available for the diagnosis of incomplete saphenous varicosity.

Secondary popliteal and femoral vein insufficiency is rarely observed in the setting of incomplete saphenous varicosity. It occurs only in severe Dodd's perforator type cases where there is decompensation of the reflux circuit. Thus the global values of venous hemodynamics, i.e., the pump function, venous capacity and venous drainage, only occasionally show pathologic changes in patients with incomplete great saphenous varicosity.

Therapeutic Implications

183 In view of the incompetent transfascial connections, *surgery* is the treatment of choice. The procedure involves resecting the incompetent transfascial communicating vessel at its junction with the deep venous trunk and stripping out the varicose portion of the great saphenous vein between the proximal and distal points of incompetence. In cases of the perforator type, a knowledge of the special hemodynamic situation will help to avoid needless dissection in the groin. The inadvertent avulsion of a large Dodd's perforator that is overlooked at operation or undetected preoperatively will provoke heavy bleeding from the stripping tract whose source can be difficult to locate. Also, the surgeon should be careful not to leave a long perforator stump, as this would lead rapidly to recurrent varicosity. In cases of the posterior type, the procedure should not be limited to partial saphenectomy but should include removal of the small saphenous venous sinus.

Short Saphenous Varicosity

Varicosity of the small saphenous trunk is by no means rare. Though its prevalence relative to great saphenous varicosity is about 1:6, it is frequently 184
undiagnosed or misinterpreted.

The pathogenesis of small saphenous varicosity, like that of great saphenous varicosity, is based on

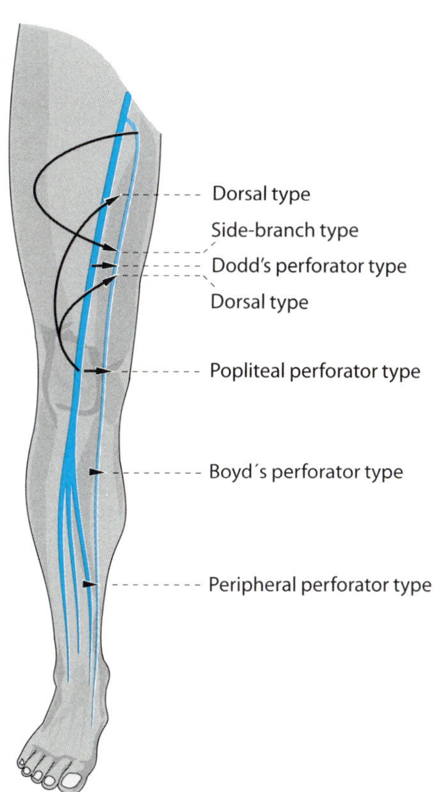

183. Incompetent transfascial communicating veins and the location of the proximal points of incompetence in incomplete great saphenous varicosity

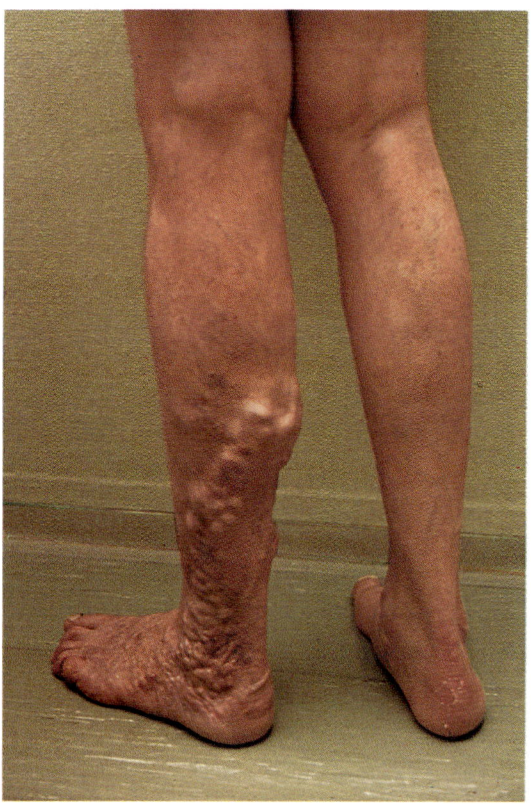

184. Stage II small saphenous varicosity with chronic venous stasis and secondary popliteal and femoral vein insufficiency. Decompensated type II reflux circuit. A large varix is seen at the distal point of incompetence at midcalf where the vessel pierces the fascia. Cutaneous changes are pronounced below the lateral malleolus. Typical presentation in a 60-year-old woman with a more than 30-year history of inadequately treated varicose veins

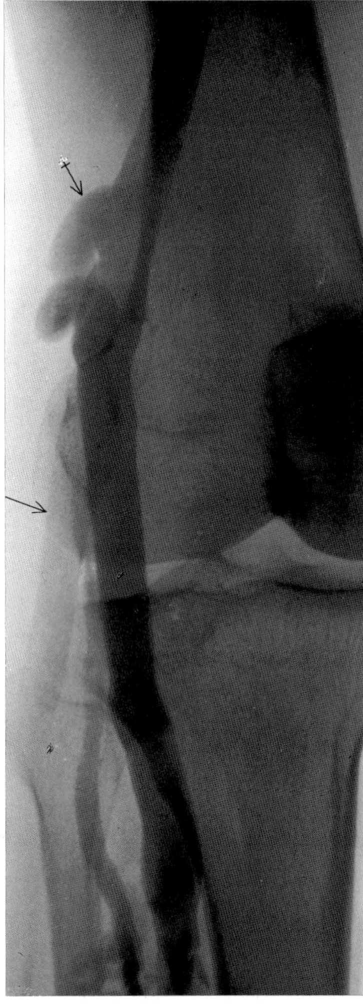

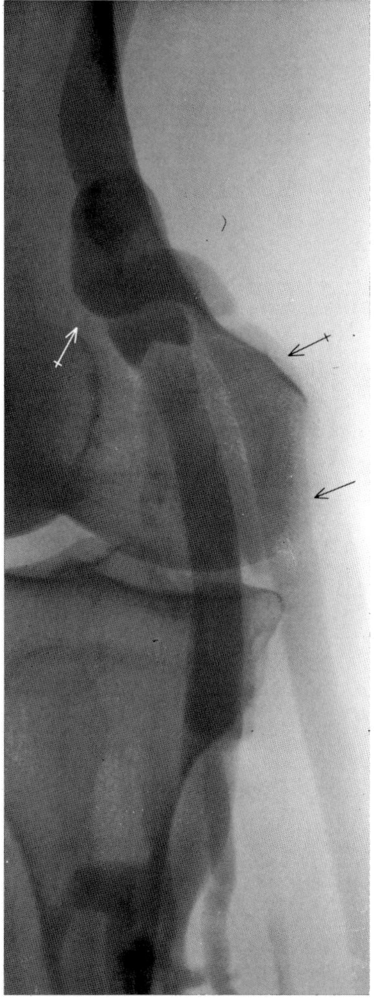

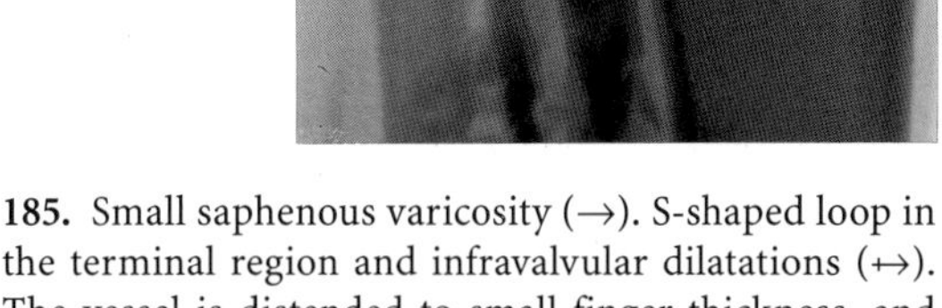

185. Small saphenous varicosity (→). S-shaped loop in the terminal region and infravalvular dilatations (↔). The vessel is distended to small-finger thickness, and there is reflux to the ankle consistent with stage III disease. Ascending pressure phlebography, internal rotation (*left*) and lateral view (*right*)

a primary incompetence of the terminal valve. This accounts for the tendency of the disease to progress in a proximal-to-distal fashion.

Clinical Symptoms

The average age at *onset* of clinical symptoms is 29 years, and thus somewhat later than in patients with great saphenous varicosity. There is a marked predilection for the younger and middle age groups.

In slender patients *examined in the standing position,* the dilated vein is palpable at the center of the popliteal fossa. The proximal, subfascial portion of the vessel takes a straight course until it pierces the fascia, and conspicuous varices may
form at that site. In stage III cases the varicose 184
trunk can be traced to the lateral malleolus and the lateral border of the foot. In many cases, however, the vein cannot be identified clinically even when varicosity is pronounced.

Faint broom straws in the malleolar region are an *early* indirect symptom of small saphenous varicosity. Sites of local edema are present in 34.5% of cases (Hach 1981). In the *late stage* there may be chronic venous congestion with siderosis, dermatoliposclerosis, stasis eczema, and ulcerations; as in great saphenous varicosity, this chronic congestion signifies decompensation of the reflux circuit with secondary popliteal and femoral vein insufficiency. The statistical frequency of these sequelae is 10.9%. In keeping with the course of the small

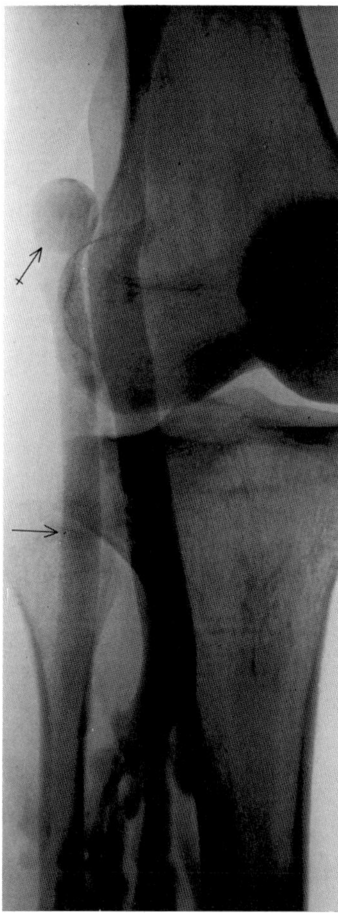
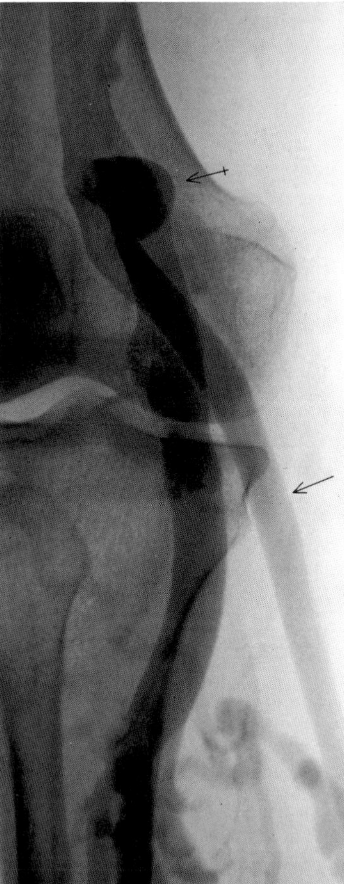
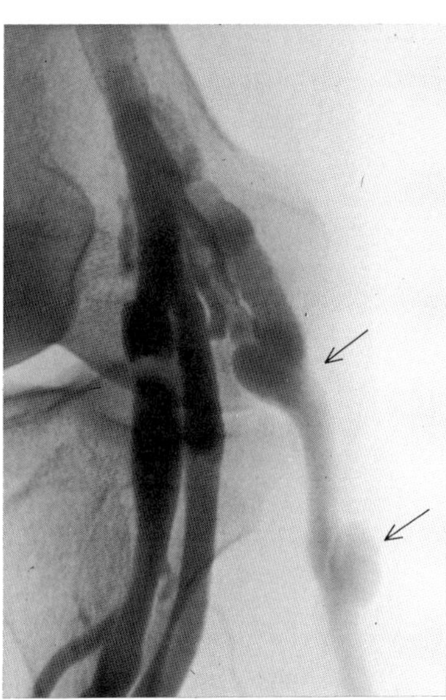

186 *(left, middle).* Stage III small saphenous varicosity (→) with an aneurysmatic dilatation in the terminal region (↔). There is secondary popliteal and femoral vein insufficiency due to decompensation of the reflux circuit. Ascending pressure phlebography, internal rotation (*left*) and lateral view (*right*)

187 *(right).* Infravalvular aneurysms (→) associated with stage III small saphenous varicosity. The popliteal vein is duplicated. Ascending pressure phlebography

saphenous vein, cutaneous changes are most pronounced on the lateral side of the foot. Involvement of the ankle and subtalar joint capsules by the inflammatory process leads ultimately to the severe complication of arthrogenic stasis syndrome.

Phlebographic Diagnosis

Ascending pressure phlebography is suitable for
the radiographic evaluation of small saphenous
varicosity. Normally the terminal valve of the small
39 saphenous vein is demonstrated as a stumplike
structure by contrast flow from the popliteal vein.
23 Sometimes the *telescope sign* is present signifying
that the subterminal portion of the vein is functionally sound. When *varicosity* is present, the terminal valve is functionally incompetent and usually is not seen. A Valsalva maneuver elicits reflux
of contrast medium down the vessel, which is dilated to pencil or finger thickness. The preterminal portion of the small saphenous vein describes
a slight laterally directed loop. The proximal por- 185
tion is subfascial and straight. In most cases the
vein pierces the fascia in the middle third of the
lower leg, where a very tortuous varix is commonly found.

Just before its union with the popliteal vein, the incompetent saphenous trunk often exhibits a circumscribed outpouching or asymmetrical infra- 186
valvular dilatation, incorrectly characterized as a 187

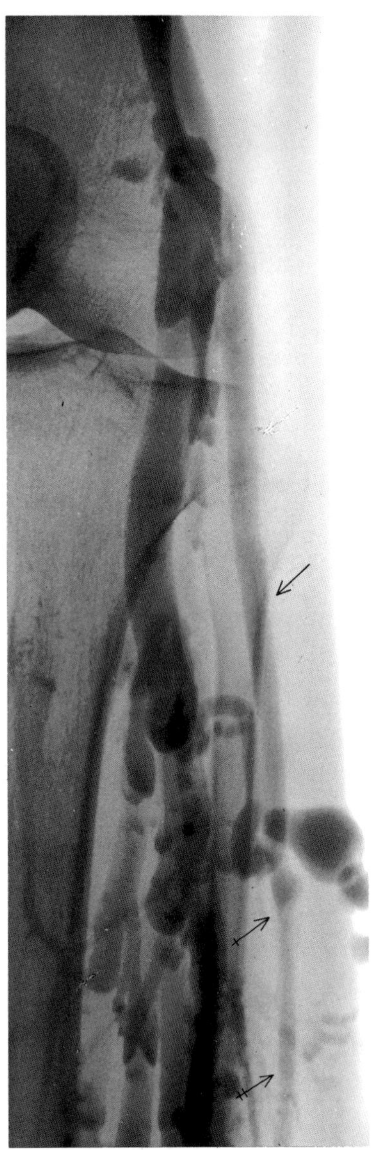

188. Stage II small saphenous varicosity in the left leg. The vein is dilated to small-finger thickness (→). +→ Distal point of incompetence with typical branch varix; ++→ competent portion of small saphenous vein

187 *"terminal aneurysm."* True ***aneurysms*** rarely occur in the small saphenous vein. This may result from the subfascial position of the vessel and its support by adjacent connective tissue structures.

Stages of Small Saphenous Varicosity

As in the great saphenous vein, varicose degeneration of the small saphenous vein commences at the incompetent terminal and sluice valves and propagates distally. The junction of the incompetent and competent venous segments is called the *distal point of incompetence,* and its location forms the basis for classifying the disease into three stages. The proximal point of incompetence corresponds to the incompetent ostial sinus.

As in the great saphenous vein, *stage I* varicosity refers to an abnormally enlarged small saphenous sinus with an atypically placed terminal valve. Accordingly, the femoropopliteal vein enters the sinus above the valve and, with varicose degeneration, forms a corresponding branch varix. This situation can give rise to the *posterior type* of incomplete great saphenous varicosity. 189

The branch varix may run distally and reconnect
with the small saphenous trunk, creating a *side-* 188
branch type of incomplete small saphenous varicosity.

In *stage II*, the distal point of incompetence is sited 190
in the calf area.

Stage III is characterized by varicose degeneration of the entire small saphenous vein. The hemodynamic conditions are generally more favorable than in the great saphenous vein, because less blood is able to reflux into the vessel. But as in the great saphenous, the recirculating flow eventually leads to secondary popliteal and femoral vein insufficiency with chronic venous congestion.

Primary Reflux Circuits

As in great saphenous varicosity, recirculating
flow patterns develop in association with the vari- 191
ous forms of small saphenous varicosity. Blood refluxing down the trunk reenters the deep venous system through competent perforators, where it once again drains upward. In the lower leg, the increased load is distributed among several stem veins that contain abundant valves, so the hemodynamic strain is well tolerated. As the disease progresses, however, the popliteal vein responds by expanding its lumen so that its valves can no longer close, and secondary popliteal vein insufficiency ensues. The changes then spread to involve the superficial femoral vein, though to a lesser degree than in great saphenous varicosity.

A ***type I recirculation pattern*** through the varicose femoropopliteal vein moves only a small volume of blood, so it remains compensated. The ***type II circuit*** also tends to remain compensated except when the varicosity is exceptionally severe. A ***type***

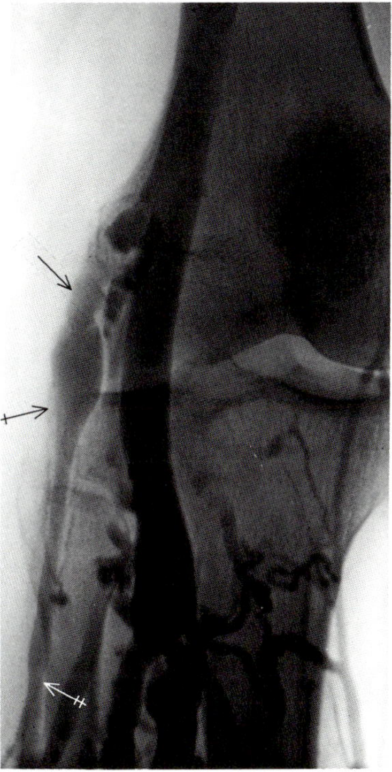

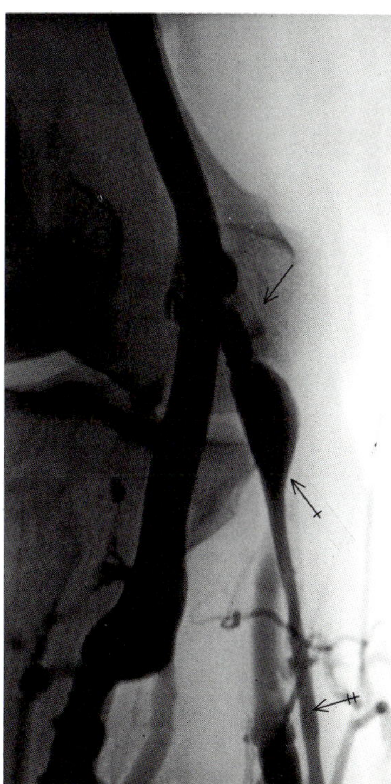

189. Early stages of small saphenous varicosity (stage II). There is no telescope sign in the region of the terminal valve (→); infravalvular dilatation at the sluice valve (+→); slight enlargement of the vascular stem (++→)

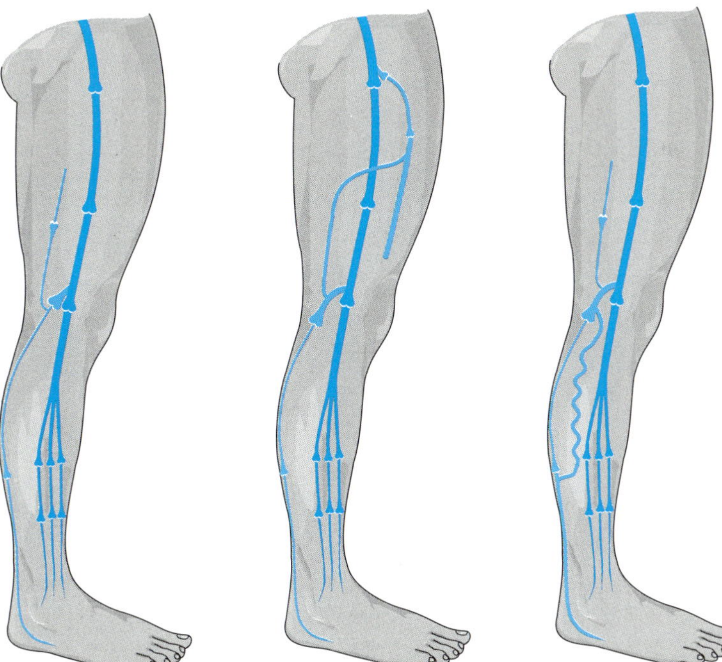

190. Terminal region of the small saphenous vein. *Left,* normal situation. *Middle,* side-branch varicosity of the femoropopliteal vein with a pathologically enlarged saphenous sinus (*stage I small saphenous varicosity*); transition to incomplete dorsal great saphenous varicosity. *Right,* unnamed side-branch varicosity with a pathologically enlarged saphenous sinus *(stage I small saphenous varicosity*); transition to incomplete small saphenous varicosity

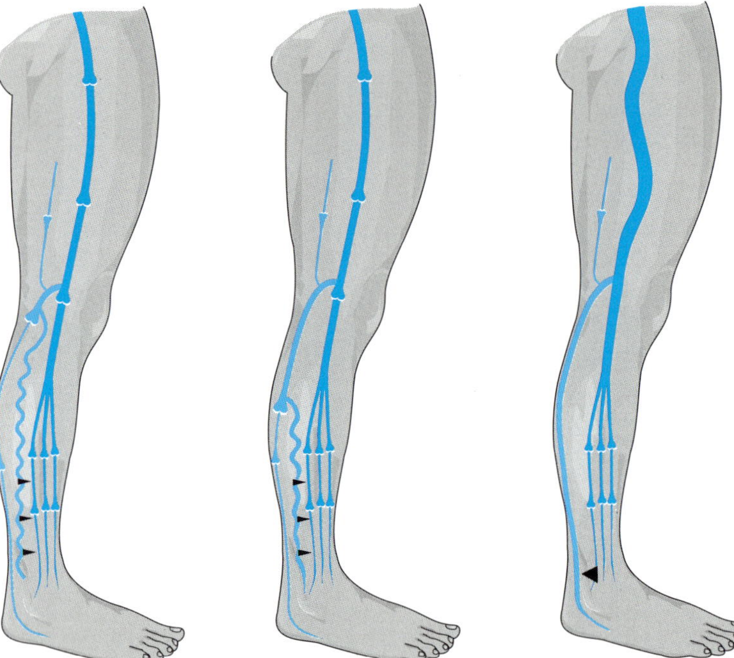

191. Schematic diagram of reflux circuits associated with small saphenous varicosity. *Left,* compensated type I reflux circuit with a long branch varix. *Middle,* compensated type II reflux circuit with a branch varix and competent perforators. *Right,* decompensated type III reflux circuit with secondary popliteal and femoral vein insufficiency. Small valve-bearing segments or side branches are interspersed from the groin to the periphery. There is an incompetent Cockett's, lateral, or other perforator in the lower leg

III reflux circuit can decompensate after a decades-
191 long course through *secondary popliteal and femo-*
184 *ral vein insufficiency*. But once any degree of valvu-
186 lar incompetence has developed in the superficial femoral vein, the disease progresses with great hemodynamic vehemence, much as in stage IV great saphenous varicosity. The venous hypertension leads to Cockett's perforator varicosity and chronic venous insufficiency.

Special Problems and Pitfalls

Retrograde contrast flow from the popliteal vein down the varicose small saphenous vein is induced by having the patient perform a Valsalva maneuver. During this time the valves in the deep venous trunks are closed, blocking contrast access both proximally and distally to the segment of the popliteal vein from which the saphenous varicosity arises. This distinguishes the examination of the small saphenous vein from that of the great saphenous, in which there are no further valves past the junction of the saphenous vein with the deep venous system, so that a large blood volume is available for reflux. These special hemodynamic conditions explain the relative weakness and time delay of opacification even in a severely dilated small saphenous vein. Sometimes the saphenous varicosity cannot be clearly visualized until late in the examination, when it is filled by the *overflow*
effect. For this reason it is recommended that a 192
steep table tilt be used. Experience has shown that a *high anomalous entry* of the small saphenous vein is easily missed, even with severe varicosity. This site is consistently visualized during the concluding fluoroscopic observation, however.

Sometimes it is difficult to distinguish early incompetence of the small saphenous vein from regressive changes in the *gastrocnemius veins*. The 364
two vessels enter the popliteal vein separately or
by a common trunk. Biplane views of the terminal 24
region and the observation of contrast flow into the peripheral venous segments will help to make
a correct interpretation. A *varicose popliteal perfo-* 220
rator is recognized by the development of large varices in the popliteal region.

The communication of a varicose small saphenous vein with peripheral branches of the great

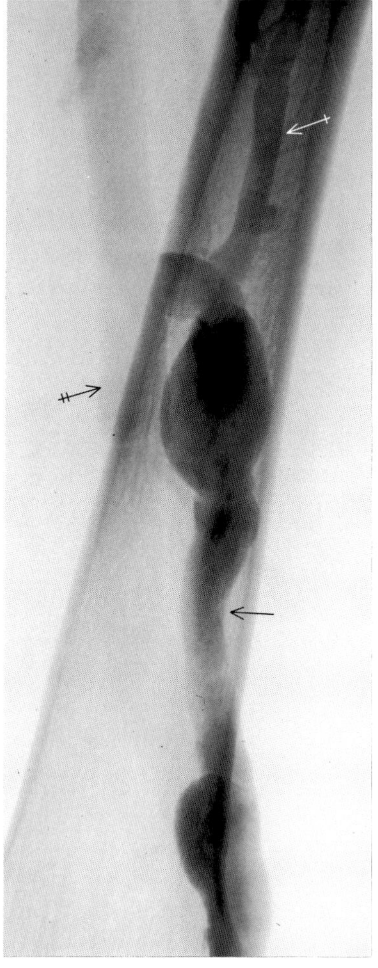

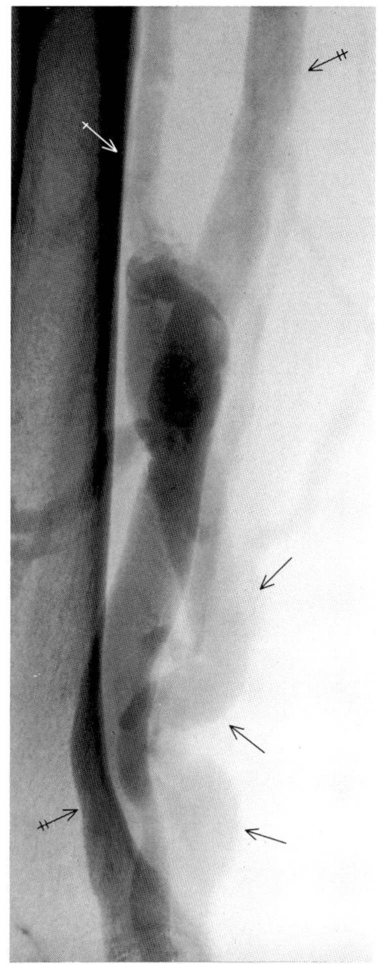

192. Small saphenous varicosity (→) in the left leg with termination of the vessel at the superficial femoral vein (high anomalous entry). Decompensated reflux circuit. +→ Incompetent femoropopliteal vein; ++→ superficial femoral vein. Secondary popliteal and femoral vein insufficiency. Demonstrated by varicography, internal rotation (*left*) and lateral view (*right*)

saphenous vein can assume major practical importance. The pressure and flow waves impinging on the medial malleolar region can precipitate the
193 development of an *anterior ulcer* above the medial
malleolus. Without phlebographic examination, this lesion can pose formidible problems of differential diagnosis.

Comparison of Phlebography with Other Diagnostic Methods

Clinical symptoms are relatively insensitive in the diagnosis of small saphenous varicosity. The most important clinical examination, *palpation of the vein in the popliteal fossa,* has a sensitivity of only 40.6% when compared with the "gold standard" of ascending pressure phlebography (Hach 1981). This accounts for the high rate of misdiagnoses (>50%) and the high incidence of recurrent varicosities following inadequate therapy.

The *Doppler examination* appears to be a suitable screening procedure. Retrograde flow signals can be recorded during the calf decompression test. Sometimes the small saphenous vein is difficult to locate, especially when it takes an anomalous course about the lateral gastrocnemius head in the
popliteal fossa. Real-time sonography and duplex 194
scanning can easily detect a severely varicose saphenous vein and demonstrate its junction with the popliteal vein. In less pronounced cases, how-

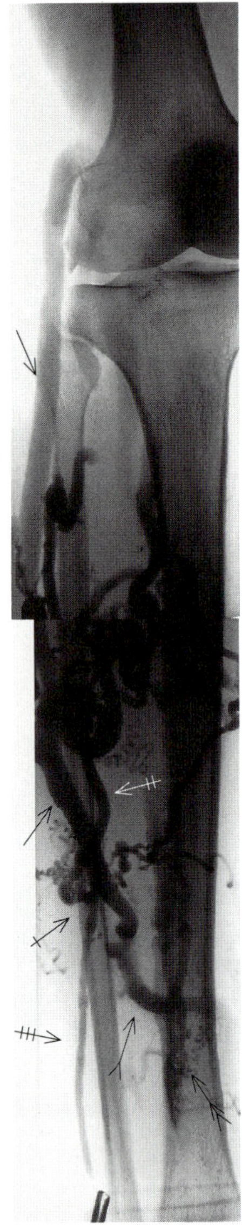

193. Stage II small saphenous varicosity with an anterior ulcer. Varicose degeneration of the proximal portion of the small saphenous vein (→). The distal point of incompetence is at the junction of the middle and lower thirds of the lower leg (+→) with branch varices (++→) and a large venous trunk on the medial side of the leg (>→). The peripheral segment of the small saphenous vein is competent (+++→). Ulcer pad (»→)

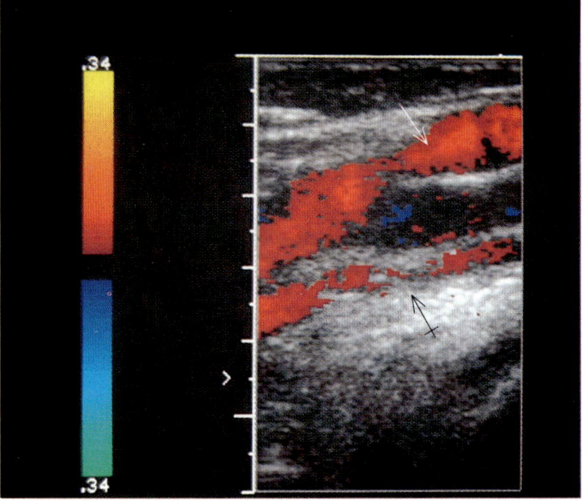

194. Small saphenous varicosity (→) at the junction with the popliteal vein. Demonstrated by color-coded duplex sonography (*red* in the upper part of the image). Examination carried out using the calf decompression test with the patient standing. Popliteal artery (+→). (Acuson, 7-MHz transducer)

ever, the diagnosis is unclear. Sensitivity has been
estimated at 90%, specificity at 67% (Wupper-
194 mann 1991). These methods cannot provide detailed information on recirculating flow patterns.

Global function studies demonstrate practically no abnormalities in patients with type I and II reflux circuits. The major change measured in a decompensated type III circuit is a reduction in the pump function of the leg. Peripheral phlebodynamometry indicates a reduced delta-P pressure fall and a shortened venous refill time. Corresponding results are provided by light reflection rheography. Venous occlusion plethysmography can demonstrate an increase of venous capacity and drainage.

Therapeutic Implications

Short saphenous varicosity in stages II and III is an indication for surgical treatment with resection of the vessel at its junction with the popliteal vein. The surgeon must tailor his incision to the topographic relationships in the popliteal fossa. If the termination of the small saphenous vein is higher than 8 cm from the joint line of the knee, additional incisions are required. A relatively low termination can easily lead to confusion and thus to operative errors.

Stages I and II are adequately managed by crossectomy or *partial saphenectomy*. A decompensated reflux circuit necessitates a *complete extrafascial ablation* with resection of the venous trunk and branch varices and selective perforator dissection. If secondary popliteal and femoral vein insufficiency and Cockett's perforator varicosity have led to chronic venous congestion in the *medial* supra-

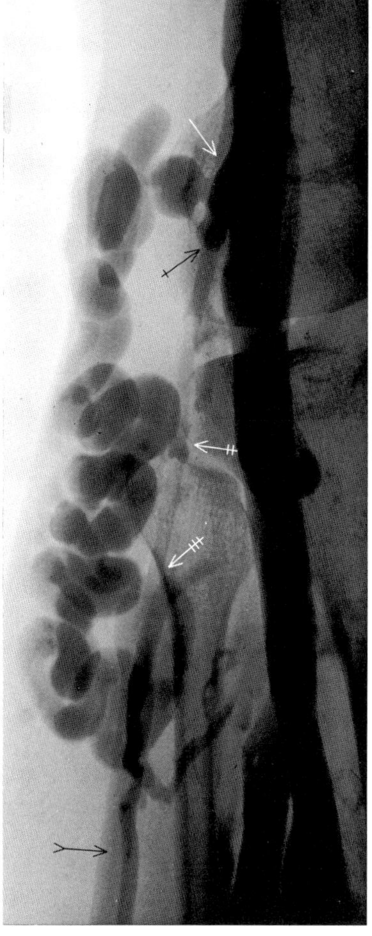
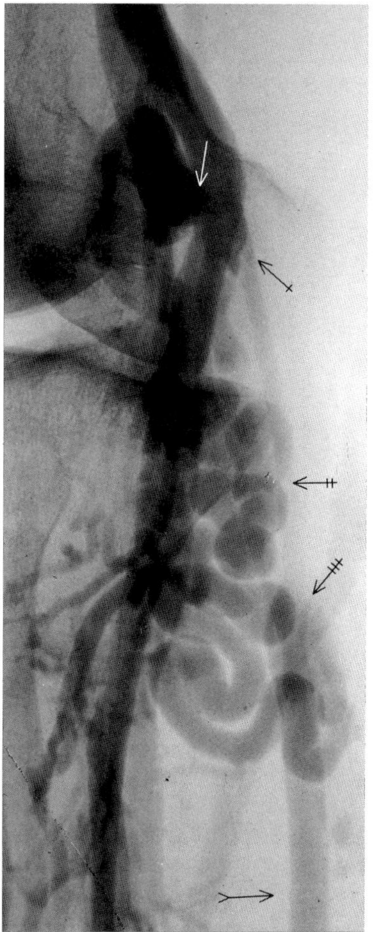

195. Side-branch type of incomplete small saphenous varicosity. Abnormally large ostial sinus (→) with the origin of an (unnamed) branch varix. The terminal valve is competent (+→), and the telescope sign is preserved. The proximal segment of the small saphenous vein is also competent (++→). Proximal point of incompetence (+++→) is at the termination of the side branch. The peripheral portion of the small saphenous vein is dilated to small-finger thickness (>→). *Left,* internal rotation; *right,* lateral view

malleolar region, paratibial fasciotomy should also be considered; if a chronic crural ulcer is observed on the outside, lateral muscle transposition may be considered in some cases (Hach and Hach-Wunderle 1994). Sclerotherapy is a viable alternative to surgery only in elderly patients.

Incomplete Small Saphenous Varicosity

190 The small saphenous vein may be involved by var-
195 ious types of incomplete varicosity. The *side-branch type* is analogous to that in the great saphenous vein, with an (unnamed) branch varix arising from an enlarged ostial sinus and reentering the small saphenous trunk to form the proximal point of incompetence. This condition is rarely observed, however.

The *perforator type* is based on an incompetent May's perforating vein, so the proximal point of incompetence is at the midcalf level. Varicose degeneration of the saphenous vein progresses distally from that site. The treatment of choice for incomplete saphenous varicosity is surgery.

The junction of the incompetent ostial sinus of the small saphenous vein with the varicose femoro-popliteal vein is directed proximally. Usually there
is a connection with the great saphenous vein 176
above the knee via Giacomini's anastomosis or 177
unnamed transfascial varices, giving rise to an incomplete *great* saphenous varicosity (see p. 112). The surgeon must take this into account when

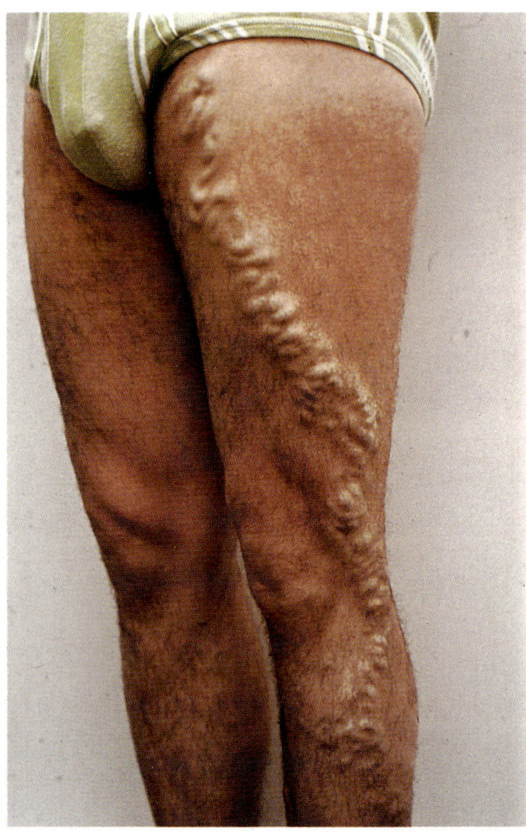

196. Varicose lateral accessory saphenous vein with inguinal termination in a 33-year-old man

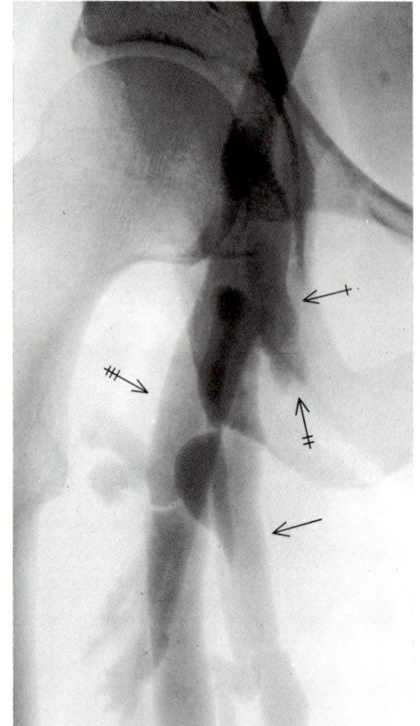

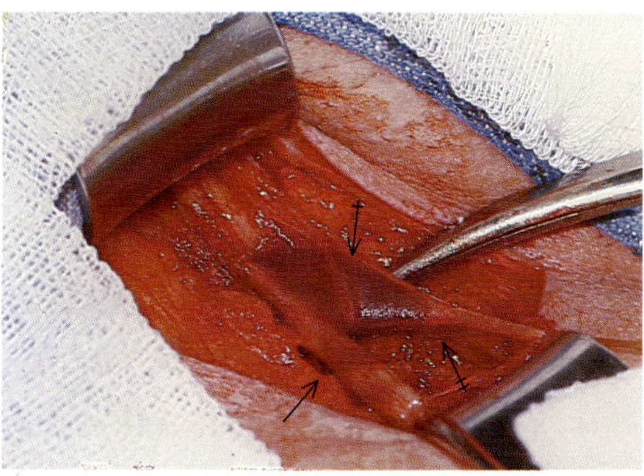

197. Varicose lateral accessory saphenous vein (→) with a large ostial sinus (↔) of the great saphenous vein. *Top,* demonstrated by ascending pressure phlebography. ⇸ Terminal valve of great saphenous vein. ⇻ Superficial femoral vein. *Bottom,* appearance at operation

planning his operative strategy. Ascending pressure phlebography is practically the only study that can define the specific roentgen morphologies of these disease entities.

Branch Varicosities

The large side branches of the great saphenous vein can undergo varicose degeneration due to an incompetent communication with the deep venous system (transfascial form) or primary damage to the vessel wall (extrafascial form). Differentiation is accomplished by ascending pressure phlebography.

Varicosity of the Lateral Accessory Saphenous Vein

Varicosity of the lateral accessory saphenous vein
196 is easily diagnosed by its typical clinical presentation. The extremely tortuous varix decends along the lateral side of the thigh and in pronounced cases can be traced distally past the knee.

The mode of termination of the lateral accessory saphenous vein can be characterized radiographically as transfascial or extrafascial. The ***inguinal type*** is of greater importance because it generally is amenable to surgical treatment. The special anatomic relationships were discussed earlier in connection with the type I reflux circuit of great saphenous varicosity (see p. 101). Due to the ab-

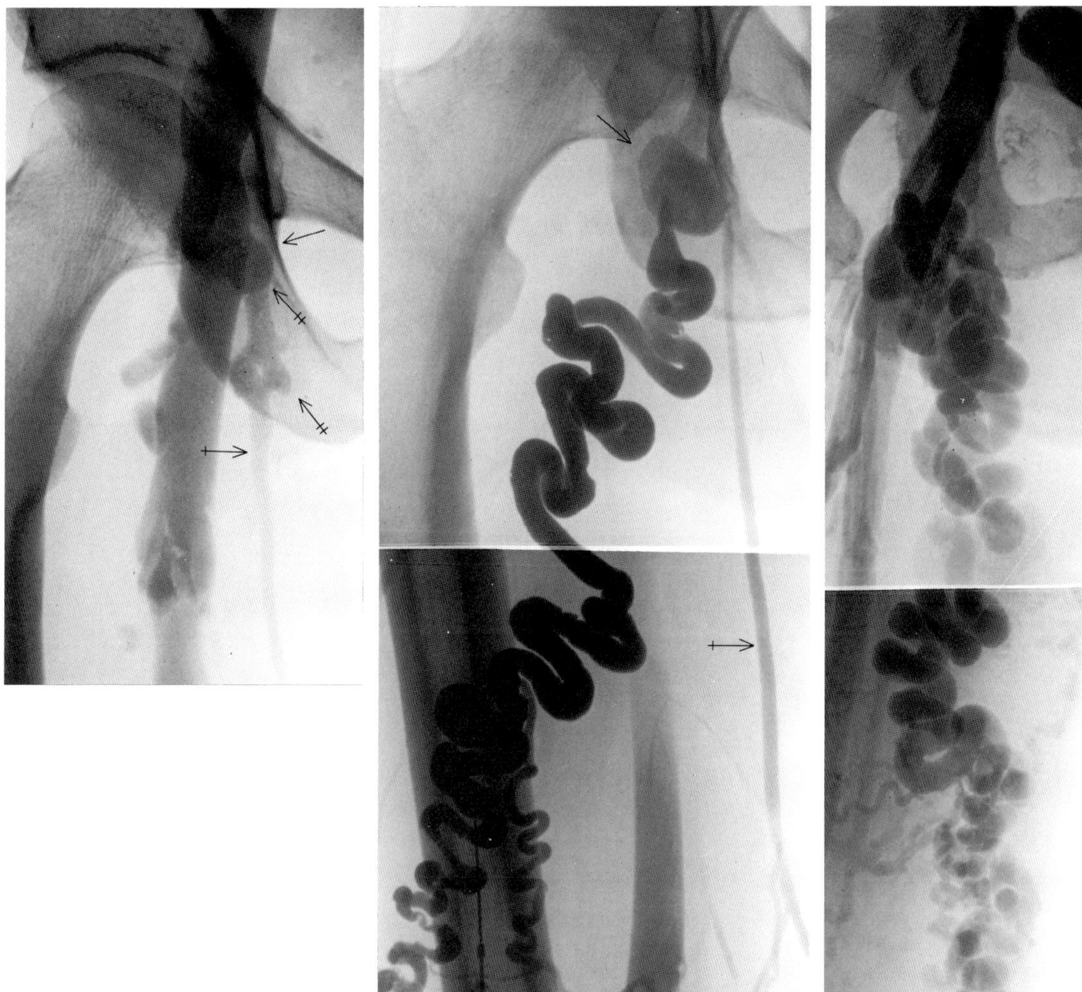

198 *(left).* Varicose lateral accessory saphenous vein with an infravalvular termination. Normal ostial sinus of great saphenous vein (→). Origin of lateral accessory saphenous vein (+→) between competent sluice valves (++→). Opacified by overflow effect in ascending pressure phlebography

199 *(middle).* Varicose lateral accessory saphenous vein with inguinal termination. The vessel shows marked sacculation in the groin (→) resembling an aneurysm. +→ Great saphenous vein. Demonstrated by varicography

200 *(right).* Varicose lateral accessory saphenous vein showing an unusual degree of tortuosity. Demonstrated by ascending pressure phlebography

normal size of the ostial sinus, the terminal valve of the great saphenous vein is separate from its actual site of entry into the common femoral vein. As a result, the lateral accessory saphenous vein does not enter the great saphenous vein in the usual fashion between the sluice valves but con-
197 nects directly with the abnormal sinus.

The varicose lateral accessory saphenous vein is a component of the type I reflux circuit in great 161
saphenous varicosity. In pronounced cases the 199
blood flows back from the groin to the lower leg, 200
where it reenters the deep venous system through competent perforators. The tortuosity of the varix greatly slows the retrograde flow rate, so the hemodynamic effects on the venous circulation are mild. Decompensation of the type I reflux circuit

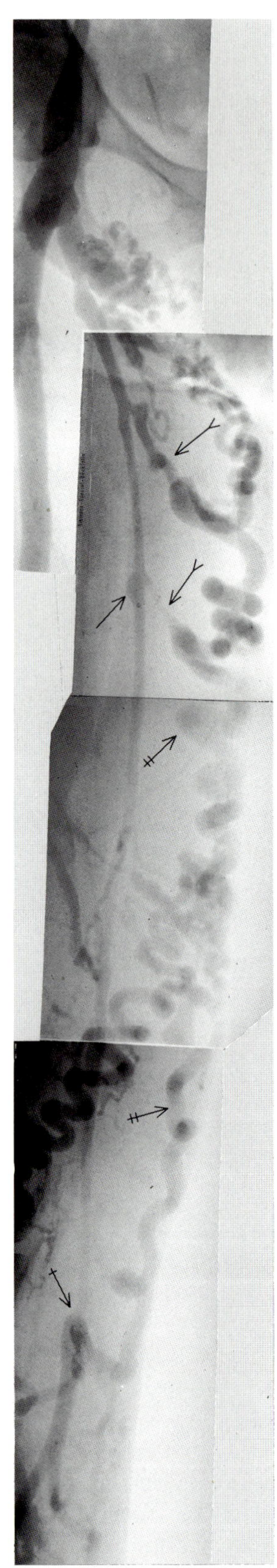

◁ **201.** Complete great saphenous varicosity with multiple sites of infravalvular dilatation (→). The caliber is enlarged in the distal thigh (↦) by the entry of a varicose lateral accessory saphenous vein (⧻→), which also has multiple connections with the great saphenous trunk (↣)

is very rarely observed, although there may be associated congestive complaints, eczematous skin changes, and pigmentation.

Rarely the lateral accessory saphenous vein enters the 198
great saphenous vein below the terminal valve, between the two sluice valves, while the ostial sinus is normal. In this case there is no incompetent transfascial communication. The two modes of termination can be differentiated as the *supravalvular* or *infravalvular* type. The infravalvular form is detected only incidentally by ascending pressure phlebography.

The varicose lateral accessory saphenous vein
with an *inguinal termination* is easily identified by 199
ascending phlebography with a Valsalva maneuver. The vessel exhibits a more or less tortuous course. In terms of the reflux circuits, the distal point of incompetence corresponds to the (atypically situated) terminal valve of the great saphenous vein. Aneurysms do not form in a branch va- 200
rix, but the tortuosities and sacculations are sometimes so pronounced that they present as a tense mass in the groin of the standing patient. A connection with the great saphenous trunk can develop distally from the saphenous sinus via the varicose lateral accessory saphenous vein and the accessory anastomosis and produce a side-branch
type of *incomplete saphenous varicosity*; the proxi- 201
mal point of incompetence is located at the junc- 170
tion with the great saphenous trunk. 172

The treatment of choice is surgical and consists of *crossectomy*. The large varices can then be removed by *subcutaneous exeresis* or obliterated with sclerosing injections. Sclerotherapy alone does not afford a permanent cure, however. With an isolated side-branch varicosity, the great saphenous vein is left alone.

Modes of termination seen in varicose lateral accessory saphenous veins
Inguinal mode
Supravalvular type
Infravalvular type
Femoral mode

A varicose lateral accessory saphenous vein with a ***femoral mode*** of termination has no direct con-
18, 20 nection with the deep venous system. The vari-
202 cose vein enters the great saphenous vein within the thigh. It is not visualized by ascending pressure phlebography, and roentgen diagnosis must rely on varicography or noncompression phlebography. Since there are no incompetent transfascial connections, patients should be managed nonoperatively.

Varicosity of the Medial Accessory Saphenous Vein

17 Normally the medial accessory saphenous vein
67 enters the great saphenous trunk between the sluice valves or at a more distal level. Thus, when varicose degeneration is present, ascending pressure phlebography can provide retrograde contrast filling of the vessel only if there is coexisting varicosity of the great saphenous trunk. This form
203 of disease is very rare.

It is more common to have a direct union of the varicose femoropopliteal vein with the medial ac-
21 cessory saphenous vein via *Giacomini's anastomosis*. This establishes a communication from the sinus of the small saphenous vein to the great
176 saphenous trunk which can incite a posterior type
177 of incomplete great saphenous varicosity (see p. 112). The treatment of choice is always surgery.

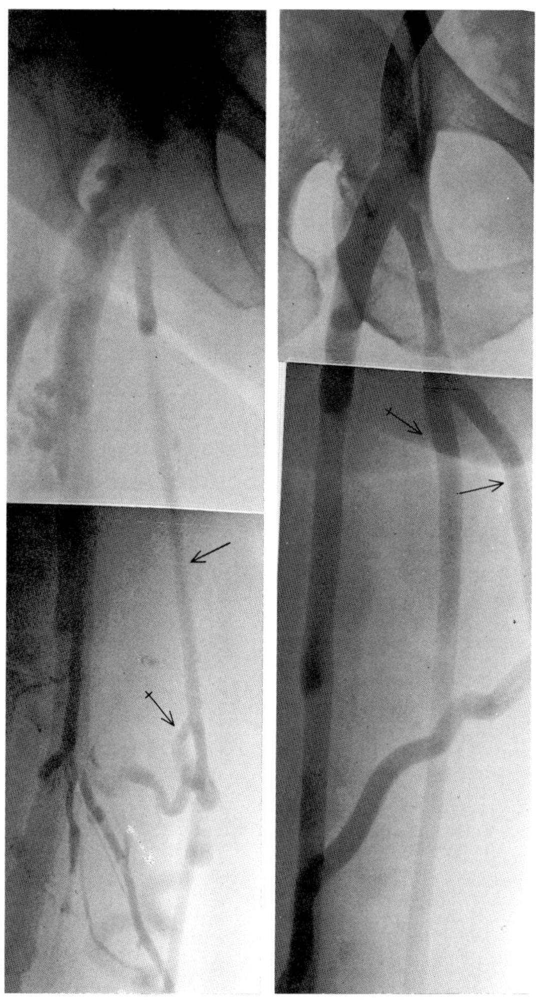

202 *(left).* Varicose lateral accessory saphenous vein with femoral mode of termination. → Competent great saphenous vein; ↦ termination of the side branch. Demonstrated by superficial phlebography

203 *(right).* Varicose medial accessory saphenous vein (→) in stage III great saphenous varicosity (↦)

Varicosity of the Posterior Arch Vein

Varicose degeneration of the posterior arch vein is
48 of major practical importance. It results from an incompetent Cockett's perforator, which allows blood to reflux under high pressure from the posterior tibial vein into the posterior arch vein. With passage of time the vessel is transformed into an extremely tortuous varix. It can no longer adequately drain the plexuses of the superficial tissues, especially when there is coexisting saphenous varicosity. As a result of the venous stasis, symptoms of *chronic venous insufficiency* develop
204 over the site of emergence of the perforating vein and in the vicinity of the posterior arch vein.

The disease can frequently be diagnosed clinically. It occurs predominantly in the setting of a decompensated reflux circuit in saphenous varicosity. Ascending pressure phlebography demonstrates the varicose posterior arch vein as a tortuous, pencil- to small-finger-thick vessel on the medial side of the calf. It is filled at the start of the examination by
antegrade flow from the incompetent *Cockett's per-* 205
forator. In severe cases the contrast flow into the extrafascial venous system through the incompetent perforator is so copious that the deep veins cannot be evaluated. The films show an undecipherable jumble of vessels that may prompt an erroneous diagnosis of post-thrombotic syndrome. For optimum visualization, the tourniquet should always be tightly placed distal to a blow-out or a varicose

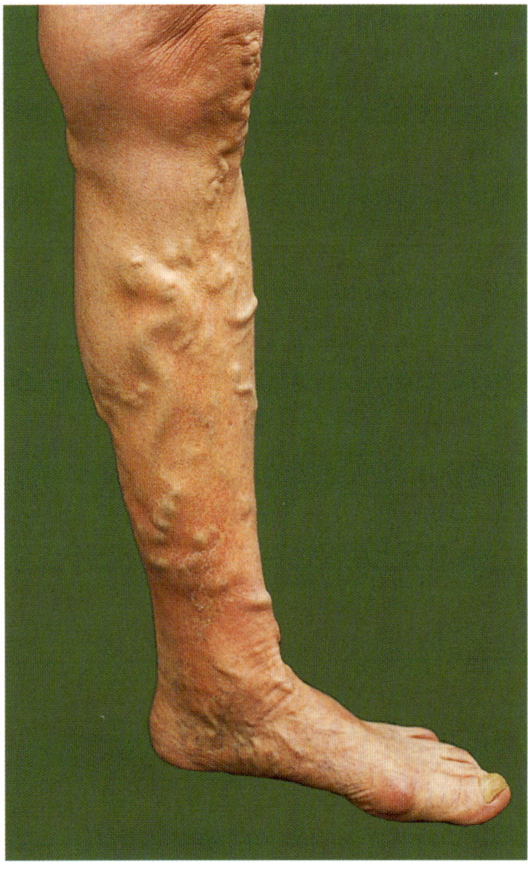

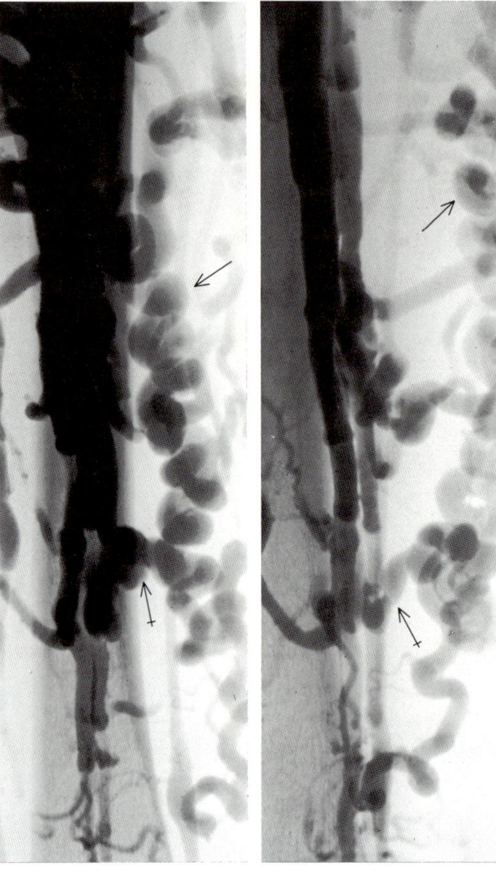

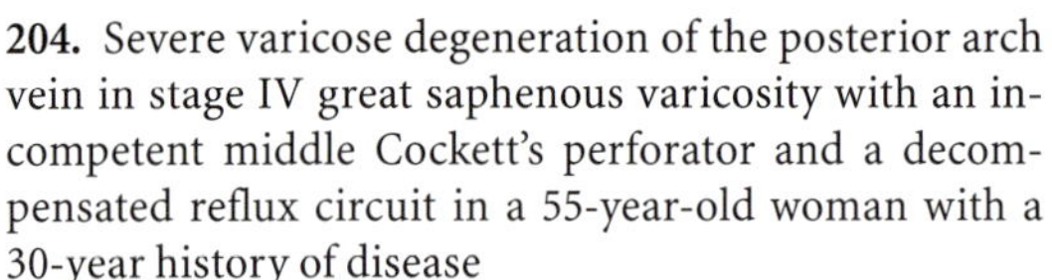

204. Severe varicose degeneration of the posterior arch vein in stage IV great saphenous varicosity with an incompetent middle Cockett's perforator and a decompensated reflux circuit in a 55-year-old woman with a 30-year history of disease

205. Varicose degeneration of the posterior arch vein (→) due to an incompetent middle Cockett's perforator (↔). Ascending pressure phlebography, internal rotation (*left*) and lateral view (*right*)

205 ulcer. Applying a pressure bandage before the contrast medium is injected is recommended in order to achieve better visualization of the deep veins.

The *treatment* of choice is complete obliteration of the extrafascial venous system to eliminate the decompensated reflux circuit. The incompetent perforator is ligated subfascially, then the posterior arch vein is surgically exstirpated or sclerosed. Today we recommend the endoscopic method adding pretibial fasciotomy when trophic skin disturbances are present.

Varicosity of the Anterior Arch Vein

17 Isolated varicosity of the anterior arch vein is diagnosed clinically. The highly tortuous varix runs
206 up the anterolateral side of the lower leg from the malleolar region to a handswidth below the knee, where it crosses over the tibia and enters the great saphenous vein.

Treatment is nonoperative, so there is rarely an indication for phlebography. Varicography appears 207
to be the best roentgen study.

Varicose Perforators

Incompetence of a perforating vein occasionally occurs as a separate entity but more commonly coexists with other forms of primary and secondary varicosity in the setting of decompensated reflux circuits and angiodysplasias. This particularly applies to Cockett's perforators.

It has been estimated from anatomic studies that there are between 90 and 150 communicating

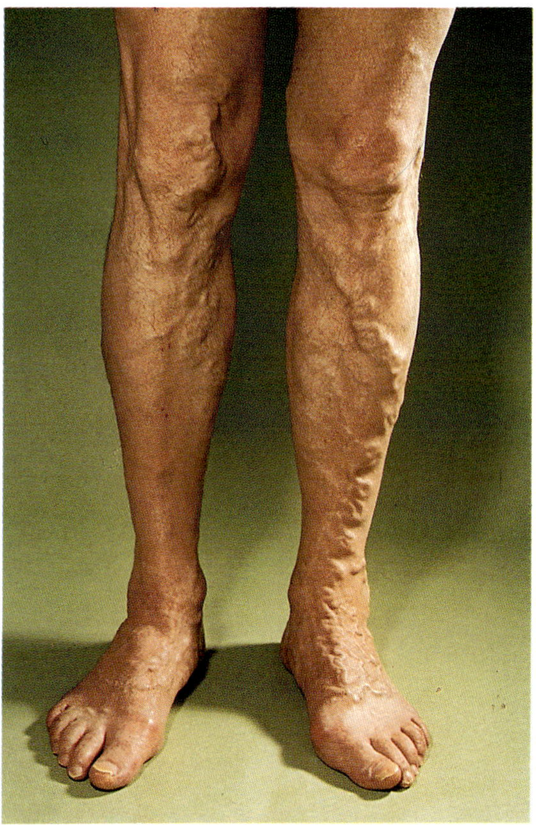

206. Varicose anterior arch vein in the left leg

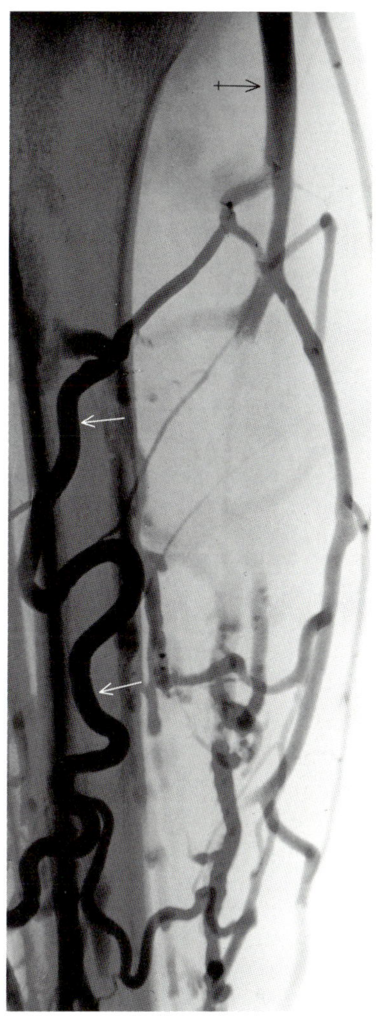

207. Varicose degeneration of the anterior arch vein ▷ (→). Great saphenous vein (↔). Demonstrated by varicography

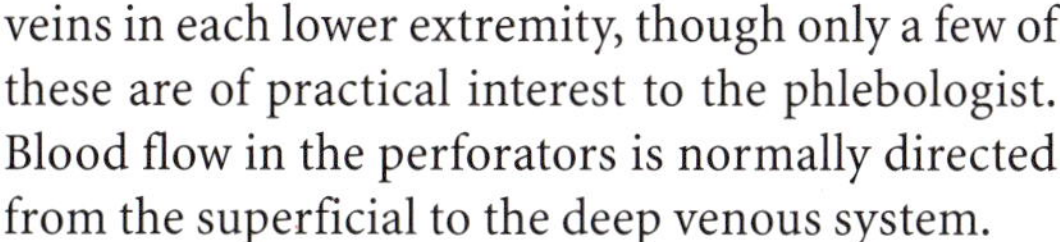

veins in each lower extremity, though only a few of these are of practical interest to the phlebologist. Blood flow in the perforators is normally directed from the superficial to the deep venous system.

Special forms of varicosity resulting from perforator incompetence	
Incompetent perforator	Possible result
Cockett's veins	Incompetent posterior arch vein, tortuous varix
Boyd's vein	Incomplete great saphenous varicosity, tortuous varix
Dodd's vein	Incomplete great saphenous varicosity
May's vein	Incomplete small saphenous varicosity
Hach's profunda perforator	Lateral thigh varicosity

Varicosity of Cockett's Veins

48 The three groups of Cockett's veins are located behind the medial malleolus, a hands width above the malleolus, and level with the junction of the middle and lower thirds of the lower leg (see p. 29). The vessels in the middle and upper groups most frequently become incompetent. Each of these two venous groups consists of three vessels.
209 The medial and anterior veins are of greater importance because they perforate the fascia with a short, perpendicular segment that has considerable hemodynamic potential. The posterior vessel

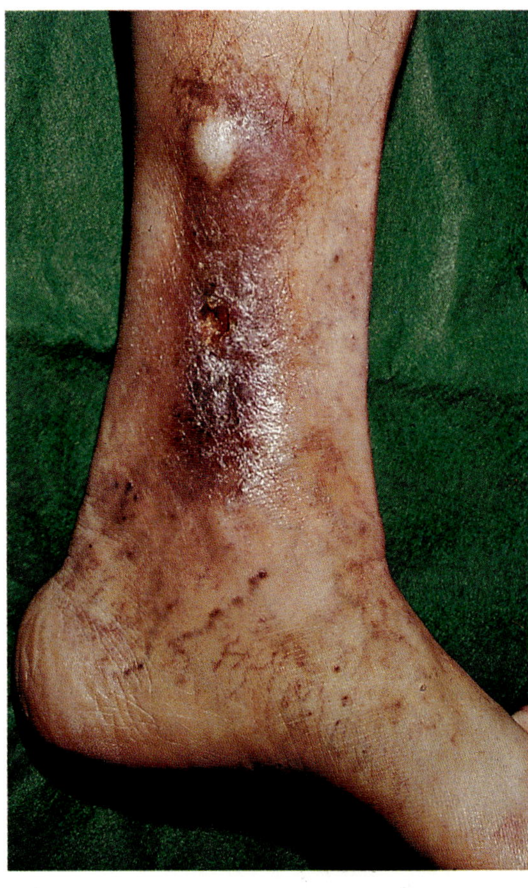

208. Varicosity of upper Cockett's perforator with chronic venous insufficiency. Great saphenous varicosity with type III decompensated reflux circuit

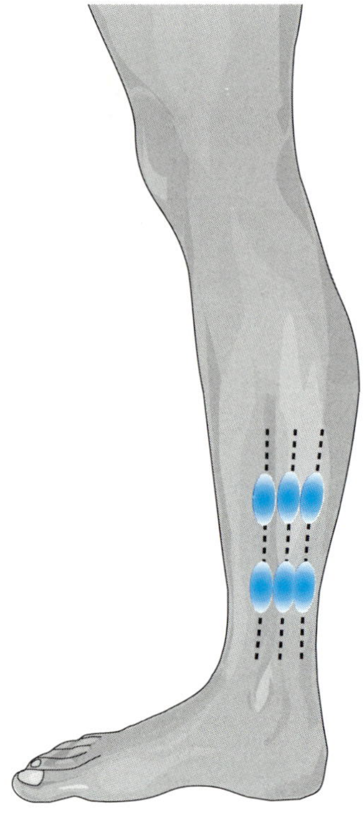

209. Imaginary projection lines of the middle and upper Cocketts venous groups. Anterior projection line at the dorsal edge of the tibia. Middle projection line between the dorsal edge of the tibia and the Achilles tendon. Posterior projection line between the middle projection line and the Achilles tendon

of the middle and upper Cockett's perforator groups takes a tortuous course through the musculature, is relatively long, and is constricted by surrounding tissues, so it tends to suppress the jet effect during activation of the calf muscle pump.

When the leg is inspected in the standing patient, the
208 *blow-out* appears as a bulge over the incompetent perforator. This site is often marked by abnormal pigmentation, scarring, eczema, or even ulceration. *Palpation* for incompetent perforators is done in the supine position with the leg externally rotated. A pit can be felt over the affected site. This depression represents a *"canyon effect"* in the subcutaneous tissue rather than the fascial defect itself. These changes can be especially pronounced in the presence of dermatoliposclerosis, or they may be effaced by induration or a venous ulcer.

Projection lines provide convenient references for locating the anterior, medial, and posterior vessels of the middle and upper Cockett's groups. The *anterior projection line* runs along the posterior tibial border; there the anterior perforator of the middle and upper groups runs directly upon the tibial periosteum as it exits the
intrafascial space. The medial vessels of these groups lie 209
on the *middle projection line*, which corresponds to Linton's line midway between the posterior tibial border and the Achilles tendon. The *posterior projection line* with the posterior vessels runs between the middle projection line and the Achilles tendon. This distinction cannot be made on a phlebogram.

Perforator varicosity begins with a failure of clo- 210
sure of the valves within the vein. Usually the 211
deeper valve fails first, perhaps relating to a congenital disposition. The valvular incompetence is precipitated by a rise of dynamic venous pressure during muscular effort and by the increased flow volumes that occur in the setting of various venous disorders. The perforator becomes dilated, and flow through it is reversed. The physiologic spindle shape of the perforator, caused by the greater distensibility of the vascular segment
between the two valves, becomes *cylindrical*. The 212

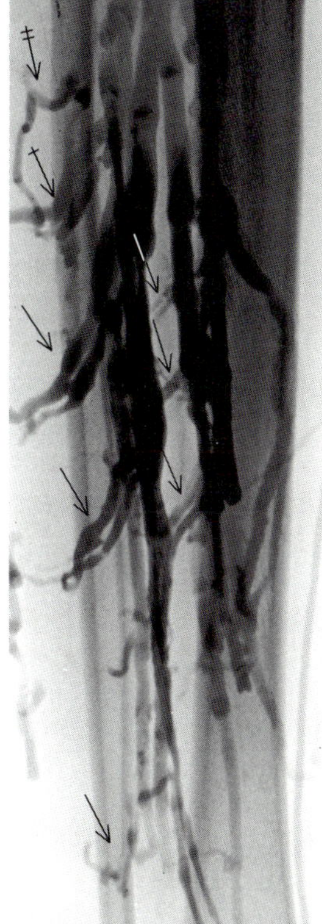

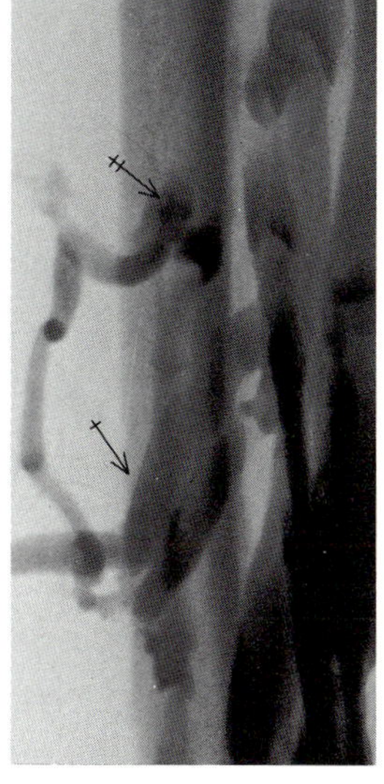

210. Competent (!) perforators in the lower leg (→) demonstrated by ascending pressure phlebography. *Left,* general view. *Right,* close-up view of two lateral perforator groups. The *lower* vessels (↛) pass upward to the deep veins at an acute angle, each displaying two closed valves, a spindle shape, and smooth wall contours. The more distal of the paired vessels in the *upper* group shows stumplike opacification as far as its inner valve (⇸)

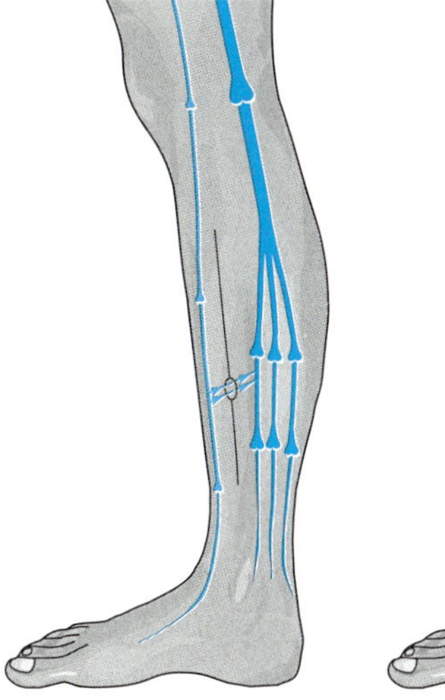

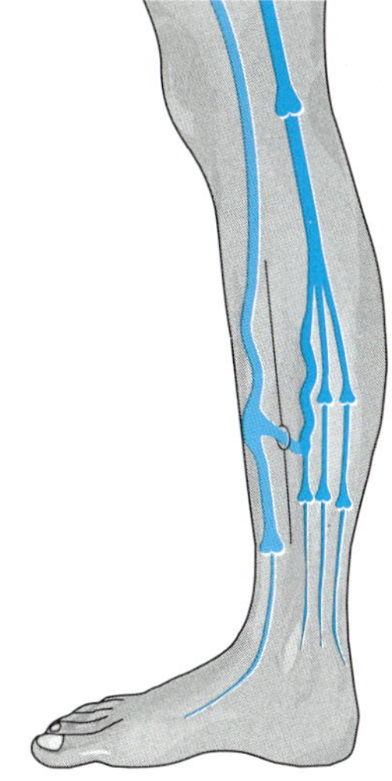

211. Changes associated with perforator varicosity in the lower leg. *Left,* normal perforators with competent valves are paired and enter the deep vein at an acute, ascending angle. *Right,* the incompetent perforator is unpaired and passes downward to the deep vein, which shows signs of secondary insufficiency

Criteria for diagnosing below-knee perforator incompetence by ascending pressure phlebography
Unpaired vessel
Junction angle with deep vein >60°
Straightened course
Cylindrical shape
Loss of competent valves
Reversal of flow direction

vein develops slightly *irregular wall contours* as evidence of structural damage to the vessel wall secondary to varicose degeneration and perhaps inflammatory changes. The *venous valves* are no longer visible on radiographs.

Every communicating vessel adapts its course to the prevailing direction of flow. Normally the blood drains proximally and centrally, the perforator joining the deep vein at a slightly ascending, acute angle. The average junction angle is 29° and is always less than 60°.

Like all venous return from the leg, blood refluxing from an incompetent perforator into the extrafascial venous system must be routed toward the groin. Over time the vessel adapts to the flow reversal, doing so initially in the region of the intrafascial communication. The *junction angle* with the deep vein increases and in severe cases may reach or surpass 90°. The average value is 81° but is consistently greater than 60° (Hach 1981 b).

Normally the perforating veins in the lower leg are paired. An *unpaired* perforator is an important radiographic criterion for incompetence. As the disease progresses, the delicate, functionally sound 213
adjacent vein becomes strangulated within the fascial opening by its incompetent, dilated twin.

Even a functionally competent twin vein may not appear on phlebograms due to physical causes (Bernink 1971). As the pressure rises in intercommunicating cylindrical vessels that have equal wall thicknesses and elastic moduli but different diameters, only the vessel with the larger radius will be

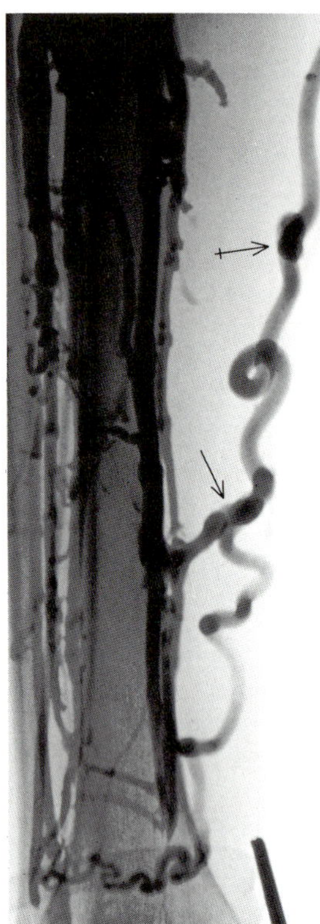

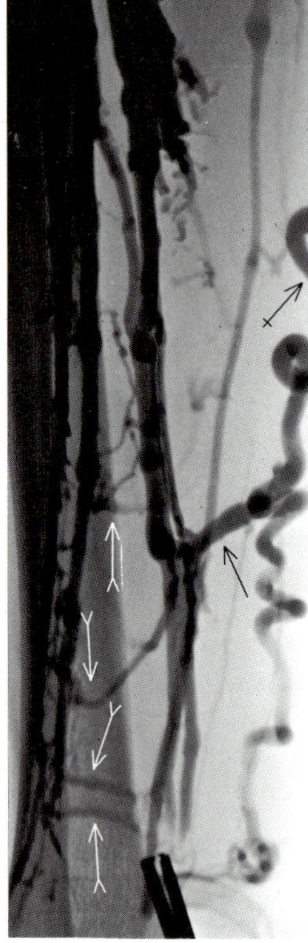

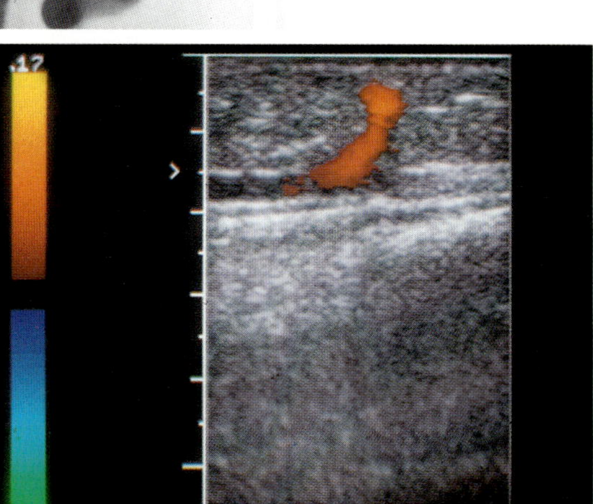

212. Incompetent upper Cockett's perforator (→) with varicose degeneration of the posterior arch vein (↦) demonstrated by ascending pressure phlebography. ↣ Bridging veins. *Left,* view in internal rotation. *Top right,* close-up view shows the unpaired perforator passing downward to its deep vein, entering at an obtuse angle. The incompetent perforator is cylindrical with slightly irregular contours, is valveless, and carries retrograde flow. *Bottom right,* color-coded duplex sonography. (Acuson, 7-MHz transducer)

distended. Moreover, the pressure and flow velocity in an incompetent communicating vein, regardless of flow direction, are significantly higher than in a healthy vessel; this further increases the chance of contrast filling.

The unfavorable projection of two incompetent
214 perforators arising from *different* deep veins can be a source of misdiagnosis. As in determinations of the junction angle, close scrutiny should be giv-
215 en to the central portion of the perforators to establish whether or not the veins connect to the same trunk.

The *caliber* of the perforator in itself is not a useful diagnostic criterion (Hach 1981b). It has pathologic significance only when combined with other radiographic signs of incompetence, especially cylindrical shape distortion. The maximum diameter ranges from 0.5 to 9 mm under physiologic conditions (Hach 1981b).

Retrograde blood flow in Cockett's perforator incites varicose degeneration of the posterior arch vein. A circumscribed sacculation called *Dow's* 215
sign is frequently visible at the extrafascial communication. It corresponds to the blow-out that is noted clinically, which is also characterized by hyper- or depigmentation, eczema, and spider webs.

Below a *chronic venous ulcer,* the incompetent perforator sometimes opens into a dense network of small and minute varices. The term *ulcer pad* is applied to the characteristic phlebographic appearance of this lesion. Often the perforating vein 216
can no longer be clearly identified within the varicose cluster, and varicography may be needed for further clarification.

215. Severe varicosity of a middle Cockett's perforator (→) with secondary tibial vein insufficiency (↦). Stage IV varicosity of the great saphenous trunk (⇸) with a decompensated reflux circuit. *Left,* internal rotation view. *Right,* lateral view ▷

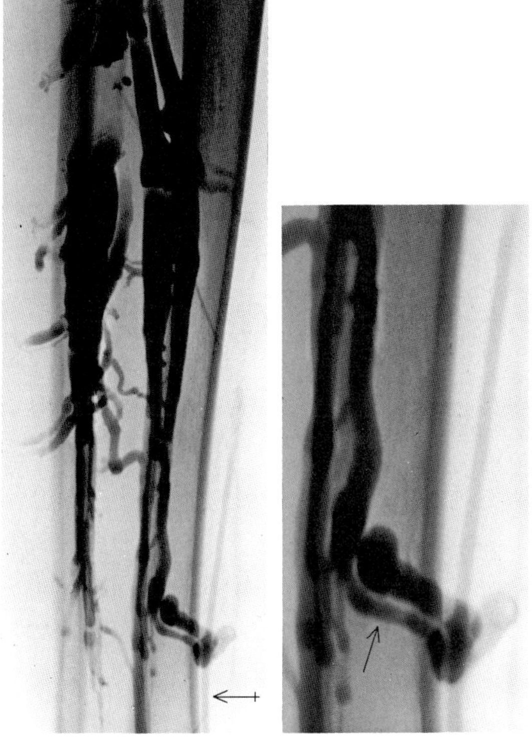

213. Progressive incompetence of the middle Cockett group (→) demonstrated by ascending pressure phlebography. *Left,* general view in internal rotation. +→ Great saphenous vein. *Right,* close-up view of Cockett's group. The upper perforator shows cylindrical dilatation and irregular contours. The lower vein is still competent but is markedly displaced and constricted within its fascial opening

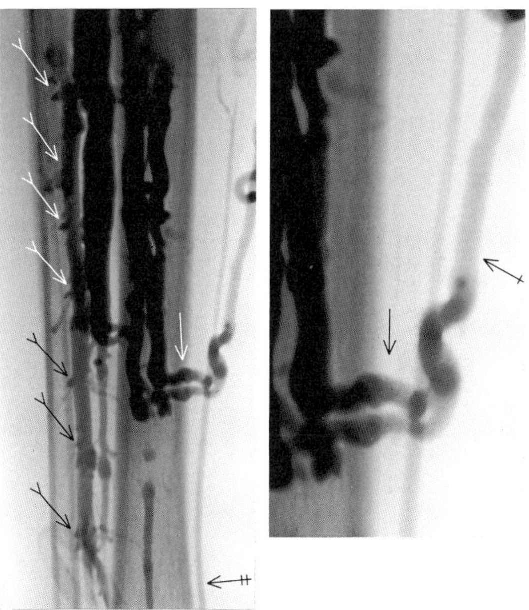

214. Incompetence of middle Cockett's perforators (→) with varicose degeneration of the posterior arch vein (+→). The perforators look paired, but each enters a different trunk of the posterior tibial veins. Incompetence is manifested by a large junction angle, cylindrical shape, irregular wall contours, and retrograde flow. The outer valve plane is poorly defined. ++→ Great saphenous vein. Ascending pressure phlebography demonstrates several competent perforator groups with paired, partially opacified vessels (>→). *Left,* general view in internal rotation. *Right,* close-up view

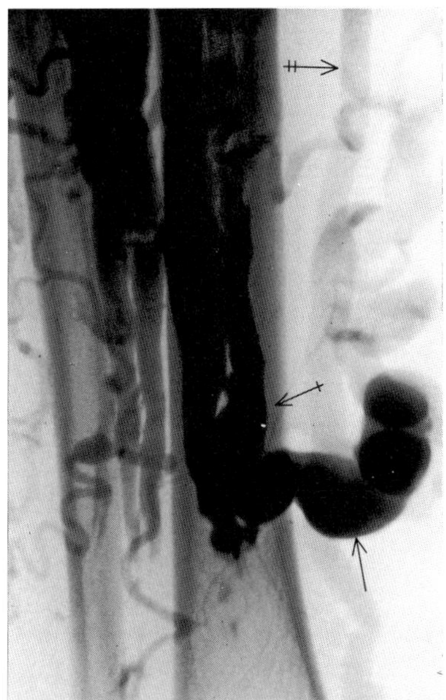

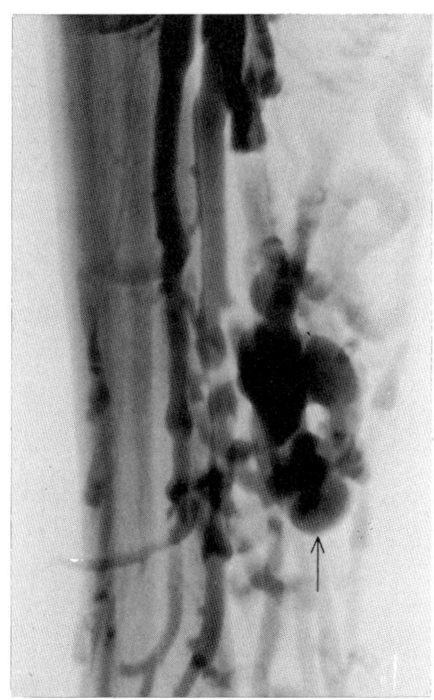

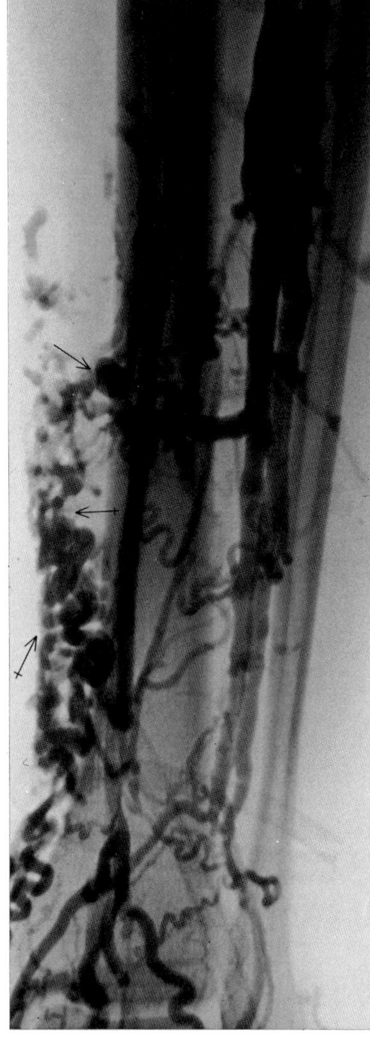

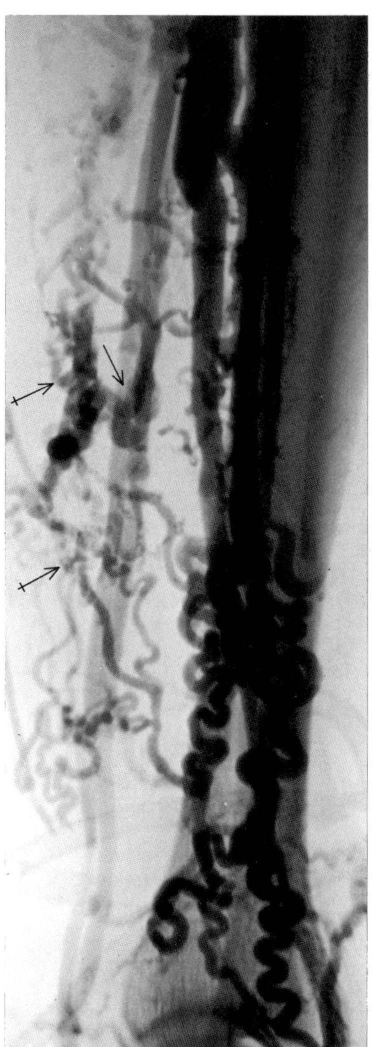

216. Incompetent upper Cockett's perforator (→) in the left leg with a distal ulcer pad (↦) demonstrated by ascending pressure phlebography. *Left,* internal rotation view. *Right,* lateral view

The pathophysiology of the flow reversal can account for the secondary effects of severe perforator incompetence on the associated deep venous
217 groups, which respond with varying degrees of dilatation and tortuosity. The changes always occur above the level of the affected perforator, so there is a limited region of retrograde flow. Involvement of *both* posterior tibial veins is attributable to the small rung veins that bridge between
35 the vascular trunks. This ***secondary tibial vein insufficiency*** (Hach 1981 b) is analogous to the secondary popliteal and femoral vein insufficiency arising in severe saphenous varicosity. According to Thomas' law (1893), the blood vessel responds to the increased flow velocity with luminal enlargement. Apparently this mechanism, which is operative within the arteries, is also applicable to the venous system. It is not known whether the adaptive changes are regressive following eradication of the incompetent perforator.

Ascending pressure phlebography is only 70% sensitive in the diagnosis of Cockett's perforator incompetence, based on intraoperative measurements. Accordingly, there is *no* strict indication for roentgenography if the *sole* object is to detect incompetent communicating veins. On the other hand, identification of the foregoing radiographic changes does furnish objective evidence of the funtional incompetence in all cases.

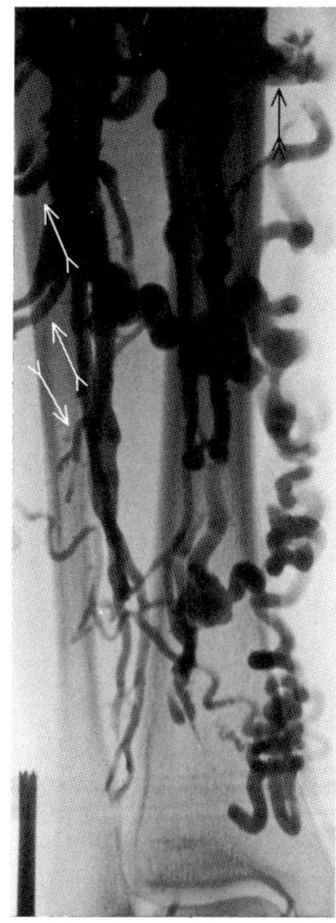
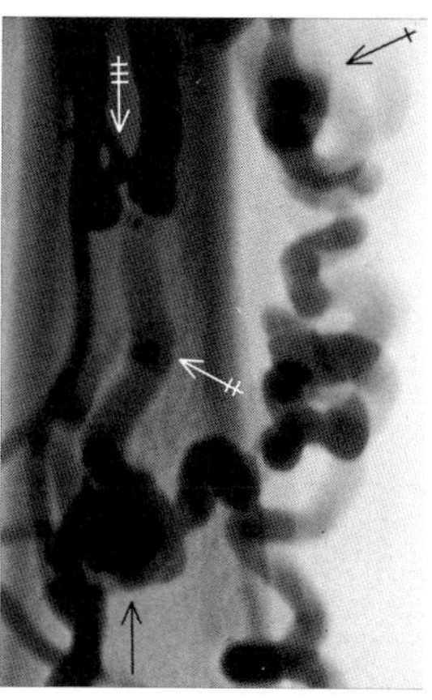

217. Incompetent middle Cockett's perforator showing central aneurysmatic dilation (→). Varicose degeneration of the posterior arch vein (↦). Secondary insufficiency of the posterior tibial veins (⇸) above the incoming perforator. ⇻ Rung veins; ↣ competent perforators; ⤖ incompetent Boyd's perforator. Demonstrated by ascending pressure phlebography. *Left,* general view in internal rotation. *Right,* close-up view

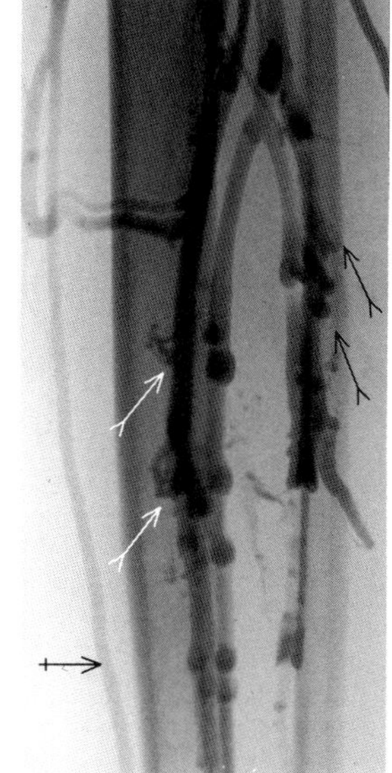
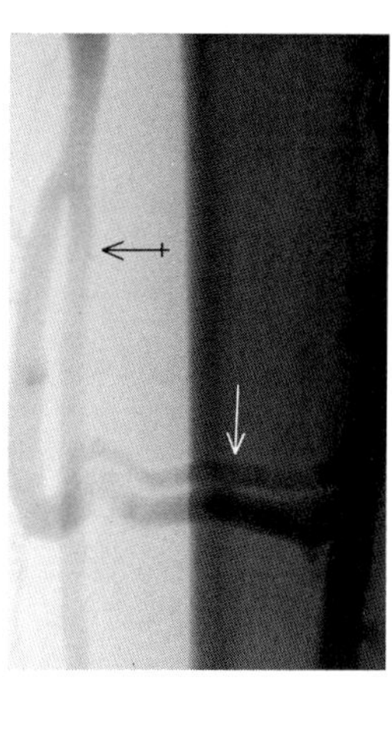

218. Incipient incompetence of Boyd's perforator in the left leg, demonstrated by ascending pressure phlebography. *Left,* general view in internal rotation. → Boyd's group; ↦ great saphenous vein; ↣ competent perforator groups. *Right,* Boyd's veins with acute junction angle and horizontal course. The lower vein shows marked dilatation and slightly irregular contours. Retrograde blood flow with varicose dilatation of the great saphenous tributary

A basic *problem* in the evaluation of Cockett's veins has been the lack of a standard reference test. All sensitivity data are based on surgical exploration, which, as a reference method, is subject to various subjective and objective influences. Clinical examination, plate thermography after Tricoire, sonographic imaging, Doppler ultrasound, and fluorescent labeling each shows a sensitivity of approximately 70%. But the value of these procedures is compromised by the relatively high rate of false-positive diagnoses. Ascending pressure phlebography is decidedly superior owing to the 100% specificity of its radiographic criteria in the diagnosis of incompetent Cockett's perforators.

The transfascial communication with the deep venous system makes surgery the treatment of choice. The surgeon's task is to locate the incompetent vessel. When an experienced team is at work, we do not believe that localization is significantly aided by using a ruler with radiopaque markers.

Of the various *surgical treatments* for Cockett's perforator incompetence, selective dissection is preferred today. A stab incision is sometimes sufficient. The endoscopic procedure, if necessary with paratibial fasciotomy, is indicated for patients with severe skin changes due to chronic venous insufficiency.

Varicosity of Sherman's Perforator

The varicose Sherman's perforator occurs at about the middle of the lower leg on the medial side of the calf. It has little clinical significance, and usually only a small varix is found. Selective subfascial perforator dissection may be considered as a treatment option.

Varicosity of Boyd's Perforator

218 Boyd's perforator incompetence is uncommon; we have seen only 12 definite cases in 20000 phlebographic examinations. Since the incompetent vessel courses between the posterior tibial vein and great saphenous vein, it can give rise to an incomplete saphenous varicosity. Clinical symptoms are relatively mild, though some cases may justify recommendation for surgery.

A significantly higher incidence of Boyd's perforator varicosity has been reported in clinical series. This most likely results from confusion with the distal point of incompetence in a stage III great saphenous varicosity.

Dodd's Perforator Incompetence

The significance of incompetent Dodd's veins in
170 the thigh is based on their causal role in *incom-*
174 *plete saphenous varicosity*. The vessels establish connections between the superficial femoral vein and the great saphenous vein. An incompetent perforator may dilate to finger thickness and show
182 aneurysmatic sacculation. The retrograde blood flow creates a proximal point of incompetence at the entry of the vein into the great saphenous trunk, with varicose degeneration of the trunk progressing distally from that level. A reflux circuit is established that may decompensate with passage of time, leading to chronic venous insufficiency.

A blow-out noted clinically may suggest the correct di-
171 agnosis, but the clinical features are difficult to distinguish from those of complete saphenous varicosity. Only ascending pressure phlebography allows for reliable documentation of the hemodynamic status of the limb. Doppler ultrasound has the value of a screening test. Real-time ultrasound imaging and duplex scanning are useful for documentation only when findings are pronounced. Impairment of the musculovenous pump function of the leg and an increase in venous capacitance and drainage signify decompensation of the recirculating flow.

The treatment of choice is selective subfascial dis-
175 section of the affected vessel, combined if necessary with surgical treatment of the incomplete saphenous varicosity. If the surgeon was unaware of the incompetent Dodd's perforator before operation and tears it while stripping the great saphenous vein, a life-threatening hemorrhage can ensue. Thus, radiographic documentation of the venous morphology assumes particular significance in cases of this kind.

Varicosity of May's Perforator

May's perforator lies at the midcalf level between
the small saphenous vein and gastrocnemius ves- 219
sels. Incompetence of this perforator generally causes a conspicuous blow-out, for each calf muscle contraction acts directly on the extrafascial communicating vessel, propelling a spurt of retrograde flow. Generally a circumscribed varix is found in proximity to this "incompetent gastrocnemius point." The condition is painful but seldom causes local skin changes.

In rare cases the incompetent May's perforator gives rise to an incomplete small saphenous varicosity. The proximal portion of the vascular trunk appears competent, but there is varicose degeneration below the incoming transfascial communicating vein – the proximal point of incompetence.

Varicosity of the Popliteal Perforator

Isolated incompetence of the perforating vein in the popliteal fossa causes a large, tortuous varix and may prompt referral for phlebographic evaluation. The vessel opacifies from the popliteal vein when the patient performs a Valsalva maneuver. It is approximately level with the termination of the
small saphenous vein, so it may be difficult to dis- 220
tinguish from a saphenous varicosity that pierces the fascia at a high level. Doubts are resolved by tracing the course of the vessel to the lower leg. In pronounced cases, selective subfascial ligation of the perforator is advised.

Varicosity of Hach's Profunda Perforator

An incompetent profunda perforator has characteristic clinical features that enable a spot diagnosis to be made. The varicose vein emerges through a palpable fascial defect on the lateral side of the upper thigh and takes a very tortuous downward course. It sometimes causes pain.

We have elucidated the hemodynamics of the profunda perforator by varicography, which demon- 221
strates a large-caliber, valveless connection with the profunda femoris vein. The recommended

treatment is selective intrafascial dissection of the incompetent perforator followed by a sclerosing injection.

Reticular Varicosity

Reticular varicosities have no direct relationship to the deep venous system. They occur in isolation, within large scars, or in conjunction with any other form of primary varicose disease. Unlike

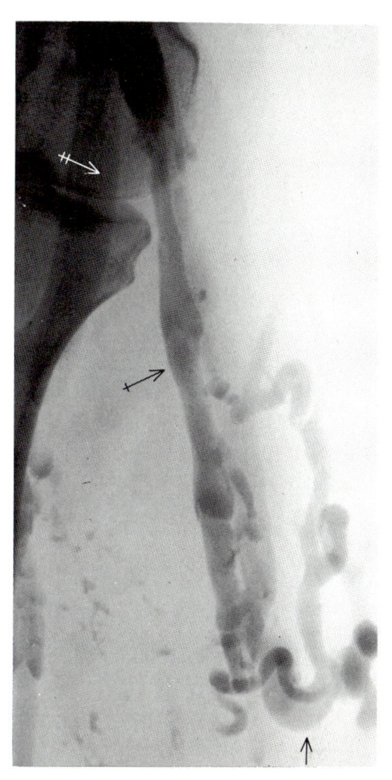

219. Incompetent May's perforator (→). ↔ Gastrocnemius veins. ⇸ Popliteal vein. Demonstrated by overflow effect in ascending pressure phlebography ▷

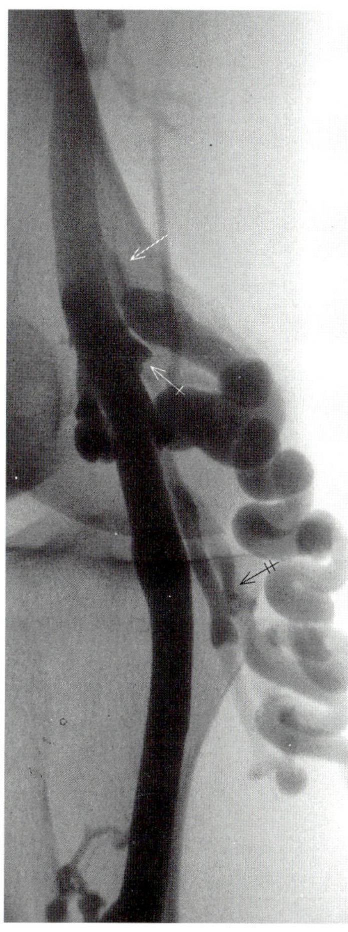

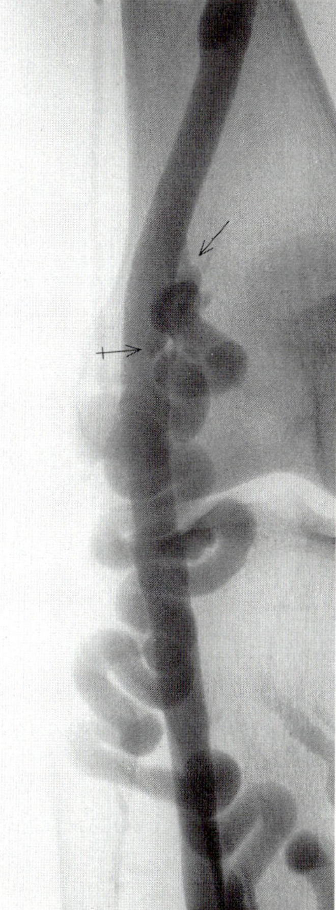

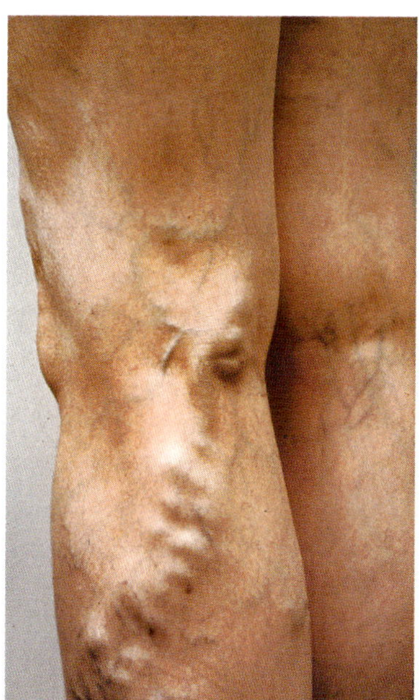

220. Varicose popliteal perforator. Junction with the popliteal vein (→). Competent terminal valve (↔) of the small saphenous vein. ⇸ Gastrocnemius veins. Demonstrated by ascending pressure phlebography; *left,* internal rotation; *middle,* lateral views; *right,* clinical appearance ▽

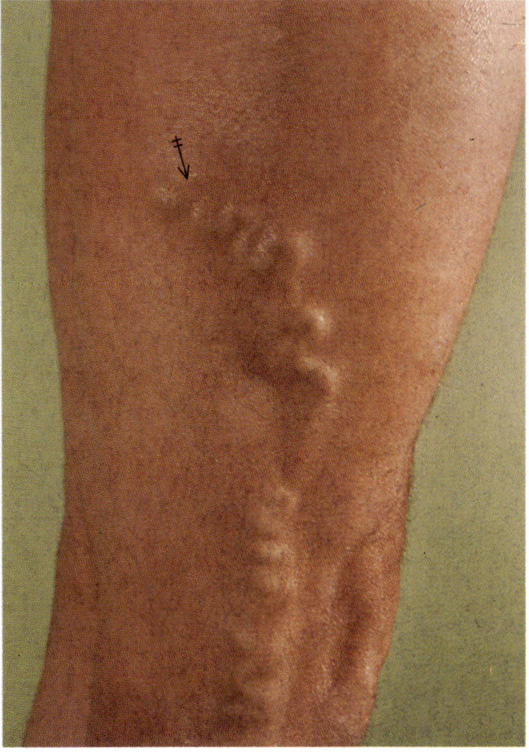

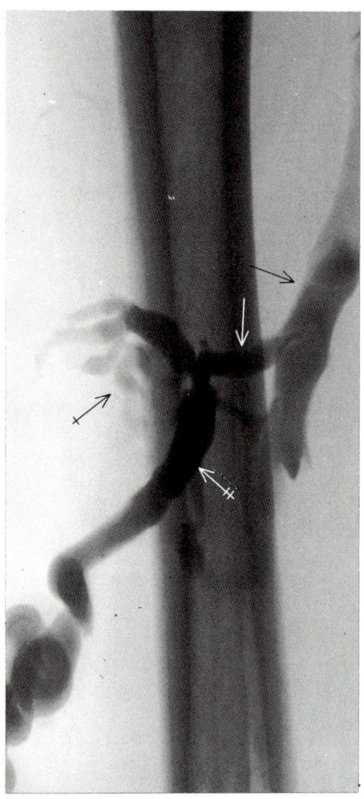

221. Incompetent Hach's profunda perforator. *Left,* clinical appearance of the blow-out (⇻). *Right,* varicogram. → Profunda femoris vein; ⇸ merging muscle branches; ⇻ profunda perforator

saphenous varicosities, they tend to form during or past middle age. They show a strong propensity for recurrence following any mode of treatment.

The radiographic visualization of reticular varicosities is indicated only in special inquiries, e.g., to locate a hidden perforator. This is best accom-
104 plished by varicography. The treatment of choice is sclerotherapy.

Recurrent Varicosity After Surgery

Varicose veins may recur only a short time after sclerotherapy or surgery. Often these are not true recurrences but residual varices that were incompletely removed or overlooked at initial treatment. Despite their protean clinical features, almost all conditions associated with these "recurrent" varicosities fit into a scheme corresponding to the primary varicose conditions and their associated recirculating flow patterns. In a control series of 102 patients examined elsewhere, the territories of the great saphenous vein were involved in 66.7%, small saphenous vein in 21.6%, and perforating veins in 11.7% (Hach 1981 b).

Of course it is possible for a new varicose condition, such as small saphenous incompetence, to develop years or even decades after the successful surgical treatment of a great saphenous varicosity or after the sclerotherapy of a varicose side branch. This no more constitutes a recurrence than, say, an umbilical hernia developing several years after the surgical repair of an inguinal hernia.

Recurrent Great Saphenous Varicosity

There can be no true recurrence of a surgically treated great saphenous varicosity in cases where an adequate extirpation has been performed. The diagnostic workup of a given case must include a precise evaluation of prevailing hemodynamic conditions so that the surgeon will have the information needed for a second intervention. Only ascending pressure phlebography is acceptable for this purpose.

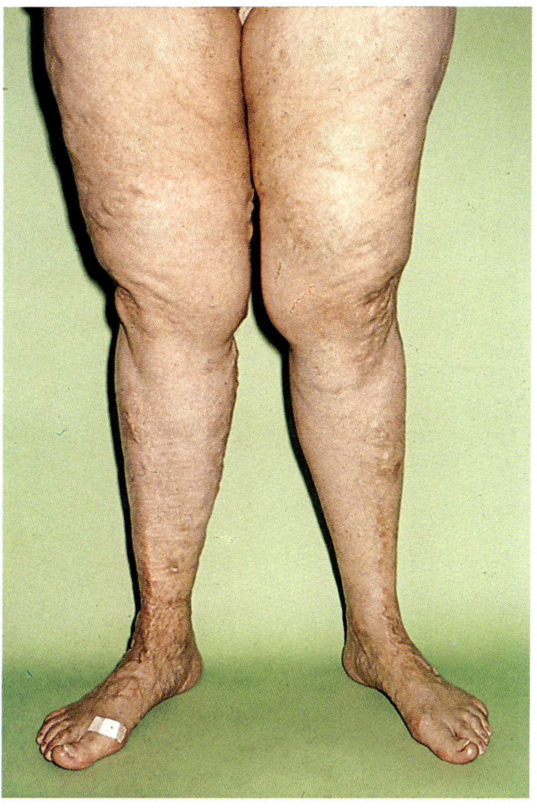

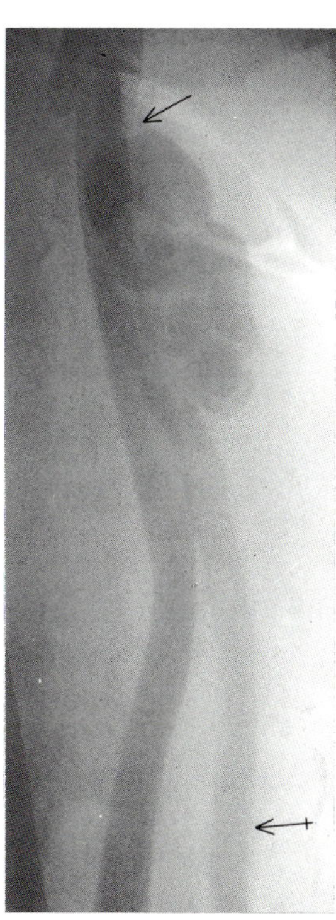

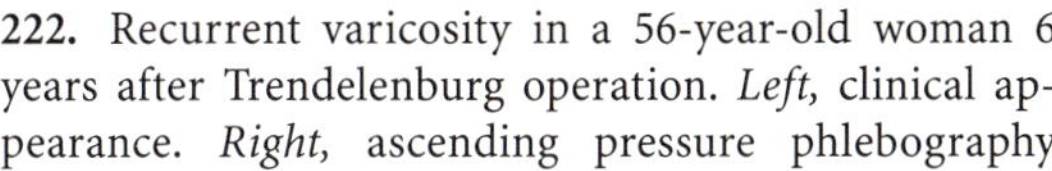

222. Recurrent varicosity in a 56-year-old woman 6 years after Trendelenburg operation. *Left,* clinical appearance. *Right,* ascending pressure phlebography shows a tortuous varix (→) below the previous ligature; ↔ great saphenous trunk

Generally the clinical presentation is a poor indi-
222 cator of the morphologic situation, although old surgical scars may help to determine where previous surgery was not performed. Real-time sonography and duplex scanning can demonstrate larger venous segments in isolation but cannot disclose the full extent of the persistent reflux circuit. The bridging collaterals that develop after an incomplete vascular resection often have a smaller caliber and a tortuous course. Even with provocative testing, this reduces blood flow below the threshold accessible to Doppler investigation.

The routine technique of radiographic examination is ascending pressure phlebography. Special care is taken to define incompetent transfascial communications that were missed in the previous operation.

The radiographic appearance of a ***residual saphenous varicosity*** is indistinguishable from that of the primary disease. In the foregoing series of patients with recurrent varicosity operated elsewhere, this finding was identified in 20.6% of the cases (Hach 1981 b). Duplicated vessels can be excluded as a cause if the crosse can be radiographically visualized.

Duplication of the great saphenous vein is not as important a factor in recurrence as is widely claimed. Once the residual "duplicated" segment has been deprived of its connections with the deep veins by crossectomy, its hemodynamic significance becomes minimal.

The ***interrupted saphenous varicosity*** results from outmoded surgical procedures that omitted crossectomy and venous trunk resection. The high
ligation of Trendelenburg or the Moskowicz tech- 222
nique of surgical ligation with retrograde injection are no longer practiced today. Sometimes
collaterals can be seen bridging between the prox- 223
imal and distal vascular stumps.

A ***long saphenous stump*** is frequently encountered 224
as a cause of recurrent varicosity. At initial operaton crossectomy was omitted, and the vein was merely stripped out. Clinical examination shows an atypical location of the surgical scar, which does not lie on the inguinal fold but a hands width

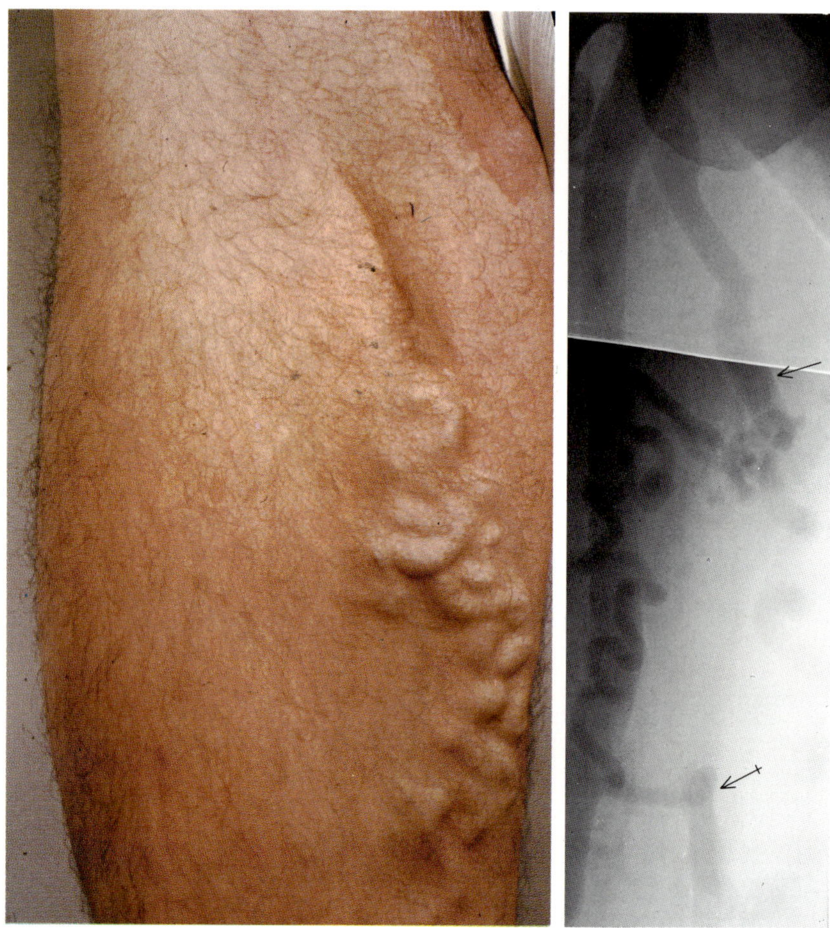

223. Recurrent varicosity after incomplete long saphenectomy in a 40-year-old man. *Left,* clinical appearance 1 year after operation. *Right,* ascending pressure phlebography shows a 13-cm-long interruption of the varicose great saphenous vein (→) with retrograde filling of the distal incompetent venous segment (↔) through bridging collaterals. Persistent type III reflux circuit with chronic venous insufficiency

below it. Large varices can arise from the lower
224 end of the saphenous remnant.

If significant portions of a decompensated reflux circuit remain intact following incomplete surgery or sclerotherapy, there will be a rapid progression of *secondary popliteal and femoral vein incompetence* with persistence of chronic venous insufficiency. Thus it is mandatory to perform a thorough reoperation with a complete extrafascial ablation whenever large varicose saphenous remnants are encountered.

225 The most common cause of postoperative recur-
226 rent varicosity is now a ***short stump.*** During the initial operation, the crossectomy was for some reason incomplete, and a very curved varicose vein stretches distally from the remaining saphenous sinus. In phlebography, the important point is to actually visualize the stump and thus to provide the surgeon with a radiomorphologic basis for the planned operation. This is particularly indicated in cases in which a decompensated reflux circuit is still present.

We feel that a short residual stump of the great saphenous vein is best managed by prefemoral stump ligation or stump dissection using the technique of Hach (1981 b). The anterior wall of the common femoral vein is exposed directly at the inguinal ligament, and the dissection is carried distally to expose the residual saphenous sinus, which is doubly ligated. This technique avoids bleeding from varicosities in the old scar region.

Inguinal varicose bed denotes a typical radio- 227
graphic appearance of recurrent varicosity that occasionally develops after a complete crossecto-

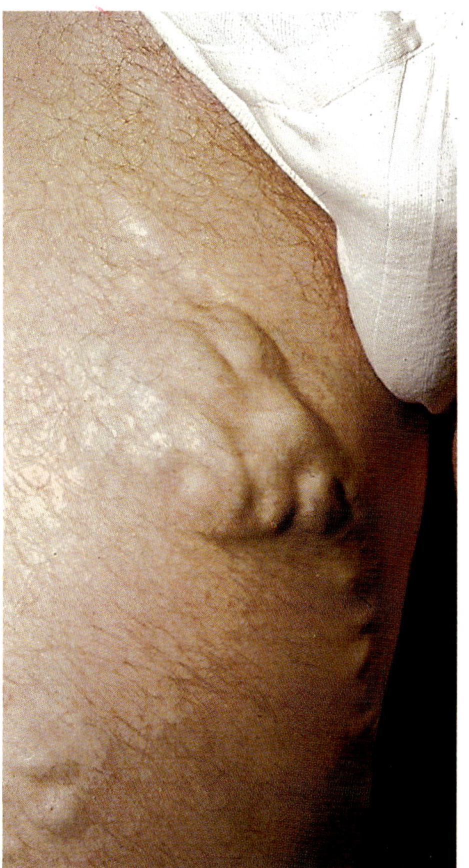

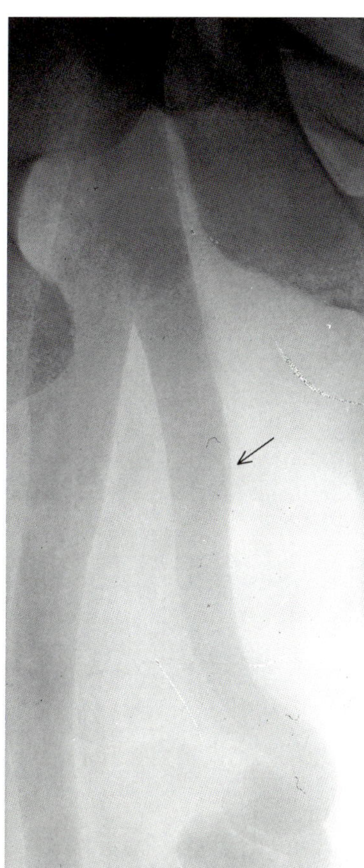

224. Severe recurrent varicosity with a great saphenous stump in a 49-year-old man. *Left,* clinical appearance 4 years after operation. The scar is a hands width below the inguinal fold. Chronic venous insufficiency. *Right,* ascending pressure phlebography shows a 12-cm-long varicose saphenous stump (→) uniting with a large, tortuous varix. Persistent decompensated reflux circuit

Potential technical causes of recurrent great saphenous varicosity			
Problem	Relative frequency (n=68)	Crossectomy	Resection
Saphenous vein left intact	20.6%	Not performed	Not performed
Saphenous vein interrupted	14.6%	Not performed	Not performed
Great saphenous stump	41.7%	Not performed	Performed
Small saphenous stump	11.8%	Incomplete	Performed
Inguinal varicose bed	11.8%	Performed	Performed

my for severe saphenous varicosity. A fine meshwork of varicose veins arises from the small varicose tributaries of the saphenous trunk.

The formation of an inguinal varicose bed can be prevented by always resecting smaller tributaries of the crosse behind their initial point of branching. Postoperative pathologic refluxes of the sonographic investigation are usually due to this phenomenen.

Recurrent Small Saphenous Varicosity

As with the great saphenous vein, a true recurrence of small saphenous varicosity is not possible following adequate surgical treatment. Severe recurrent varices are an indication for phlebographic evaluation of venous hemodynamics. *Persistent saphenous varicosity* is a relatively common finding, since involvement of the small saphenous

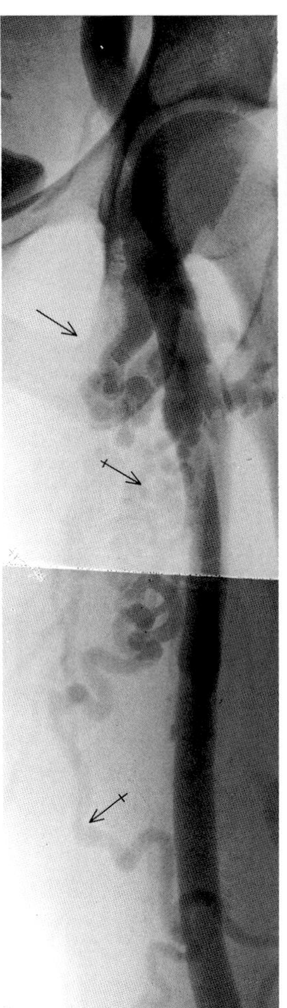

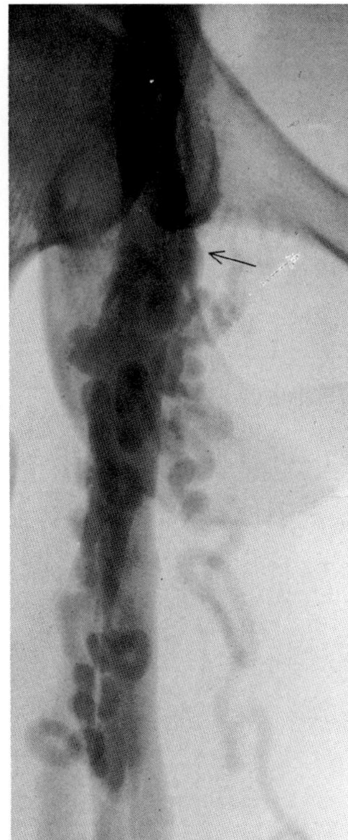

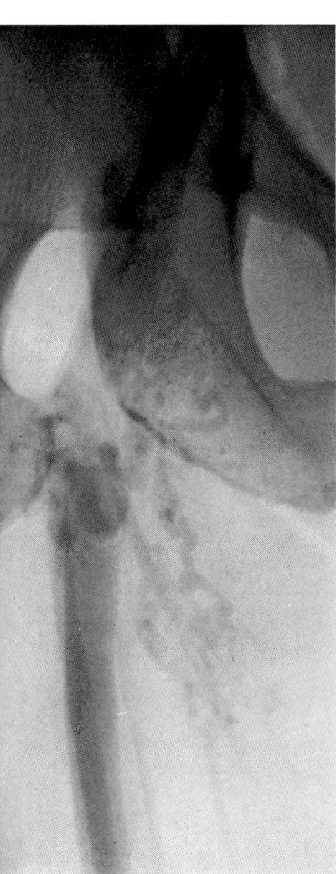

226 *(middle)*. Recurrent varicosity in a 34-year-old woman. Reappearance of varicose veins in the thigh 3 years after surgery. Retrograde pressure phlebography demonstrates the 1 cm-great saphenous stump (→)

225 *(left)*. Recurrent varicosity in a 35-year-old woman with a small saphenous stump (→) and tortuous varices distal to the old ligature (↔)

227 *(right)*. "Inguinal varicose bed." Small-caliber recurrent varicose veins in a 38-year-old woman 5 years after surgery for great saphenous varicosity. Demonstrated by ascending pressure phlebography

vein in the primary varicose condition often is not recognized by clinical examination alone.

228 Absent or incomplete crossectomy leaves behind a *saphenous stump* in the popliteal fossa that can give rise to large varices and cause complaints. Reintervention is advised (Hach and Hach-Wunderle 1994).

Recurrent Varicosity of Incompetent Perforators

An incompetent Cockett's perforator is easily overlooked during presurgical evaluation due to a lack of effective diagnostic techniques. This is especially common in obese patients. *Recurrent Cockett's varicosity* is a relatively common finding, therefore.

Persistence of chronic venous insufficiency should always raise suspicion of a persistent incompetent perforator. After surgery or sclerotherapy has been performed, varicose veins or fascial defects often can no longer be detected in the supramalleolar region by clinical examination. The varicosity may have been missed during the previous treatment or may have redeveloped in the setting of a persistent secondary popliteal and femoral vein insufficiency. At one time surgeons deliberately omitted perforator dissection initially, even in complicated cases, to avoid wound healing problems.

Before the introduction of Hach's paratibial fasciotomy (1983) and the endoscopic technique (Hauer 1985), only the very invasive procedures of Linton or Cockett were

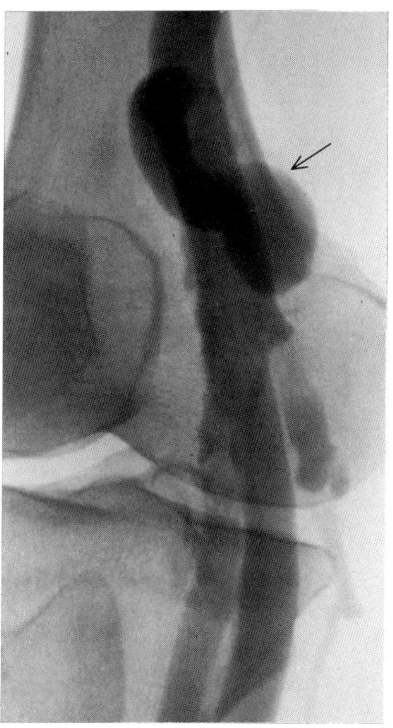

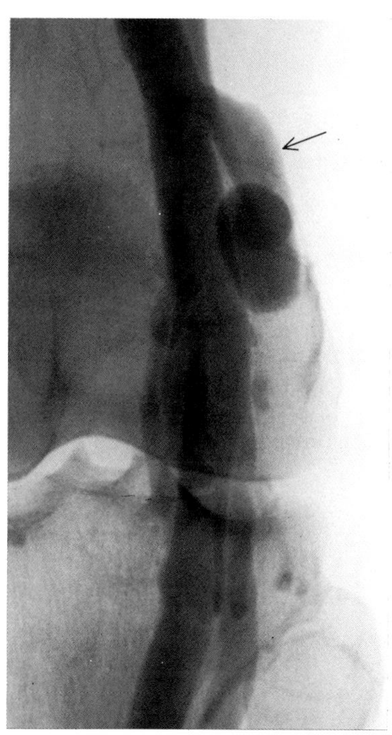

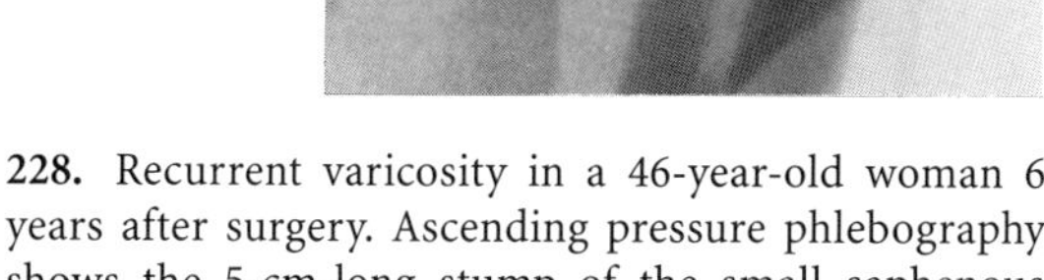

228. Recurrent varicosity in a 46-year-old woman 6 years after surgery. Ascending pressure phlebography shows the 5-cm-long stump of the small saphenous vein, dilated to finger thickness (→). Internal rotation (*left*) and lateral view (*right*)

available for the surgical treatment of chronic recurrent crural ulcers. These procedures led to serious complications in a large percentage of cases. Today, the endoscopic technique, if necessary combined with paratibial fasciotomy, can effect a surgical cure even in severe cases.

Before the repeat dissection of incompetent Cockett's perforators is commenced, the hemodynamic status of the limb should be evaluated by phlebography. It is important to identify *all* residual components of a reflux circuit, especially in patients previously treated elsewhere by various means. No other diagnostic procedure can adequately justify selection for reoperation or direct the formulation of a precise operating plan. In some cases the evaluation of the muscle pump function of the leg and data on venous capacitance and drainage can provide useful adjuncts to the X-ray morphologic diagnosis.

229 *Dodd's perforator varicosity* occasionally recurs in cases where an incomplete saphenous varicosity was managed by Babcock's operation that did not include selective perforator dissection. Again, a second operation is indicated.

Recurrence After Sclerotherapy

In principle, sclerotherapy is appropriate for all varicose veins that do not communicate directly with the deep venous system through incompetent transfascial channels, i.e., the extrafascial side-branch varicosities and reticular varicosities. Elderly patients are the only population in which these differential diagnostic considerations do not apply.

Severe varicosity of the great or small saphenous vein in young patients recurs in the central portions of the vessels within a short time after injection therapy. Due to the high fibrinolytic activity of the venous wall, recanalization proceeds rapidly after thrombosis. The injected trunk occasion- 230
ally exhibits the post-thrombotic roentgen signs of irregular contours, internal webs and islets within the vessel lumen. These changes are also well demonstrated by color-coded duplex sonography.

Only diagnostic imaging procedures can furnish reliable information on the success or failure of the nonoperative treatment of saphenous varicosity. Whenever a reflux circuit is present, a high

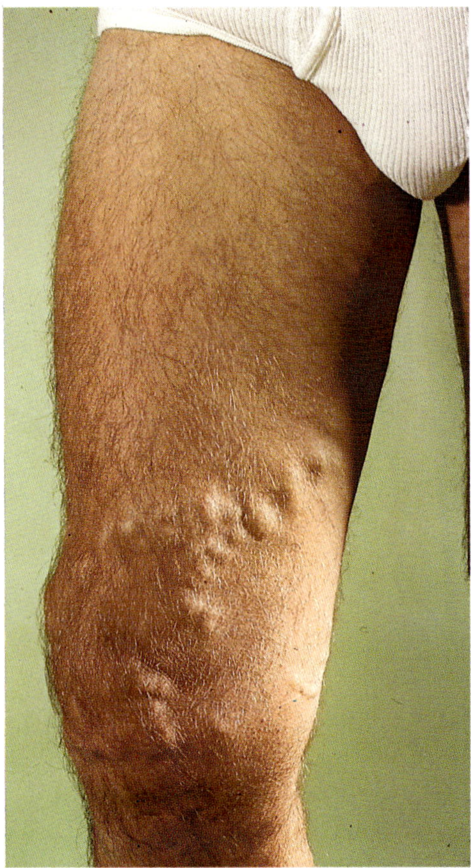

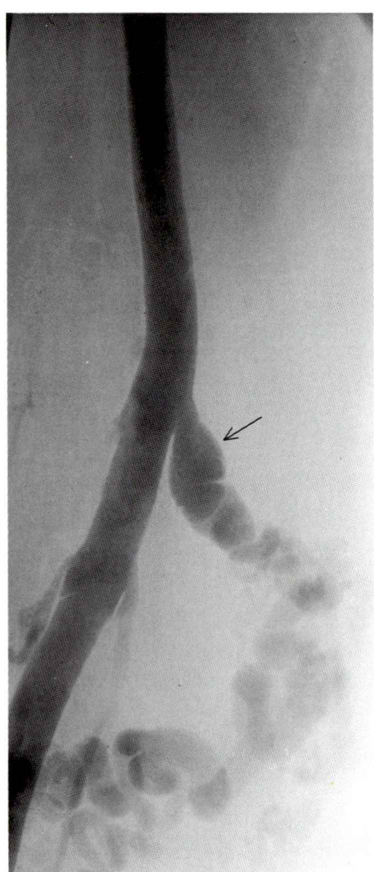

229. Recurrent varicosity in a 60-year-old man 6 months after varicose vein surgery. *Left,* clinical appearance. *Right,* ascending pressure phlebography shows a residual finger-thick stump of Dodd's perforator (→) with large associated varices

priority is attached to protecting the patient *from secondary popliteal and femoral vein insufficiency.* This can be ensured only by the methodical exclusion of the affected segments from the circulation. Once decompensation of the deep stem veins has supervened, the modern-day therapist *must prove* the complete eradication of the *entire* extrafascial venous system. It is incumbent upon the sclero-
230 therapist in this regard to document the efficacy of his measures at 1 year or later by repeat phlebography or color-coded duplex scanning.

Reticular varices have a strong tendency to recur following any type of treatment, so regular outpatient follow-ups should be scheduled. In pronounced cases a *single* follow-up phlebogram should be taken to ensure that incompetent transfascial communications are not overlooked.

References

Bernink BP (1971) Sind die phlebographisch als inkompetent gedeuteten Venae communicantes auch physiologisch insuffizient? Zbl Phlebol 10: 41

Hach W (1981 a) Die Erhaltung eines transplantationswürdigen Venensegments bei der partiellen Saphenaresektion als Operationsmethode der Stammvarikose. Phlebol Proktol 10: 171

Hach W (1981 b) Differenzierte Diagnostik der primären Varikose. Demeter, Gräfelfing

Hach W (1985) Die Varikose der Profunda-Perforans, ein typisches phlebologisches Krankheitsbild. Vasa 14: 155

Hach W (1991) Varizenoperation – Wie radikal dürfen wir vorgehen? In: Maurer PC, Dörler J, v. Sommoggy S (Hrsg) Gefäßchirurgie im Fortschritt. Thieme, Stuttgart

Hach W (1993) Die Rezirkulationskreise der primären Stammvarikose. Chir Prax 47: 319

Hach W, Hach-Wunderle V (1994) Die Rezirkulationskreise der Stammvarikose. Springer, Berlin Heidelberg New York Tokyo

Hach W, Schirmers U, Becker L (1980) Veränderungen der tiefen Leitvenen bei einer Stammvarikose der V. saphena

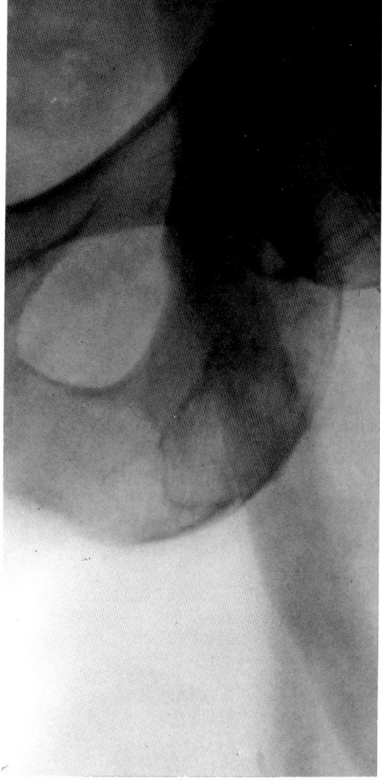

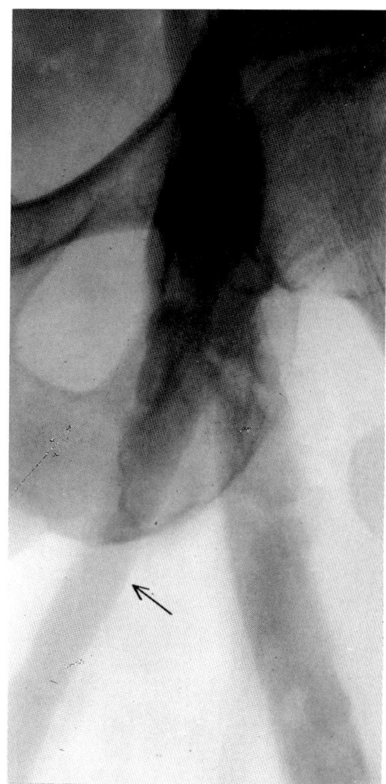

230. Recurrent varicosity in the left leg after sclerotherapy in a 56-year-old woman. Ascending pressure phlebography shows pronounced secondary femoral and popliteal vein insufficiency, causing poor opacification of the large inguinal vessels. *Left,* radiograph 2 weeks after complete obliteration of a pronounced great saphenous varicosity to groin level demonstrates thrombotic occlusion of the vessel. *Right,* radiograph at 3 years later shows complete recanalization of the varicose great saphenous vein (→). Clinically there is severe recurrent varicosity

magna. In: Müller-Wiefel H (Hrsg) Mikrozirkulation und Blutrheologie. Witzstrock, Baden-Baden
Hach W, Langer C, Schirmers U (1983) Das arthrogene Stauungssyndrom. Vasa 12: 109
Hauer G (1985) Die endoskopische subfaszerale Diszision der Perforansvenen. Vasa 14: 59
Niebes P, Laszt L (1971) Recherche sur l'activité des enzymes dans le métabolisme des mucopolysaccharides de veines saphènes humaines saines et variqueuses. Angiologia 8: 7
Schmeller W (1990) Das arthrogene Stauungssyndrom. Diesbach, Berlin
Staubesand J (1977) Matrix-Vesikel und Mediadysplasie. Med Welt 28: 1943
Stranzenbach W, Hach W (1991) Phlebographische Verlaufsbeobachtungen der sekundären Popliteal- und Femoralveneninsuffizienz bei Stammvarikose. Phlebologie 20: 25
Svejar J, Prerovsky J, Linhart J, Krumel J (1964) Biochemical differences in the composition of primary varicose veins. Am Heart J 67: 572
Wuppermann T (1991) Was können die Sonographieverfahren wirklich? In: Maurer PC, Dörler J, v. Sommoggy S (Hrsg) Gefäßchirurgie im Fortschritt. Thieme, Stuttgart

Venous Thrombosis

It is important clinically to draw a strict distinction between superficial (extrafascial) and deep (intrafascial) venous thrombosis in the lower extremity. *Superficial thrombophlebitis generally* is a mild disorder, although recurrent bouts of venous
inflammation in the setting of pronounced saphe- 231
nous varicosity can give rise to pulmonary microemboli and associated cardiopulmonary insufficiency. *Deep vein thrombosis* is *always* a serious condition whose prognosis is compromised by the risk of life-threatening complications, recurrences, and post-thrombotic deficits. It is not unusual for thrombophlebitis or phlebothrombosis to present as the initial symptom of an underlying systemic disease.

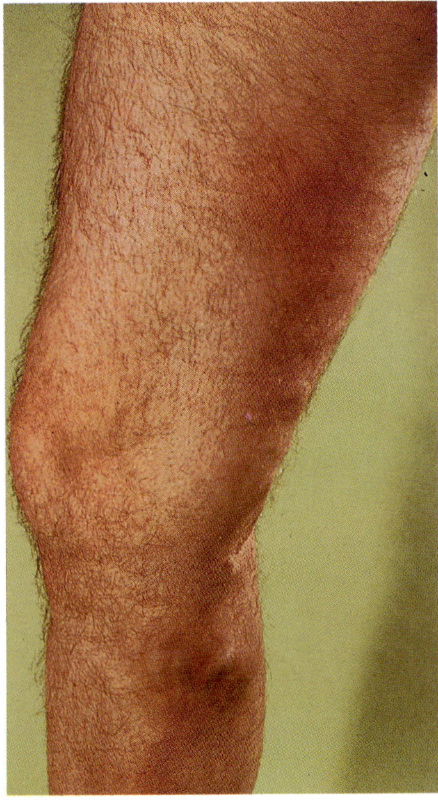

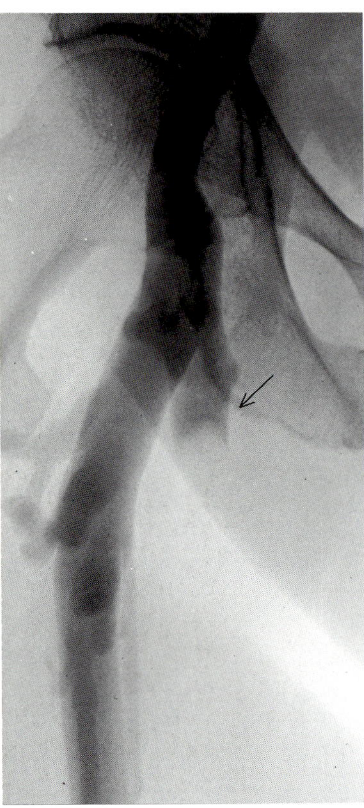

231. Varicophlebitis in the setting of severe great saphenous varicosity in a 58-year-old man with a 30-year history of varicose disease. *Left,* clinical appearance. *Right,* ascending pressure phlebography demonstrates the dome sign (→) of the thrombus tail and an eraser sign in the great saphenous vein

Thrombophlebitis

Thrombophlebitis of the extrafascial veins gives rise to various disease states that can be diagnosed clinically by their characteristic features. Generally, then, phlebography is indicated only if there is question of deep venous involvement.

Clinical Symptoms

231 The affected veins are indurated, tender to pressure, and accompanied by a more or less pronounced periphlebitic tissue reaction. *Varicophlebitis* often incites a severe local inflammation. Fever and systemic effects are occasionally seen.

Cordlike thrombophlebitis and *thrombophlebitis saltans* sometimes occur in the setting of a paraneoplastic syndrome, and patients should be referred to internal medicine for a comprehensive workup.

Phlebographic Diagnosis

Fresh thrombus in a superficial vessel is an occasional incidental finding during phlebography. The principal radiographic signs are the dome
sign, contour sign, and eraser sign. 231

During reading of the phlebogram, particular attention is given to the detection or exclusion of transfascial progression of thrombosis into the
deep venous system. *Collar-button thrombosis* de- 232
notes propagation through a perforating vein. Extension of the thrombus tail past the termination of the saphenous trunk into the common femoral
vein (saphenofemoral progression thrombosis) 233
represents a serious complication of great saphenous varicosity, with risk of pulmonary embolism. The therapeutic implications should be discussed at once with the attending physician. Surgical thrombectomy with concomitant removal of the saphenous varicosity is recommended.

In patients with recurrent pulmonary embolism, phlebography is used to search for *the source of*

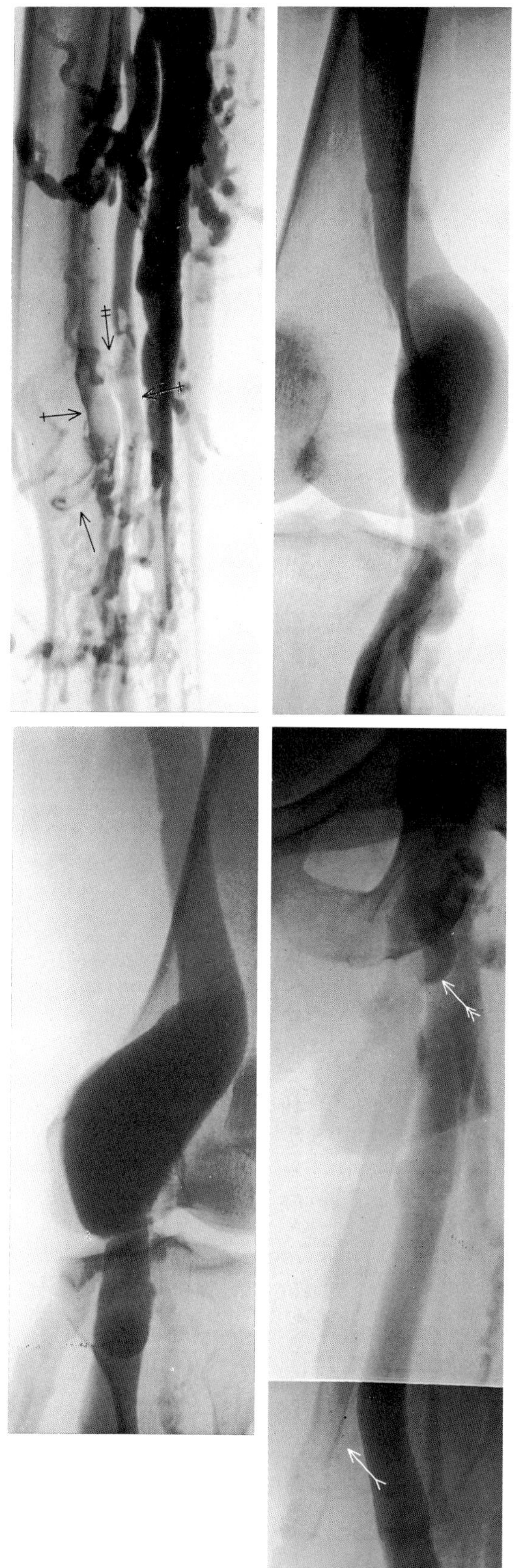

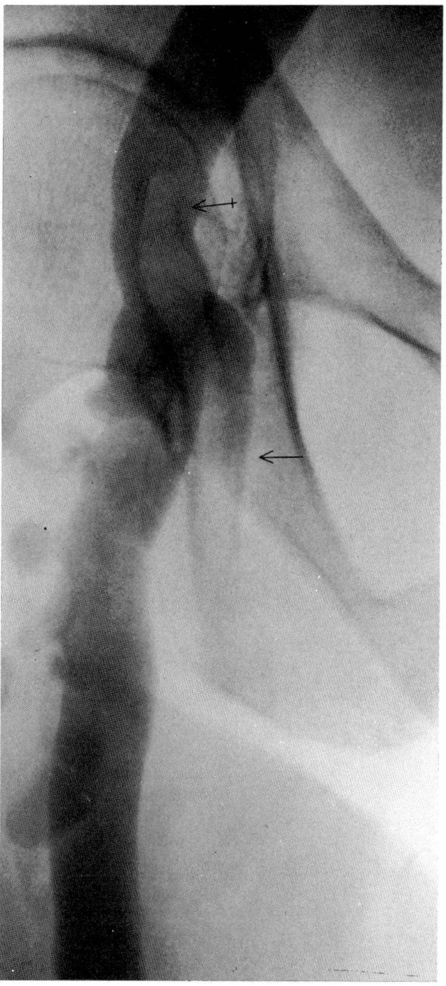

233. Varicophlebitis in a varicose great saphenous trunk. The thrombus tail extends past the saphenofemoral junction (→) into the common femoral vein (⇸). Demonstrated by ascending pressure phlebography

◁

232. Varicophlebitis and collor-buttom thrombophlebitis in a 46-year-old woman. Demonstrated by ascending pressure phlebography in the left leg. *Top left,* incompetent upper Cockett's perforator with thrombus (→), which extends well into the posterior tibial vein (⇸). Spread to second vascular trunk through rung veins (⇻). Patient had an old tibial fracture. *Top right, bottom left,* secondary popliteal and femoral vein insufficiency with a congenital valvular anomaly. No signs of phlebothrombosis. Internal rotation (*top right*) and lateral view (*bottom left*). *Bottom right,* secondary popliteal and femoral vein insufficiency. Severe stage IV great saphenous varicosity with an extensive thrombus (↣) whose tail extends into the terminal aneurysm (⤖). Contour sign

Forms of Thrombophlebitis
Varicophlebitis
Thrombophlebitis saltans
Cordlike thrombophlebitis

the emboli. Thrombi can easily develop within a varicose great saphenous vein or its aneurysms and embolize through the large lumen of the ostial region. Ascending pressure phlebography is not 100% successful in detecting these thrombi. The finding of saphenous varicosity with a normal-appearing deep venous system in the lower limb is sufficient in these cases to warrant surgery.

Sonographic Diagnosis

Varicophlebitis in the setting of saphenous varicosity is well demonstrated by real-time sonography and color-coded duplex scanning, especially in the thigh and groin region. The principal indirect sign is a negative venous compression test. If the process is more than 6 days old, scans will show increasing echogenicity of the thrombus with a marked thickening of the vein wall. On col-
234 or-coded duplex scanning, the echo-free tail of the
thrombus is well delineated with respect to adjacent unobstructed lumen.

The patient is examined in the supine position with slight external rotation of the leg using a linear 5-MHz transducer. Venous compression should be applied with care, because we know of previous published reports of clot dislodgement and pulmonary embolism induced by this procedure.

Deep Vein Thrombosis

Thrombosis of the deep veins of the pelvis and lower extremity is an acutely life-threatening condition due to the potential for pulmonary embolism. It can develop in the setting of any immobilizing illness. There has been a severel-fold rise in the prevalence of thromboembolism since the turn of the century. The incidence of iliofemoral venous thrombosis alone has risen from 2.7% to 27.7% in postmortem series (Rotter and Röttger 1976). Autopsy statistics also show a rise of lethal pulmonary embolism from 1% to 8% during a corresponding period. It is estimated that 5 million patients suffer from post-thrombotic syndrome in the Federal Republic of Germany, but the true incidence is probably much higher (Hach 1989).

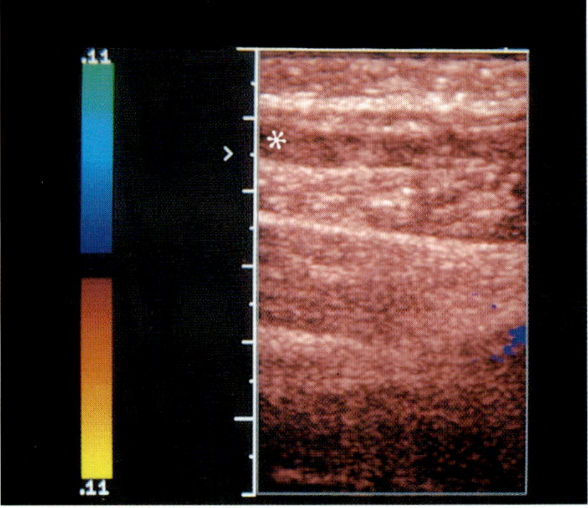

234. Thrombophlebitis in the small saphenous vein (*). Duration of disease, 7 days. Incompressibility of the vessel. Intravascular structures clearly demonstrated by sonography. Slight increase in thickness of the vascular wall. Duplex sonography with color coding. (Acuson, 7-MHz transducer)

These figures underscore the major importance of phlebothrombosis in modern medicine. With prompt diagnosis, many patients can be cured and thus spared the hazards of pulmonary embolism and post-thrombotic syndrome. Contrast phlebography and ultrasonography are the mainstays of early diagnosis.

Thrombogenesis

Virchow in 1856 correctly identified the *triad* of factors involved in the pathogenesis of acute deep vein thrombosis: changes in the composition of the blood, reduced blood flow velocity, and damage to the vessel wall.

Endothelial damage is an essential factor in thrombogenesis. Platelets adhere to subendothelial structures at the damaged site and form aggregates. Through the activation of plasma clotting factors, a fibrin network is deposited within the platelet thrombus. Further growth of the thrombus is subject to the influence of hemostaseologic and hemodynamic factors.

The smallest thrombi demonstrable by phlebography occur in the pockets of the valve cusps (*mono-* 235

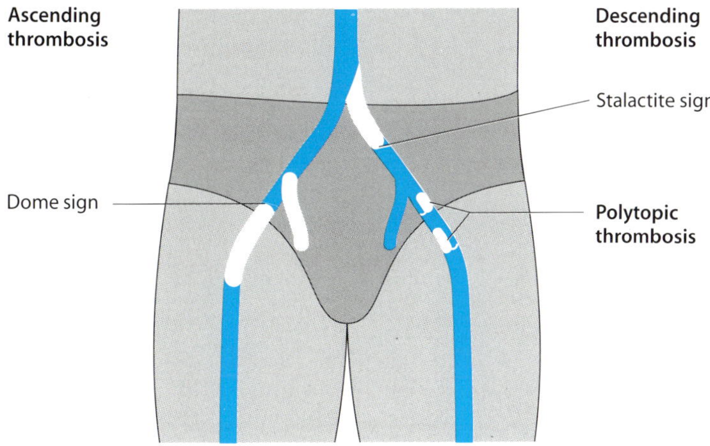

235. Radiographic signs of venous thrombi

240 *cle sign, eyeglass sign*), where they form as a result of secondary flow phenomena and turbulence. The white conglutination thrombus enlarges until
238 an occluding head is formed (*eraser sign*). Following obliteration of the vessel lumen, stasis occurs
255 (*back-up sign* in descending iliofemoral venous thrombosis), and a red coagulation thrombus develops within the stagnant column of blood, form-
238 ing the tail of the thrombus (*dome sign, contour sign*).

As soon as clot material is deposited, fibrinolytic factors are activated. Clotting factor XII A2 is also an activator of fibrinolysis. A major role is played by tissue activators, which are especially abundant in the intima of the vein wall. A reduction in the release of these substances has been implicated as one of numerous biochemical causes of venous thrombosis (Hach-Wunderle 1990).

For the first few days the thrombus is only loosely adherent to the vein wall, its tail floating freely in the lumen. But the morphologic processes of organization commence within just 24 h, characterized by a cellular response of the surrounding tissue and a homogenization of the thrombus. This is accompanied by surface endothelialization, which is complete in only 5 days. Capillary buds invade the thrombus between the first and tenth days, anchoring it firmly to the vein wall. By 42 days connective tissue transformation of the thrombus is complete (Benecke 1976), and phlebography shows the features of post-thrombotic syndrome. The spectrum of radiographic changes from acute thrombosis to post-thrombotic syndrome is continuous, and phlebographic criteria provide an

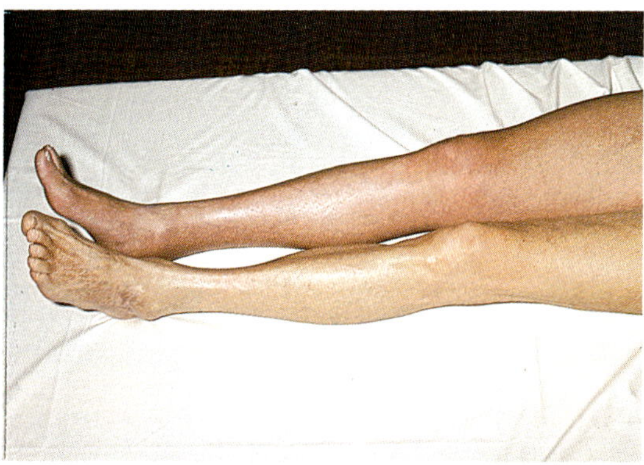

236. Thrombosis of the pelvic and leg veins in a 63-year-old man

uncertain basis for determining the age of the process. Real-time sonography and duplex scanning are more useful for estimating thrombus age.

Clinical Symptoms

Deep vein thrombosis can be extremely difficult to
detect in its early stage. Sometimes a presumptive 236
diagnosis is made less from the clinical picture than from a knowledge of risk factors in the patient's history.

The main clinical symptoms of deep vein thrombosis are *pain, edema,* and *cyanosis.* All other signs and symptoms are of lesser importance due to their high association with false-positive and false-positive results. The same is true of the countless tests that have been repeatedly described over the last 100 years.

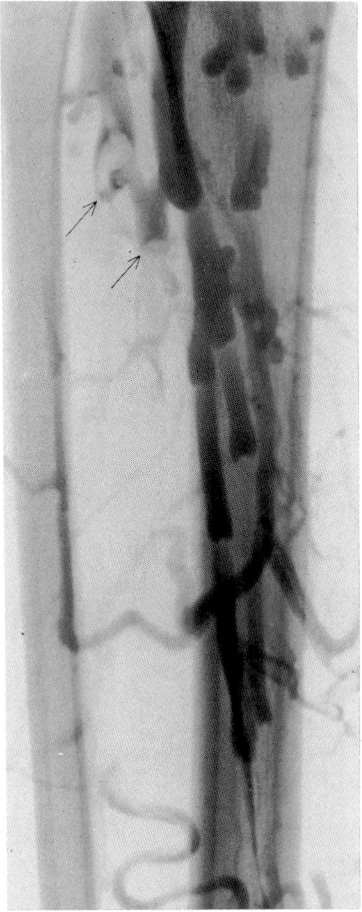

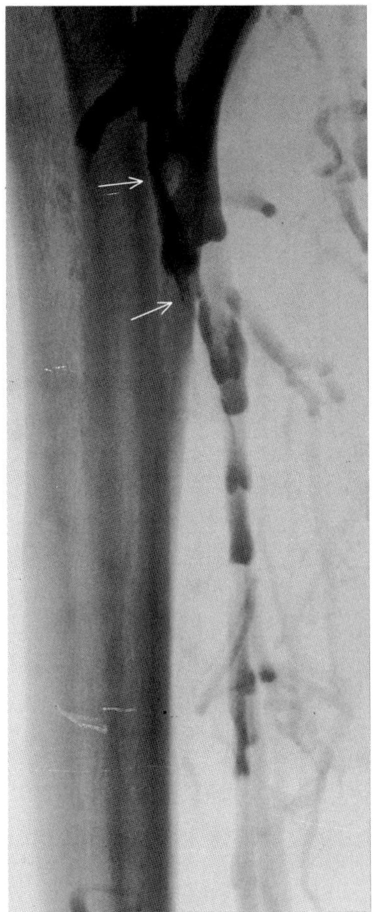

237. Thrombosis of the anterior tibial veins and fibular vein in a 33-year-old woman. Nonvisualization of the affected vessels; dome sign and contour sign at the entry to the popliteal vein (→). Demonstrated by ascending phlebography in semiupright position utilizing the overflow effect; internal rotation (*left*) and lateral view (*right*)

Thrombosis of the leg veins usually causes no symptoms in ***bed-confined patients.*** Pelvic vein thrombosis is associated with a dull pressure in the lumbar region that initially directs suspicion toward renal disease. Not infrequently, pulmonary embolism is the incident that first draws attention to the correct diagnosis.

The ***ambulatory patient*** presents with a typical set of complaints that include bursting pain in the foot and calf during exercise. A careful examination will always reveal some degree of edema. Pronounced swelling suggests occlusion of narrow venous channels in the territory of the popliteal vein, common femoral vein, or pelvic channels. Pale blue discoloration of the skin is an important symptom that is best appreciated in the relaxed, dependent limb. Prominence of the superficial veins (*signal veins*) is an additional sign.

A special form of the disease, *phlegmasia alba,* is marked by a blanched appearance of the leg (*milk leg*) due to arterial spasm. In *phlegmasia cerulea dolens,* the most severe form, all the peripheral veins are thrombosed, and there is imminent risk of venous gangrene. Most such cases result from a metastatizing malignant tumor accompanied by a severe systemic coagulation disorder.

When combined, the three cardinal symptoms
provide a high index of suspicion for deep vein
thrombosis. Nevertheless, they raise a wealth of
differential diagnostic problems. Venous com- 365
pression syndromes are of central importance in
this regard (see p. 231). For this reason alone, findings must be objectified by phlebography and duplex scanning before any type of invasive treatment is undertaken.

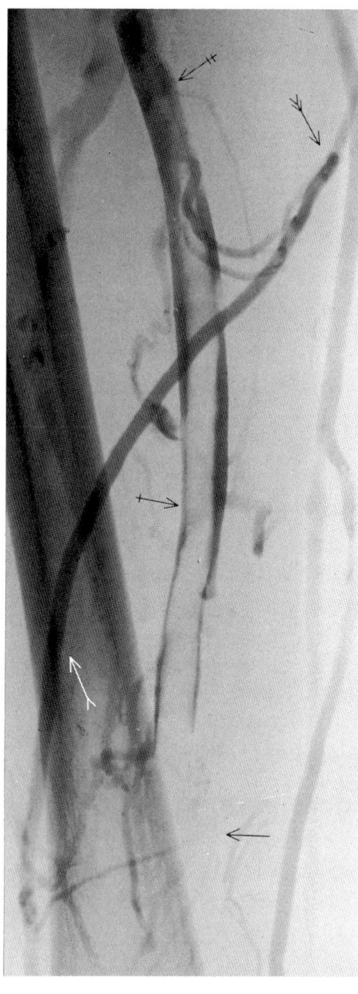

238. Thrombosis of the popliteal vein and superficial femoral vein in a 62-year-old man. Nonfilling of the popliteal vein produces an eraser sign (→). The head of the thrombus is directed downward, the tail upward, with an associated contour sign (↔) and dome sign (⇸). There is collateral flow through the femoropopliteal vein (↣) to the Giacomini anastomosis (⤖)

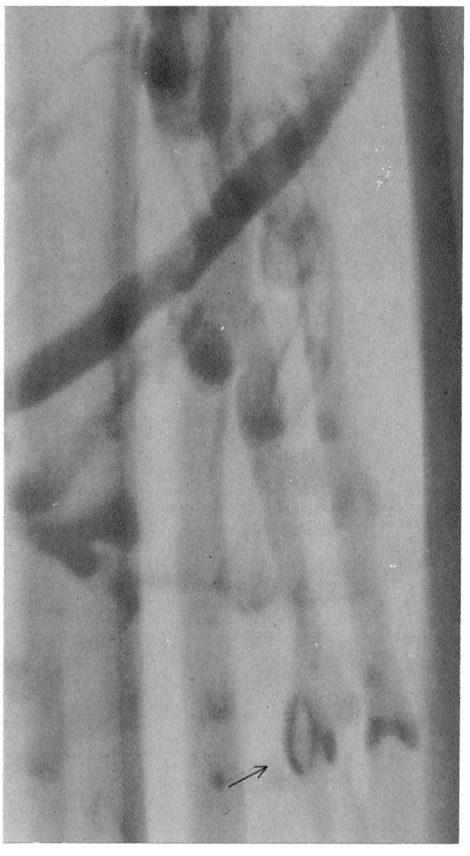

239. Thrombi in the proximal portions of the posterior tibial veins in a 30-year-old man. → Monocle sign on delayed film

Phlebographic Diagnosis

Ascending pressure phlebography is suitable for the diagnosis of deep vein thrombosis. The slightest clinical *suspicion* is sufficient ground for radiography, although real-time sonography and duplex scanning offer viable alternatives. Early detection of the disease should prompt immediate therapeutic measures consisting of anticoagulation, fibrinolysis or thrombectomy in addition to embolic prophylaxis.

Due to the danger of pulmonary embolism, *particular care* must be taken when moving the patient from a bed or stretcher to the X-ray table. Foot baths are contraindicated. Puncture of the dorsal toe vein is more easily accomplished in the sitting position. We first place a warm, damp washcloth over the forefoot for several minutes; this will make the vein prominent even when there is pronounced edema.

With severe thrombosis, the examination is performed with a slight table tilt (approximately 10°). Isolated visualization of the muscle veins is not
possible in this position, however, so a sharp foot- 237
down tilt is needed to define very small thrombi by the *overflow effect* of the contrast medium.
Sedimentation of the medium will give fine delin- 239
eation of the venous valves and their sinuses. The body position of the patient and his ability to support himself on the lateral hand grips will of course depend on the severity of the thrombosis and the patient's general state of health (p. 68).

Good *opacification* of the deep veins of the pelvis and lower extremity can be achieved with a 45%

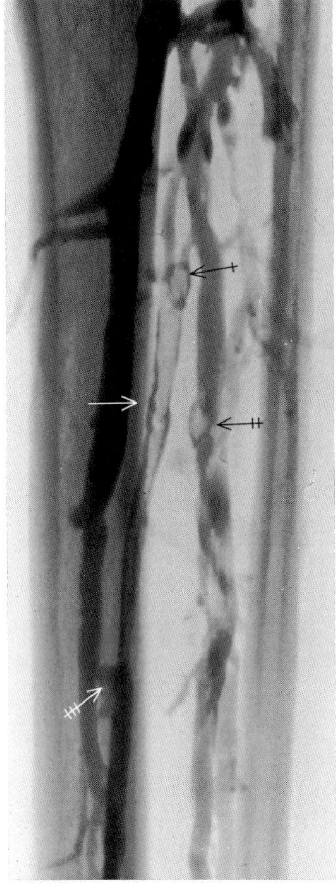

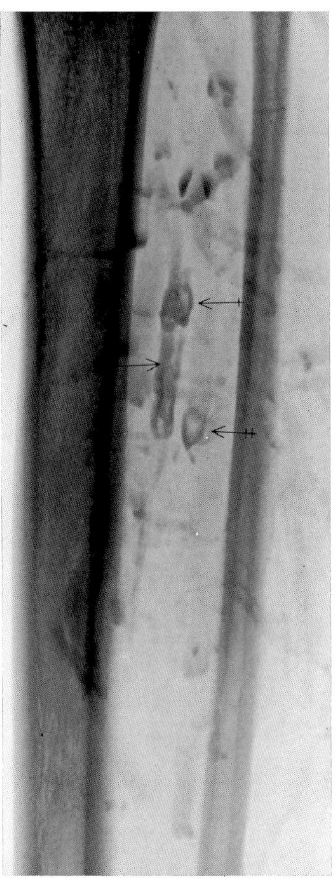

240. Circumscribed thrombosis of the veins of the left lower leg in a 52-year-old man. Clinical symptoms commenced 24 h prior to phlebography. Ascending phlebography with the patient suspended semiupright shows a 10-cm-long thrombus in a posterior tibial venous trunk with a contour sign (→). Eyeglass sign (⇸) from thrombi in the valve pockets, monocle sign (⇻) from thrombus in the fibular vein. Nonopacification of the anterior tibial veins. Collateral flow through a rung vein (⧻→). Internal rotation (*left*) and lateral view (*right*)

contrast solution injected in a dose of 70–100 ml or more. There is no danger of masking of small thrombi located in the valve pockets, although contrast density is easily lost in the more proximal venous channels, especially when thrombosis is extensive.

Injection of the contrast medium is painless when a modern, nonionic agent is used. So far there is no known instance of contrast phlebography inducing thrombus detachment, since manual instillation of the solution does not alter the peripheral venous pressure.

In all cases the thrombus should be filmed on *two planes* to avoid confusion with flow artefacts. A second, *delayed film* is sufficient for documentation of the iliofemoral region. Subtle or ambiguous findings can often be clarified by taking additional films since different aspects are presented as flow conditions change. Given the potential for multifocal occurrence of thrombosis, the examination should always cover the whole venous system, including the pelvic vessels, even in patients with an isolated occlusion.

The phlebographic signs of deep vein thrombosis may be direct or indirect. The direct signs are produced by the form of the thrombus itself, while the indirect, secondary signs relate to associated hemodynamic changes and collateralization.

The ***direct radiologic signs*** function as proof for the diagnosis.

The peripherally located head of the thrombus 240
sometimes presents indistinct contours. The head 242
is usually outlined better in the below-knee stem veins than in the vessels of the iliofemoral region, because opacification tends to be denser in the periphery and because the contrast medium is transported directly to the thrombus by numerous vascular connections. Frequently the origin of the 237

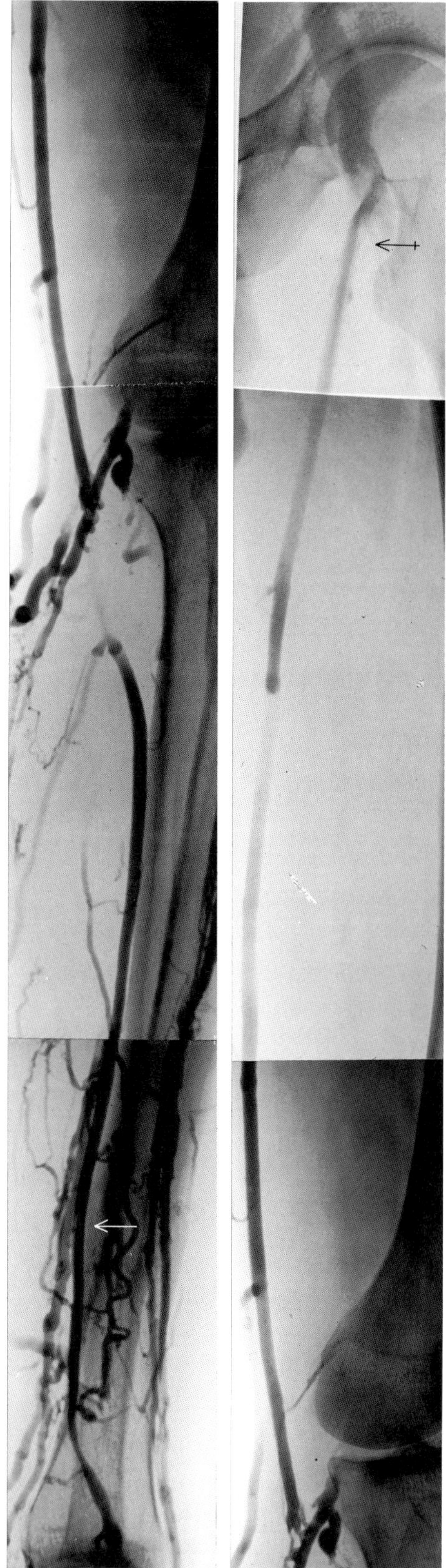

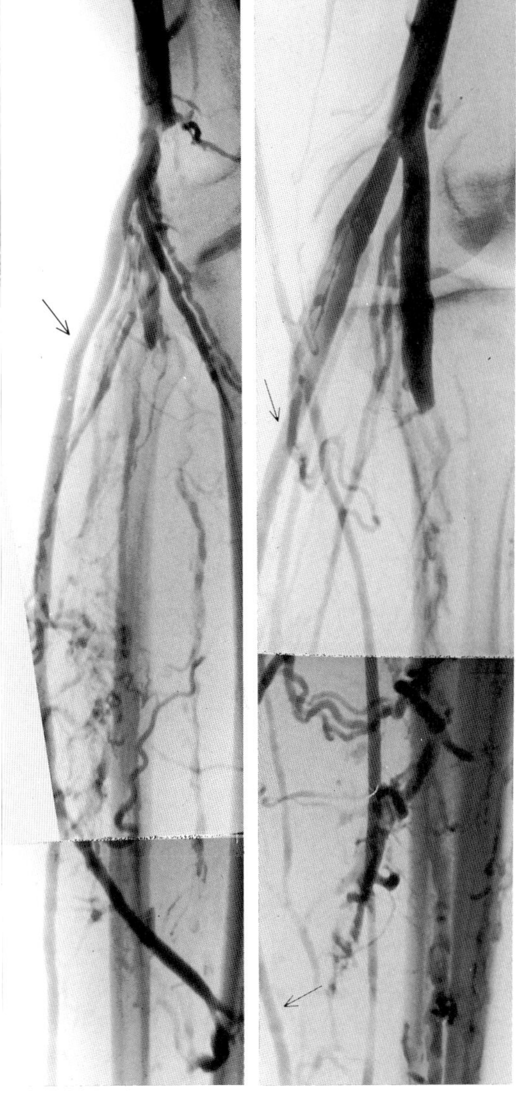

242. Thrombotic occlusion of the stem veins of the lower leg in a 42-year-old man. Main collateral flow is through the small saphenous vein (→). Demonstrated by ascending phlebography in semiupright position, internal rotation (*left*) and lateral view (*right*)

◁

241. Extensive thrombotic occlusion of the deep veins from the mid-lower leg to the groin in a 37-year-old man. There is collateral flow through the ectatic great saphenous vein with dense peripheral opacification of the vessel (→). The lumen is uniformly enlarged and shows no telescope sign (↔). Demonstrated by ascending phlebography in semiupright position in the left lower leg (*left*) and thigh (*right*)

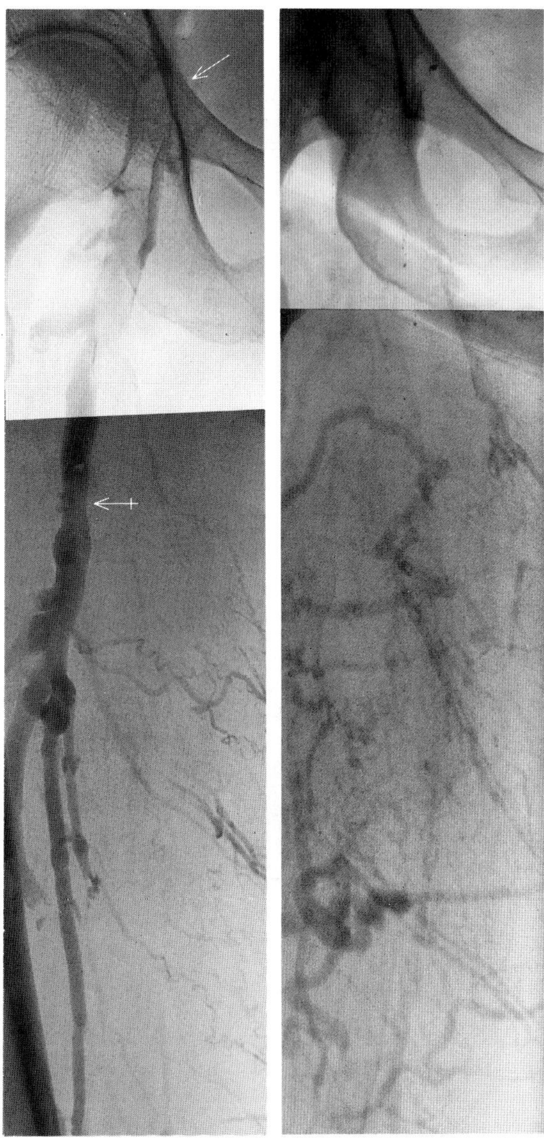

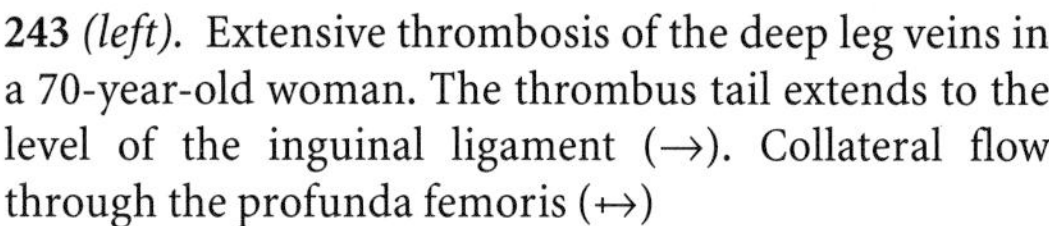

243 *(left).* Extensive thrombosis of the deep leg veins in a 70-year-old woman. The thrombus tail extends to the level of the inguinal ligament (→). Collateral flow through the profunda femoris (↔)

244 *(right).* Extensive phlebothrombosis in a 78-year-old woman. Phlebogram shows tangled networks of muscle veins and superficial vessels

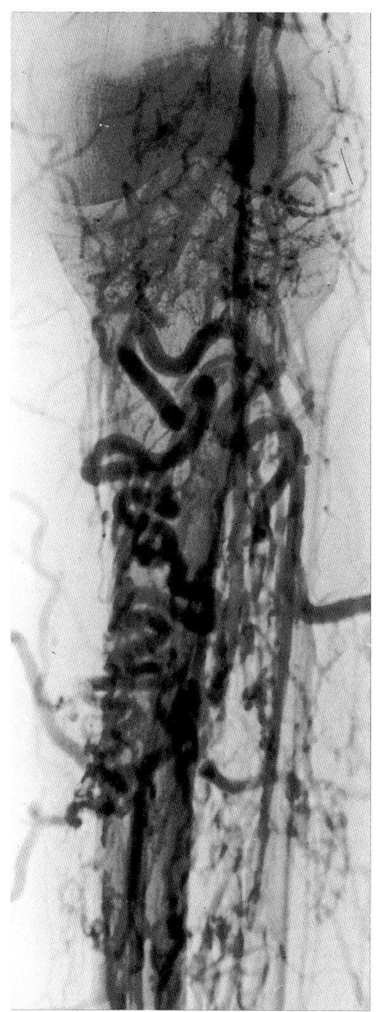

245. Severe thrombosis of the pelvic and leg veins in a 43-year-old woman with metastatic uterine carcinoma. All contrast drainage occurs through muscle veins

thrombus can be identified within a valve pocket. With occlusion of the vein, the apparent *erasure* of thrombus structures from the phlebogram produces an eraser sign.

Contrast medium diverted through superficial
238 and deep collaterals outlines the tail of the thrombus, which forms on the proximal side due to coagulation in the stagnant blood column. The *dome sign* and *contour sign* reflect the thrombus shape. These signs persist in the large stem veins for 2–6 weeks and then gradually are replaced by the features of post-thrombotic syndrome.

With meticulous technique, ascending phlebography can demonstrate thrombi as small as a millet seed. Located in the pockets of the venous valves, these lesions are manifested on phlebograms by a constant filling defect. Unilateral thrombus produces a *monocle sign,* bilateral thrombi an *eyeglass* 239
sign (Hach et al. 1983). The thrombi are particu- 240
larly well defined in the sinuses following contrast runoff from the venous trunk, so a delayed film should be obtained.

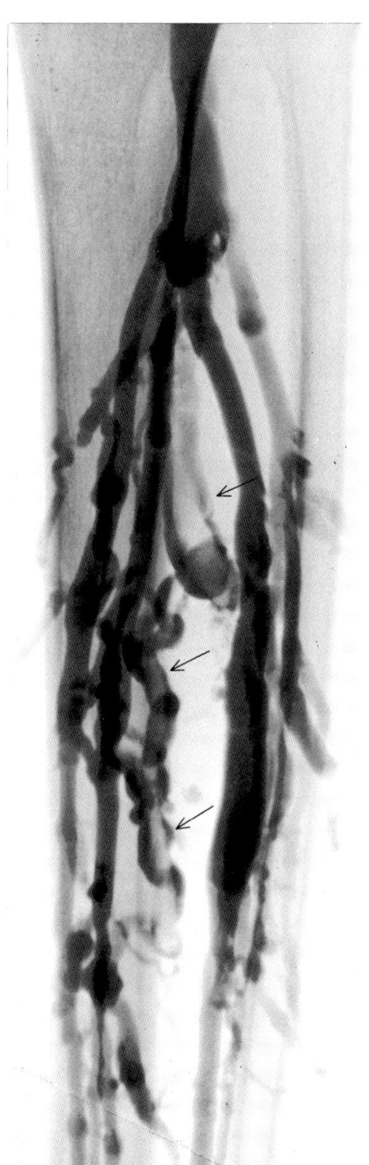

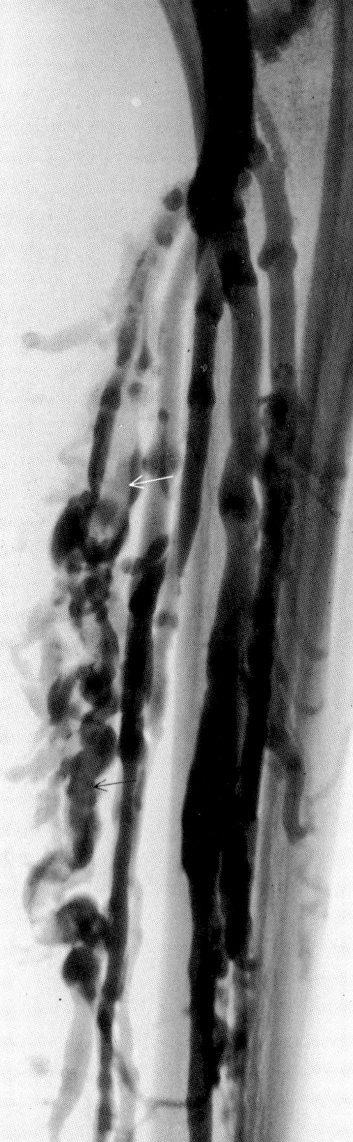

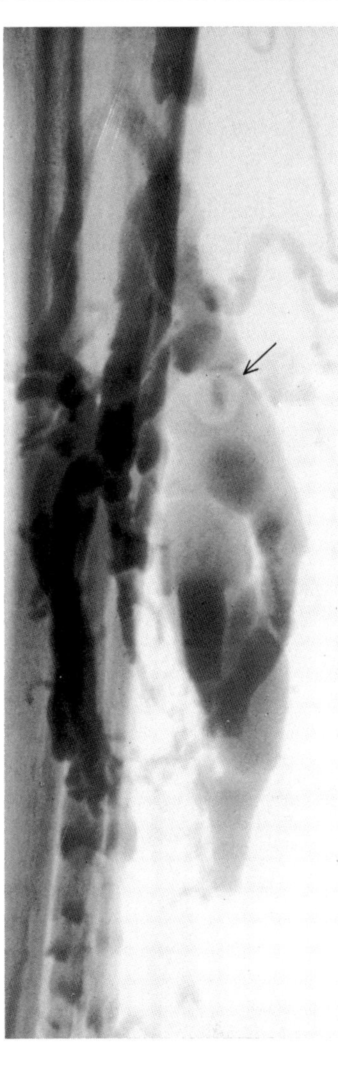

246 *(left, middle).* Thrombosis of the soleus veins (→) in a 51-year-old man. Physiologic ectasia of the fibular vein. Demonstrated by ascending phlebography in semiupright position in the left leg, internal rotation (*left*) and lateral view (*right*)

247 *(right).* Globular thrombus in a soleus vein with severe regressive changes (→) in a 53-year-old man with calf pain of unknown etiology and no clinical abnormalities. Phlebography was performed 4 days after symptom onset. Lateral view of the lower leg

Collateral channels are included among the *indirect signs* of deep vein thrombosis. In patients with extensive occlusions, all of the contrast medium drains through the extrafascial vessels, chiefly
241 the great saphenous vein. When disease is limited
242 to the lower leg, the small saphenous vein is also
available as a collateral pathway.

The *profunda femoris vein* can serve as an important collateral when the superficial femoral vein is
occluded. Communications are established through 243
muscle veins or the distal femoral anastomosis.

If all the intra- and extrafascial trunks in lower leg are occluded, a phlebogram taken after several
days shows a *chaotic pattern* of very small muscle 244
veins and superficial vessels. Associated clinical 245
symptoms are severe.

Tangled plexuses of fine intrafascial vessels appear within the lower leg only 1–2 days after onset of

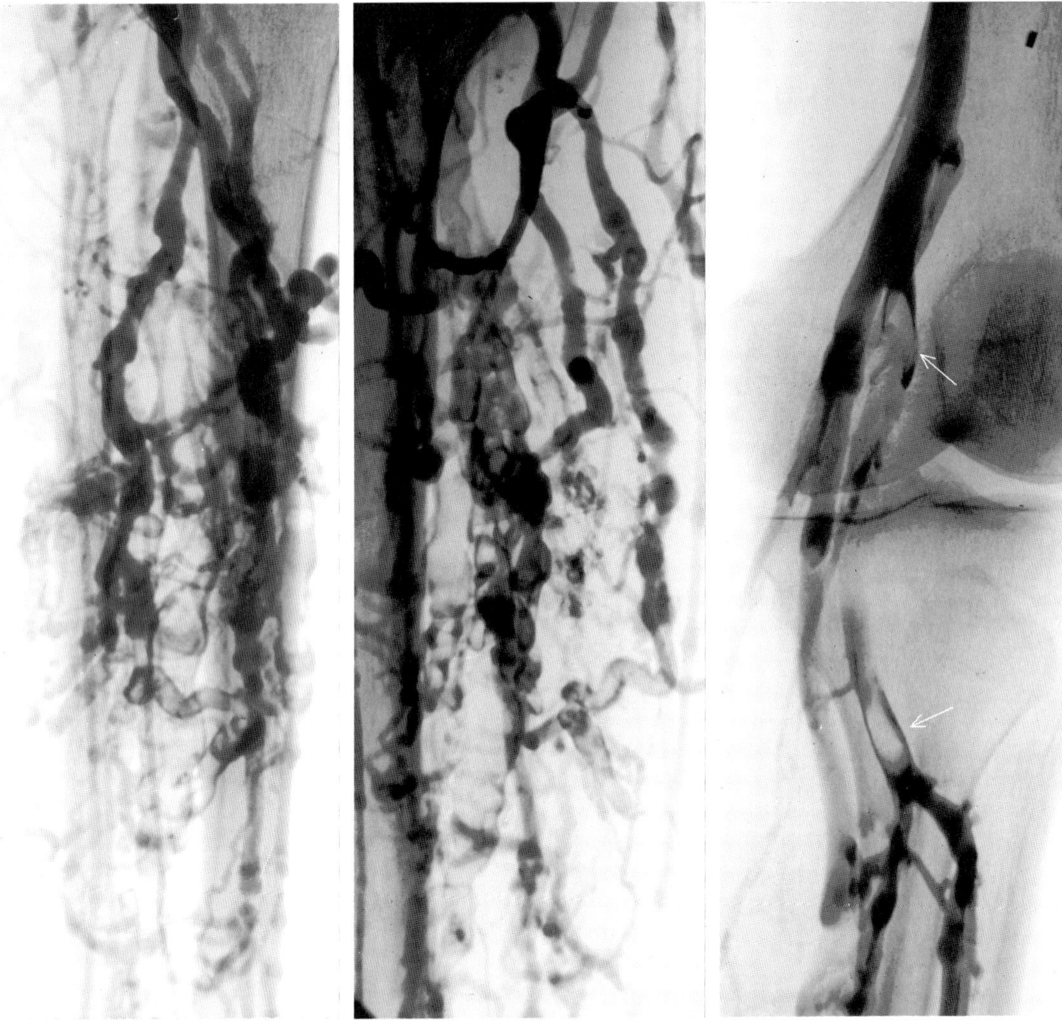

248 *(left, middle).* Extensive thrombosis of the deep stem veins and muscle veins in a 43-year-old woman with metastatic uterine carcinoma. Demonstrated by ascending phlebography in semiupright position, internal rotation (*left*) and lateral view (*right*)

249 *(right).* Thrombosis in one trunk of paired popliteal veins (→) with no apparent cause in a 64-year-old man. Demonstrated by ascending phlebography in semiupright position in the left leg, lateral projection

the disease. Unimportant as collateral pathways, these vessels occur even with very circumscribed thromboses that have no hemodynamic significance. They can persist for months or years following the complete dissolution of a blood clot in the lower leg veins.

Thrombosis in Specific Vascular Regions of the Lower Extremity

246 Isolated thrombosis of the *calf muscle veins* is often obscured on phlebograms by superimposed vessels. It is demonstrated to best advantage by the overflow effect. Thrombi in the dilated sinuses sometimes have a globular shape, similar to that 247
of a thrombus in the cardiac atrium. The cause is probably based on hemodynamic factors. Tiny thrombi are common incidental findings in the veins of the calf and lower leg and may produce no symptoms. They appear to have no clinical relevance.

Deep vein thrombosis in the *lower leg* has various presentations. With total occlusion, the phlebogram initially shows no contrast filling except in extrafascial collaterals. Within a few days, however, a chaotic pattern of small veins appears with 248
little or no evidence of larger vessels.

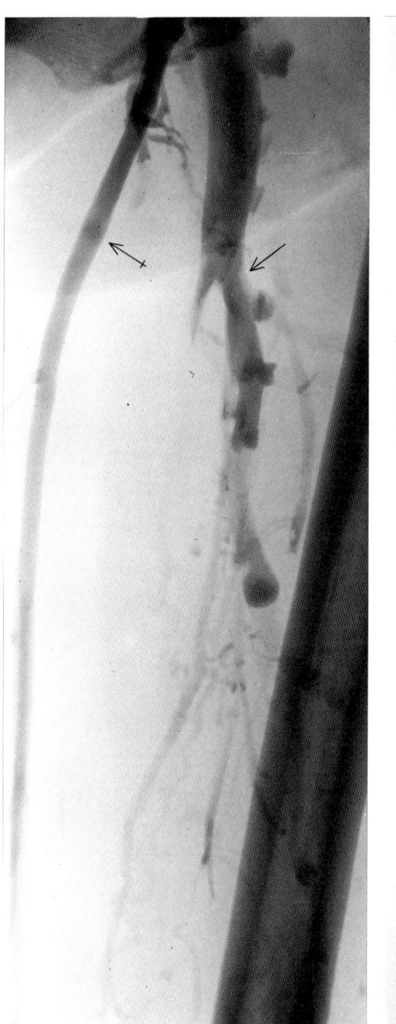

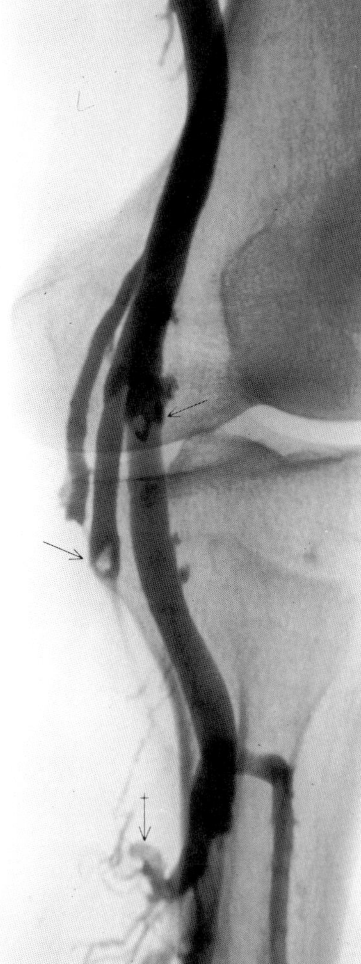

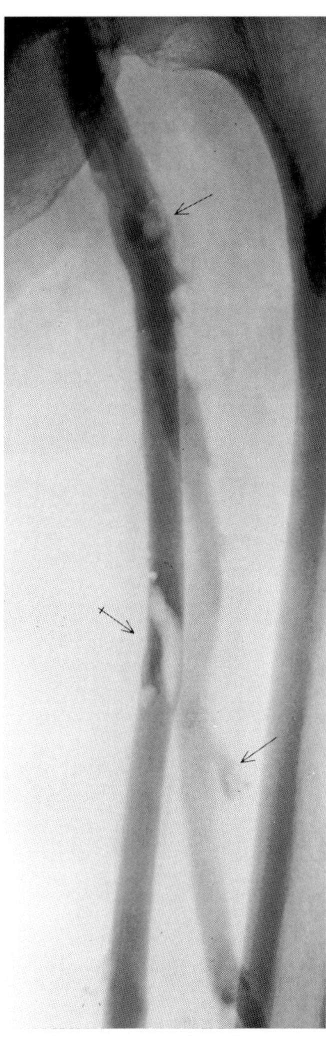

250 *(left).* Ascending thrombosis of the superficial femoral vein in a 52-year-old woman. No apparent cause. The thrombus tail terminates at the entry of the profunda femoris vein (→). Phlebectasia of the great saphenous vein (↔). Demonstrated by ascending phlebography in the left leg

251 *(middle, right).* Multiple thrombi in the valve pockets of the lower extremity veins in an 81-year-old man with metastatic pancreatic carcinoma. → Monocle sign; ↔ thrombi propagating into the lumen. Phlebograms of the left leg. *Left,* lateral film of the popliteal vein. *Right,* superficial femoral vein

249 Thrombosis of the *popliteal vein* has considerable practical significance. It often occurs as an "exertional thrombosis" (thrombose par effort; Schmitt 1977) or "weekend thrombosis" in younger individuals unaccustomed to strenuous recreational activity. It is known as "economy class syndrome" or "tourists thrombosis" following long-distance flights. Mechanical endothelial damage is the most likely nidus for thrombus formation. After a long period of sitting down, the hematocrit in the vessels of the legs increases, leading to unfavorable changes in the regional hemodynamics.

The thrombus usually propagates into the *superficial femoral vein* from below. It often terminates at 250
the entry of the profunda femoris vein due to the
inceased blood flow velocity at that site. But
thrombosis can also arise within the femoral veins 251
themselves or descend into them from a more 252
proximal level. 253

Sites of origin of deep vein thrombosis in the lower extremity	
Common iliac vein	10 %
Femoral vein	50 %
Popliteal vein	20 %
Calf veins	20 %

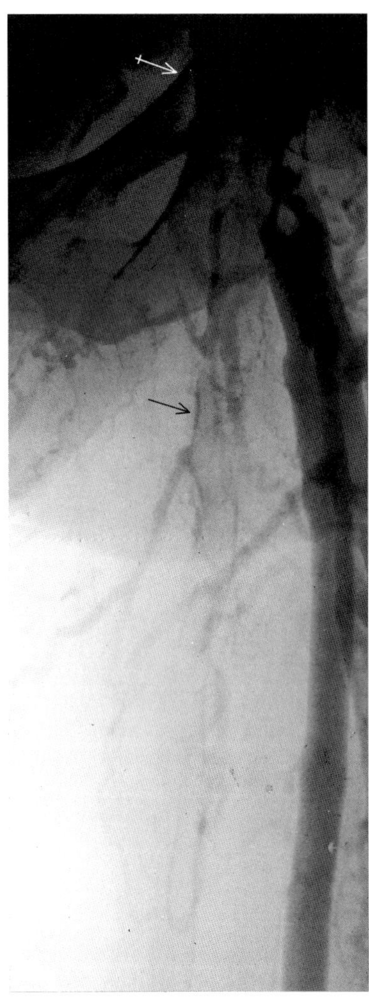

252. Ascending transfascial pelvic vein thrombosis on the left side in a 72-year-old woman with severe varicosity of the great saphenous vein. Ascending phlebography was performed 6 days after onset of varicophlebitis with severe swelling of the leg. The film shows thrombi in the great saphenous vein, dilated to finger thickness (→), and occlusion of the pelvic veins upward from the saphenous termination (↔)

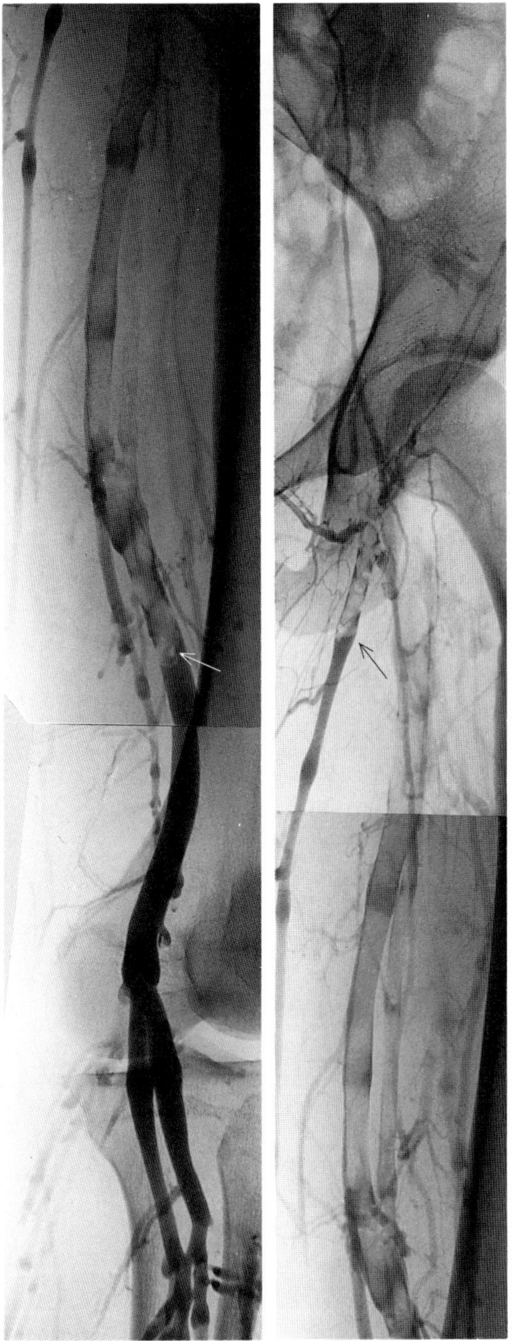

253. Descending left iliofemoral vein thrombosis in a 20-year-old woman, probably secondary to a pelvic venous spur. Ascending phlebography in semiupright position was performed 2 days after symptom onset. Typical pattern with occlusion of the proximal channel and normal filling of the periphery; stalactite sign (→). *Left,* peripheral veins. *Right,* iliofemoral veins

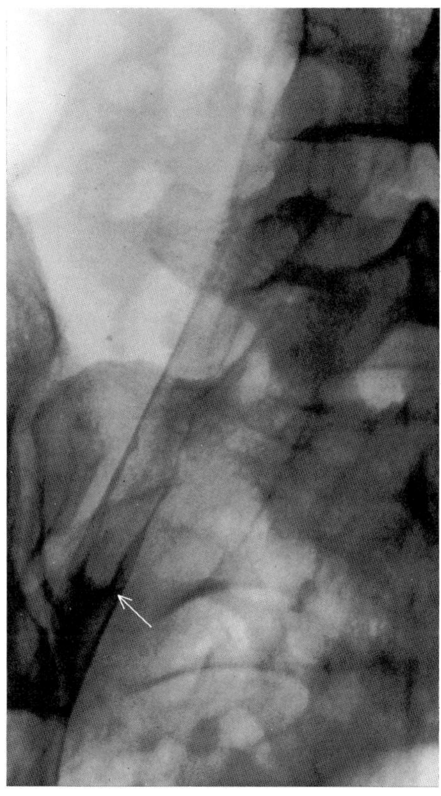

254. Stalactite sign (→) from a 5-cm-long occlusive thrombus in the external iliac vein of a 31-year-old woman with venous compression syndrome due to perivascular fibrosis (see also Fig. 267)

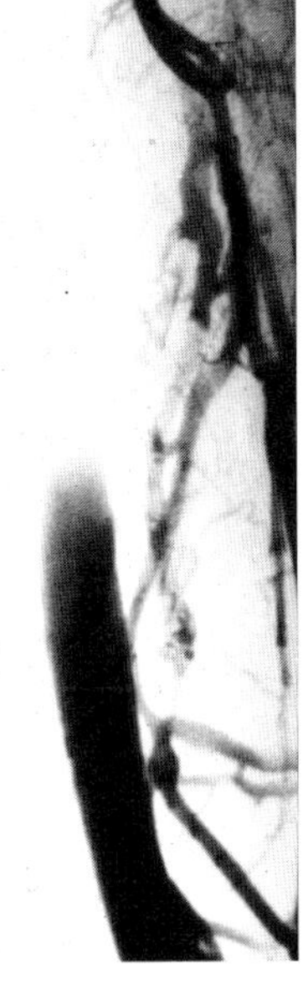

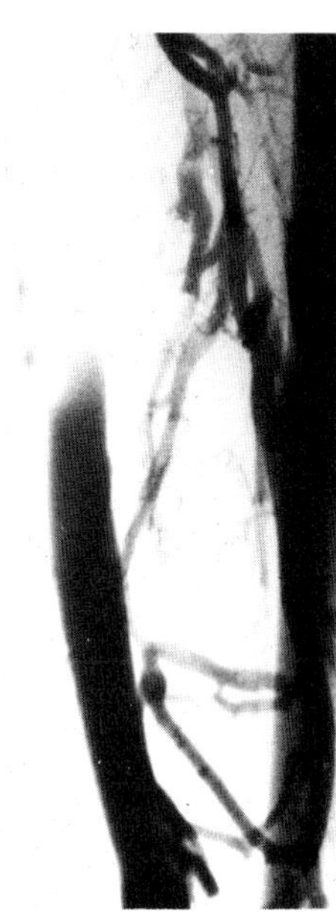

255. Back-up sign of descending iliofemoral venous thrombosis in a 24-year-old woman, probably caused by a pelvic vein spur. The stagnant opaque column is below the occlusion of the superficial femoral vein. Ascending phlebograms with the patient in a semiupright position taken about 1 min apart during fibrinolysis show almost identical findings in the left thigh

Forms of Iliofemoral Venous Thrombosis

Under unfavorable conditions the phlebothrom-
235 bosis will propagate in an antegrade or retrograde direction. This can have important therapeutic implications in the iliofemoral region, so it is useful to distinguish between the ascending and descending forms on phlebograms whenever possible.

250 ***Ascending iliofemoral venous thrombosis*** begins as a unifocal or multifocal thrombosis within the crural or popliteofemoral circulation. It is plainly manifested by the dome and contour signs on phlebograms.

From a *varicophlebitis* of the great saphenous
252 vein, the thrombus can occasionally propagate transfascially past the saphenous termination into the common femoral vein. Once again, assessment of the direct radiographic signs will permit a specific diagnosis to be made.

253 Recognition of the ***descending form*** is of considerable therapeutic importance. It is usually based on an intra- or extravascular outflow obstruction in the iliofemoral pathway. *Intravascular occlusion* may be caused by a pelvic venous spur. This contrasts with the *extrinsic occlusion* produced by compression syndromes, which can occur at all levels of the lower extremity and retroperitoneal space (see p. 231).

Descending iliofemoral venous thrombosis presents characteristic *phlebographic features* (Hach et al. 1983). An important indirect sign is the *typical* location of the occluding thrombi in the proximal venous segments while the below-knee vessels remain patent (*local pattern sign*).

A pathognomonic feature is the *stalactite sign*. The
tail of the thrombus is directed distally, contrasting 254
with the dome sign seen in the ascending forms.

The *back-up sign* also can appear in the large stem
veins under certain conditions. Stagnation of 255
blood flow in front of the occlusion leads to a damming back of the opaque column. Marked by lack of change on serial films, this situation is occasionally seen in patients receiving effective anticoagulant or fibinolytic therapy.

In selected cases, descending iliofemoral venous thrombosis initially requires reopening of the flow

path by distant embolectomy followed by removal of the causal outflow obstruction through direct vascular reconstruction or a bypass procedure.
251 The polytopic form is typical of paraneoplastic syndrome with severely disturbed blood clotting.

Special Problems and Pitfalls

101 The most common source of misinterpretation in
237 the diagnosis of thrombosis is the *eraser sign.* Lacking direct evidence of thrombosis, the non-opacification of a vessel does not necessarily signify an occluding thrombus. Nonfilling or delayed filling may be observed even in normal veins. This is especially true in the lower leg veins when the
102 supramelleolar tourniquet is placed too tightly or the contrast medium was injected not into the dorsal toe vein but at the ankle or lateral side of the foot. Venous spasms in proximity to an inflammatory process can simulate an occlusion. An *arteriovenous fistula* also causes an empty phlebogram distally. The eraser sign is *conclusive only* when combined with the dome and contour signs and perhaps with the monocle or eyeglass sign.

Dilution and sedimentation of the contrast medium in larger veins can occasionally produce *flow*
387 *artefacts,* especially at the outlets of small tribu-
389 taries, that may be mistaken for thrombi (see p. 244).

256 The *superimposition* of several veins in the lower leg can sometimes mimic the contour sign of thrombus. This error is quickly resolved by scrutinizing the course of the vessel and obtaining biplane projections. With extensive pelvic and lower limb venous thrombosis, ascending phlebography is usually not sufficient to permit a differentiated assessment of the pelvic vessels. These can be defined more clearly by injecting additional contrast medium into a superficial vein of the groin region. Transfemoral pelvic phlebography appears to be indicated only if the common femoral vein is free of thrombi. *Digital substraction angiography* can be a very useful adjunct in these cases.

It is important for therapeutic and especially pre-
267 operative planning to know whether a thrombus extends into the inferior vena cava, as this would imply an increased *risk of embolization.* This involvement can be confirmed or excluded by pelvic phlebography on the opposite side, by digital subtraction angiography, and of course by computed tomography or magnetic resonance imaging. In all cases the apparently healthy limb should also be examined radiographically. It is not uncommon for the opposite leg to harbor a circumscribed thrombosis whose symptoms are masked by the predominant disease in the other leg.

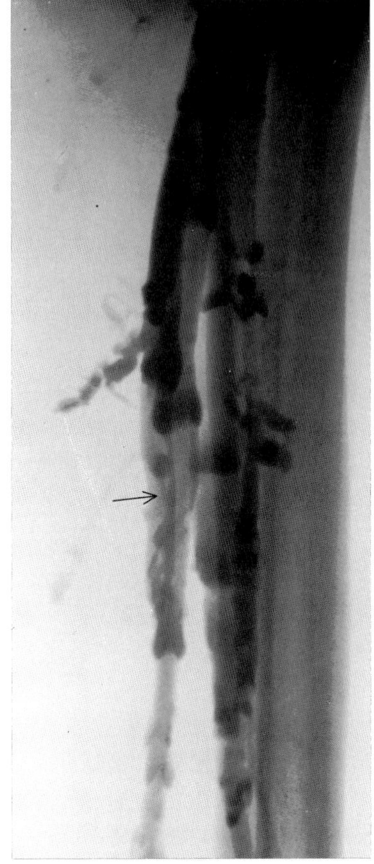

256. Superimposition of the posterior tibial veins and fibular vein mimics a thrombus (→). Demonstrated by ascending pressure phlebography, lateral view of the left leg

The relationship between the X-ray morphologic substrate of a thrombus and the natural history of the disease is extremely variable in the short term. In one patient thrombi in the lower leg veins may resolve completely in a week with heparin therapy, leaving no residual signs or complaints, while phlebograms in another patient may show essentially the same appearance of a floating thrombus in the superficial femoral vein even after a month. In principle, then, the *age of a thrombus* can be estimated from phlebograms with resonable accuracy only when the process is more than about 6 weeks old. Appositional thromboses further complicate the situation.

Value of Other Diagnostic Methods Compared with Phlebography

The possibility of deep vein thrombosis in the pelvis or lower extremity is a question that arises very frequently at bedside and in the office setting. Besides the clinical evaluation, basically two types of diagnostic procedure are available: global and selective. The *global methods* furnish physiologic data on venous circulatory parameters (pressure, capacity, drainage), measure changes in skin temperature, or trace the behavior of injected radioactive substances. The *selective procedures*, by contrast, furnish precise information on the function and morphology of a specific venous segment by the use of ultrasound or by imaging the vessels with contrast media or radionuclides. Imaging procedures are indispensable for the planning of causal therapy.

The crural, popliteofemoral, and iliocaval regions of the venous circulation must be *evaluated differently* with regard to the clinical presentation of phlebothrombosis as well as the course of the disease and therapeutic implications. With the exception of phlebography, considered the reference standard, the various diagnostic methods are not equally rewarding in different regions of the venous circulation.

Methods available for the diagnostic evaluation of venous thrombosis
Clinical examinations
Global measurements
Selective and imaging procedures

Suitability of various methods for diagnosing thrombosis in the crural, popliteofemoral and iliocaval regions			
Diagnostic method	Usefulness		
	Vascular region		
	Crural	Popliteo-femoral	Iliocaval
Clinical examination			
Outpatient	++	++	+
Hospitalized patient	0	0	(+)
Physical methods			
Doppler ultrasound	0	++	++
Plethysmography	0	++	++
Thermography	+	+	0
Nuclear medicine tests	++	(+)	0
Imaging procedures			
Real-time sonography	+	++	+
Color-coded duplex	++	+++	++
Contrast phlebography	+++	+++	+++
Isotope phlebography	(+)	(+)	(+)

The ***clinical diagnosis*** of venous thrombosis is called into question by a high percentage of false-negative and false-positive cases. Vinazzer (1981) states that only 20% of deep vein thromboses in the pelvis and lower extremity are clinically detectable. Significantly, the manifestations of phlebothrombosis are quite different in ambulatory patients than in immobilized patients. The *cardinal symptoms* – bursting calf pain during exercise, acute ankle edema, and faint cyanosis in the dependent extremity compared with the opposite side – are manifested only during hydrostatic physical exertion. In patients on *strict bed rest*, thrombosis of the leg veins causes no symptoms whatsoever while pelvic vein thrombosis is associated with twinging pains in the lumbar region that initially suggest a renal cause. This impression may be reinforced by mild micturition difficulties and increased sensitivity on rectal examination. *General symptoms* include febrile temperatures of unknown origin and episodes of mild tachycardia. Then, when the patient stands upright for the first time, a pulmonary embolism strikes "from the blue." It is not surprising that embolization from an undetected thrombosis still accounts for 30% of all embolism cases (Barthels 1979).

Today ***Doppler ultrasound*** is used routinely as a screening test for deep vein thrombosis. The ex-

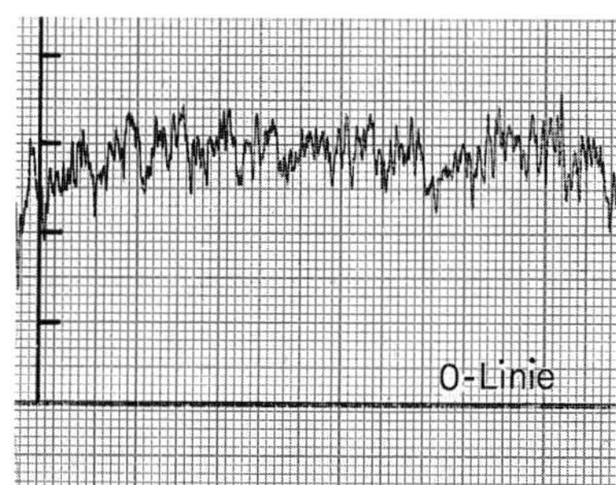

257. High-frequency continual flow noise in the groin region in thrombotic occlusion of the common femoral vein. No breathing modulation. A-sounds cannot be evoked

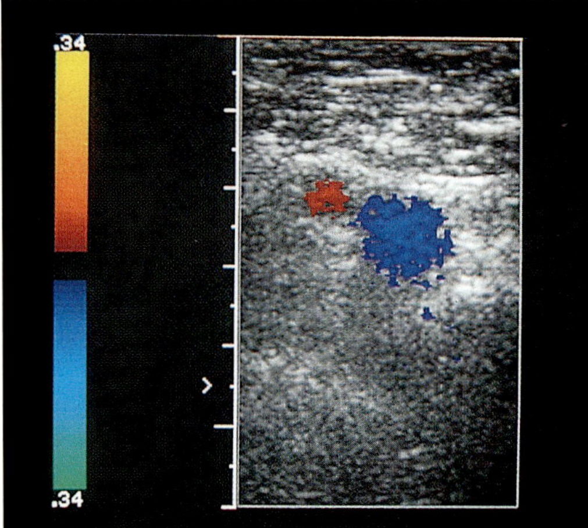

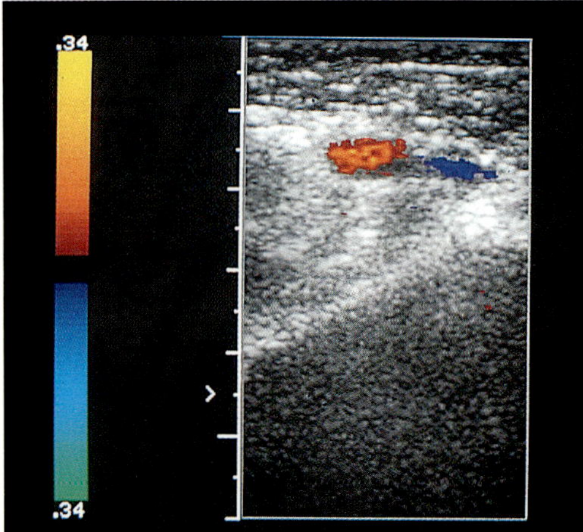

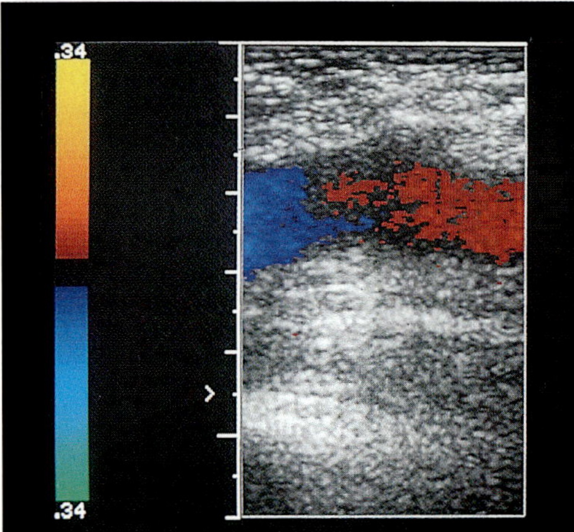

258. Compressibility of the normal common femoral vein. *Top,* cross-section of the artery and vein. *Middle,* compression of the vein (cross-section). *Bottom,* longitudinal section of the common femoral vein. Color coding: *blue,* blood flow away from the transducer; *red,* towards the transducer. Black areas in the middle due to unfavorable Doppler angle (no thrombi). (Acuson, 7-MHz transducer)

aminer may employ a simple pocket instrument or
a more sophisticated directional technique. When
a large stem vein is occluded, the peripheral venous pressure rises. Most of the blood is routed
through small collaterals, so the flow velocity in
these vessels is greatly increased. Phasic respiratory variations are abolished in favor of continuous,
high-frequency spontaneous sounds (S-sounds),
which are not disrupted even by a brief Valsalva 257
maneuver. The high blood volume is already placing a maximum load on the collateral veins, and
(careful) manual calf compression does not augment venous flow as it does under normal circumstances; augmentation sounds (A-sounds) cannot
be elicited (see p. 79).

Doppler ultrasound is not useful in the below-knee veins. At the popliteal and femoral levels, Doppler has a sensitivity of 65%–79% and a specificity of 51%–90%. It is most accurate in the diagnosis of pelvic vein thrombosis, offering a sensitivity of 91%–93% and specificity of 90%–93% compared with ascending phlebography (further references in Hach et al. 1989 and Wuppermann 1986). Important causes of false-negative diagnoses are calf muscle vein thrombosis and nonoccluding thrombi in an adjacent vessel. False-positive findings are produced by acute venous compression syndromes.

Sonographic imaging and the type-specific information it provides is now an indispensible part of the diagnostic workup of thrombosis.

Phlebography *and* sonography contribute most to the primary diagnosis of venous thrombosis when they are used jointly. In principle it does not matter which study takes precedence, although the ultrasound examination can be conducted more efficiently when the radiographic findings are known. Phlebography requires 3–5 min, while ultrasound scrutiny of the complete infrarenal venous system takes 30 min and often much longer. The examination time can be greatly shortened by concentrating the scans on the vascular regions of interest.

A fresh thrombus has the same echogenicity as
flowing blood on ***real-time ultrasound scans,*** so it
cannot be directly visualized during the examination. Nevertheless, the indirect signs of thrombosis still offer a high sensitivity and specificity. The
most important sign is lack of vein *compressibility*
in cross-section. Of course this test is of limited 258
usefulness in the pelvic veins. 260

Vascular occlusion abolishes the normal *phasic respiratory variations* of blood flow in the large

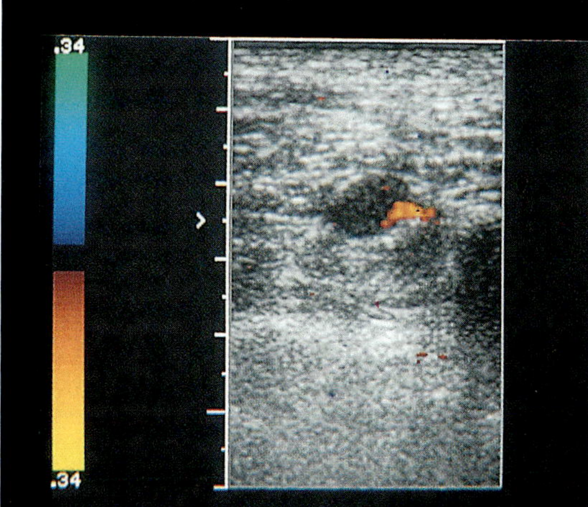

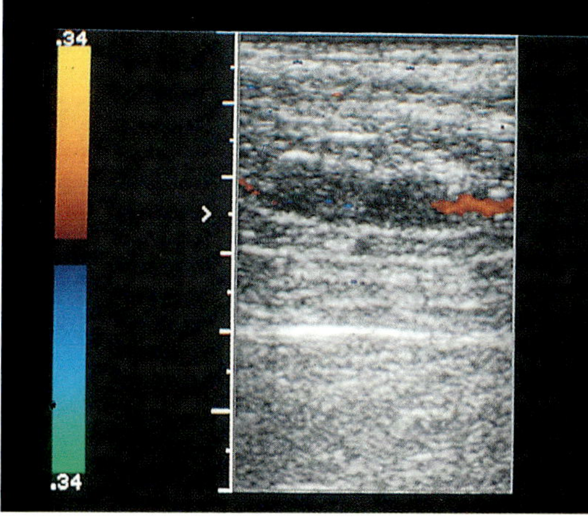

259. Thrombi in both trunks of the posterior tibial veins. Arteries coded *red. Top,* cross-section. *Bottom,* longitudinal section. (Acuson, 7-MHz transducer)

Advantages and disadvantages of phlebography and color-coded duplex scanning in the primary diagnosis of thrombosis

Criterion	Phlebography	Sonography
Direct visualization of a thrombus		
Occlusive	Reference procedure	Equivalent
Nonocclusive	Reference procedure	Easily missed
Evaluation of extent	Reference procedure	Equivalent
Evaluation of special forms	Reference procedure	Difficult
Evaluation of collaterals	Reference procedure	Not possible
Assessment of thrombus age	Imprecise approximation	Rough
Evaluation of the vein wall	Not possible	Excellent
Evaluation of perivascular structures	Not possible	Excellent
Length of examination	2–5 min	20–30 min
Risks of examination	Minimal	None
Patient discomfort	Minimal	Minimal
Documentation	Clear, comprehensive	Limited in scope
Interpretation by a second observer	Reproducible	Uncertain
Cost	Reasonable	Low

axial veins. The occluded vessel does not dilate in response to a Valsalva maneuver. The *double-stroke phenomenon* in the vena cava caused by cardiac pressure fluctuations is also lost.

A fresh thrombus causes *luminal expansion,* which is easily appreciated on comparison with the opposite side. This finding appears to be especially important in the lower leg veins. If the crural veins and muscle vein sinuses can be visualized by ultrasound and are noncompressible, a presump-
259 tive diagnosis of thrombosis can be made. The thrombosed inferior vena cava also is easily recognized by the tense, constant enlargement of its lumen.

Within a few days, foci of increased *acoustic impedance* appear within the thrombus that are easily distinguished from flowing blood. Zones of contrasting echogenicity represent areas of different age. It was originally hoped that these features would be useful for predicting the efficacy of thrombolytic therapy, but results in this area have been somewhat disappointing.

Thrombosis consistently incites an inflammatory *response in the vessel wall* and perivascular tissue. Sonography is effective for the detection and diagnostic evaluation of these changes. The vein wall appears markedly thickened and echogenic.

The introduction of ***color-coded duplex scanning*** and the ability to record slow-moving blood have greatly advanced the ultrasound diagnosis of venous thrombosis. With color-coded duplex we can define the boundary between the occluding

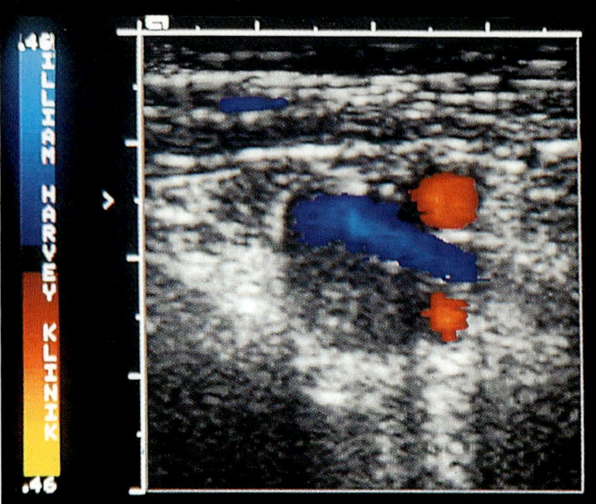

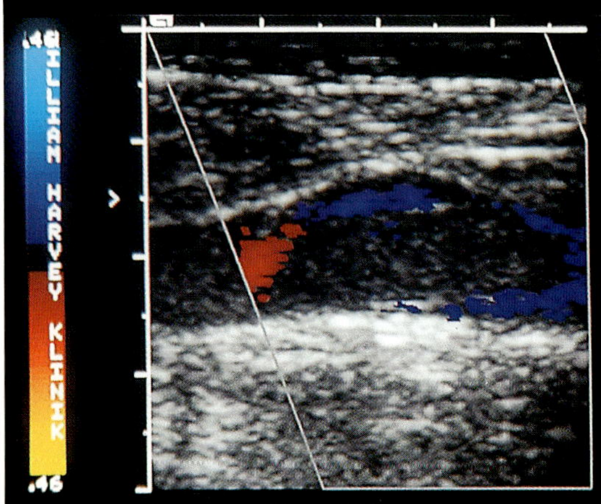

260. Nonocclusive thrombus at the level of the femoral bifurcation. Enlarged lumen at the level of the thrombus. Intravascular formation clearly shown by sonography. Increased thickness of vascular wall. *Top,* cross-section. Remaining lumen coded *blue. Bottom,* longitudinal section. Remaining lumina coded *blue* and *red.* Color-coded duplex sonography. (Acuson, 7-MHz transducer)

Real-time sonographic features of thrombosis in various vascular regions
Lack of vein compressibility
Constant dilatation of the vessel lumen
Lack of respiratory modulation and cardiac pressure fluctuations (vena cava)
Increased intraluminal echogenicity
Increased echogenicity and thickening of the vein wall

Advantages of real-time sonography and duplex scanning
Noninvasiveness
Short-term follow-ups
Immediate interpretation of findings
Assessment of the age of a thrombus and its components
Assessment of the vessel wall
Examination of perivascular tissues

thrombus and the surrounding unobstructed lumen in less time with greater precision. This ap-
260 pears to be important for the evaluation of apposition thrombi. A prospective study by Grosser et al. (1990) showed that, compared with phlebography, the procedure was 99% sensitive and 94% specific in the primary diagnosis of phlebothrombosis, regardless of the affected vascular region.

Color-coded sonography should be performed by an experienced examiner using high-quality equipment. When these conditions are met, color-coded duplex scanning can compete with phlebography in the diagnosis of thrombosis. Because it is noninvasive, it can be repeated as often as desired. The study is ideal for *short-term follow-ups,* especially during fibrinolytic therapy or after a revascularizing procedure.

A major advantage of duplex scanning over phlebography is the ability to assess *perivascular structures* and *the vein wall* itself. This makes it excellent for the prompt diagnosis of extravascular compression syndromes, which are most commonly caused by tumors, cysts, aneurysms, or perivascular callosities (see p. 231).

The disadvantageous of color-coded duplex scanning are obvious. Examination of the complete venous system is very *time-consuming.* Even an experienced examiner using meticulous technique can easily overlook nonocclusive thrombi. The iliac vessels, the adductor canal region, and the muscular veins are sometimes difficult to visualize clearly.

Real-time scanning interrogates only a small portion of the vascular system at any one time. In the evaluation of phlebothrombosis, however, consideration must be given to more general hemodynamic status of the limb, especially the presence and type of *collateral circulations,* which is an essential factor in therapeutic decision making.

One temporary problem is *lack of acceptance* of the unaccustomed format of color-coded duplex findings at many institutions, but this should change with passage of time.

The fact that color-coded sonography is noninvasive and does not require the use of contrast medium is a considerable advantage compared to phlebography. However, the modern X-ray examination technique and the development of nonionic contrast media have reduced the risk of phlebography to a statistically almost nonsignificant level. This minimal residual risk should be weighed against the advantages of a thorough morphologic diagnosis and its therapeutic consequences in each case.

As far as the costs are concerned, centers that carry out interventional treatment of vascular disorders should have both the radiographic and the corresponding sonographic types of equipment. Seen as a whole, the *operating costs* of the two methods are comparable when the cost of radiographic contrast medium and film is set off against the additional physician time required for a sonographic investigation.

Our comparison of the sonographic and radiographic modalities in no way diminishes the status of contrast phlebography as the "gold standard." When it comes to the *yes/no question* of whether or not a clinically relevant thrombosis is present, sonography can furnish an answer with extremely high confidence. Both methods are suitable for the primary diagnosis of thrombosis and appear to be interchangable *in this regard*. Beyond this, though, they supply very different types of diagnostic information which underscore their essentially complementary roles (golden partnership).

Plethysmography also appears to be a suitable screening test for popliteal and iliofemoral vein thrombosis (Hach 1981). The delay of maximum outflow rate and decrease in venous capacitance are 73 %–96 % sensitive and 80 %–99 % specific for diagnosing this disease (Wuppermann 1986). As in ultrasound flowmetry, circumscribed thromboses with slight hemodynamic effect and acute compression syndromes can lead to false-positive and false-positive findings.

The ***^{125}I fibrinogen uptake test*** is used not only as a research tool but also for the detection and localization of an established thrombosis. Today the substitution of ^{99m}Tc-labeled plasmin offers various advantages. In the lower leg, the radionuclide techniques show agreement with phlebographic findings in 90 % of cases. They are less reliable in the thigh, however, and they are unable to detect thrombus in the pelvic region (further references in Mostbeck 1981).

Phlebothrombosis is associated with a local rise in temperature. Sensitive thermal-radiation measuring instruments have revealed skin temperature discrepancies on the order of 0.2 °C. The newest instruments can record temperature profiles and analyze them numerically. ***Thermography*** in the lower leg is up to 95 % sensitive in the diagnosis of thrombosis, although its specificity is only 47 % (Jacobssen 1983). This technique has found only limited use due to high equipment procurement costs.

Sources of error in Doppler examinations of phlebothrombosis
Venous compression syndrome
Thrombi in adjacent vessels
Thrombosis in a reduplicated trunk
Nonocclusive thrombosis
Good collateralization of the occlusion
Continuous flow during thoracic respiration
Hyperemia from an inflammatory process
Faulty examination technique

Prophylaxis of Thromboembolism

When phlebography demonstrates deep venous thrombi in the pelvis or lower extremity, appropriate secondary antithrombotic measures should be instituted at once while definitive treatment is being planned. The intravenous injection of 5000 U *heparin* will reduce blood coagulability and retard progression of the thrombosis for approximately 3 h (even with contrast injection). With its short half-life, heparin will not affect subsequent therapeutic deliberations. Preliminary coagulation tests are unnecessary in patients with no prior history of excessive bleeding risk. Patients already taking *coumarin derivatives* will require no additional anticoagulant measures in the short term. Intramuscular injections are contraindicated in any case so as not to interfere with subsequent fibrinolytic therapy.

Besides secondary thromboprophylaxis, a high priority is placed on the prevention of pulmonary embolism. The *compression bandage* is a very effective appliance in this regard. The elastic band-

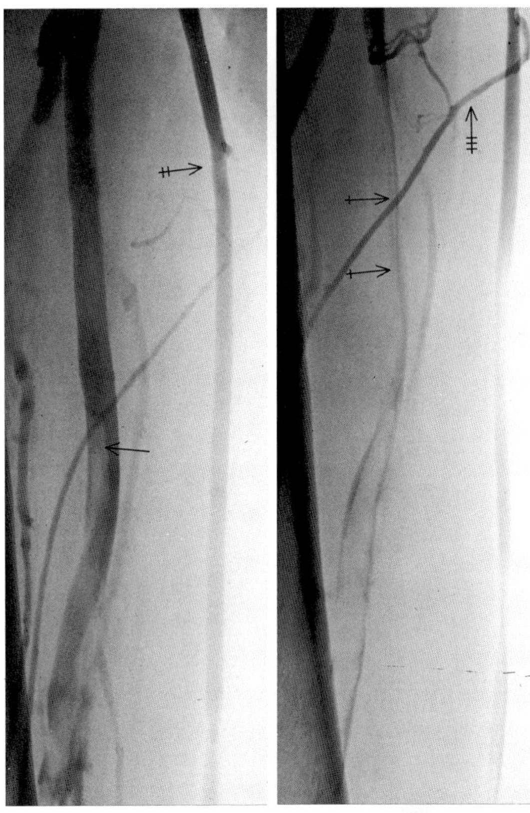

261. Effect of a compression bandage on venous hemodynamics, demonstrated by ascending phlebography in vertical position. *Left,* floating thrombus in the superficial femoral vein (→); phlebectasia of the great saphenous vein (⇸). *Right,* post-compression-bandaging film shows luminal constriction of the superficial femoral vein (⇸) with a reduced risk of pulmonary embolism. Marked acceleration of blood flow. Giacomini's anastomosis (⇻) to the great saphenous vein

age constricts the vessel lumina, thereby fixing the
261 thrombus to the vessel wall. The elastic support is so reliably effective that the patient should continue to wear it as long as the thrombose remains confined to the lower limb veins.

At institutes where phlebographic examinations are performed routinely, an assistant must master the technique of compression bandaging. This includes specialized knowledge about the material properties of elastic tapes, foam paddings, and adhesive bandages. An exchange of experience with a phlebologist may also be helpful.

In patients with *pelvic vein thrombosis,* external compression is ineffective for preventing pulmonary embolism, and it may be appropriate to place the patient on bed rest for approximately 10 days, counting from the probable onset of the thrombosis. On the other hand, strict bed rest is considered the major risk factor in thrombogenesis, especially in older patients, so the various factors must be weighed on an individual basis. The *risk of embolism is* greatest when pelvic vein thrombosis has developed in a seriously ill, bed-confined patient who has not yet gotten to his feet. In this situation, *preventive* color duplex sonography is therefore recommended. Once venous thrombosis is documented, patient care is turned over completely to the attending physician in charge.

Therapeutic Implications

The basic goal in the treatment of occlusive deep vein thrombosis in the pelvis or lower extremity is to reestablish venous patency. This can forestall the development of post-thrombotic syndrome and eliminate the nidus for recurrent thrombosis and pulmonary embolization.

Patency can be restored nonoperatively by fibrinolysis or operatively by thrombectomy. Both procedures yield optimum results only when instituted within the first 8 days, or preferably the first 4 days, after the probable onset of the thrombosis. Thus, early detection of the disease and the swift formulation of an appropriate treatment plan are
of crucial importance. *Follow-up phlebograms* are 262
routinely obtained on the fourth or fifth day after thrombectomy, when the patient will have recovered somewhat from the disease and the operation. In patients receiving fibrinolytic therapy, repeat phlebograms are taken at 2- to 4-day intervals to determine efficacy and direct further treatment
planning. With high-dosage therapy, a follow-up 263
examination is recommended after every second treatment phase.

Since the follow-up examination is confined to a specific vascular segment in most patients, *color-coded duplex scanning* appears to be particularly well suited for monitoring therapeutic response. In postoperative cases as well, it permits a rapid, reliable assessment of vascular patency.

For the common condition of ascending phlebothrombosis, there is no clear consensus favoring fibrinolytic or operative treatment. At some centers today a preference has emerged for high-dosage thrombolysis (Martin and Fiebach 1985), which is comparable to long-term lysis in its efficacy and is less harmful to the patient's physical

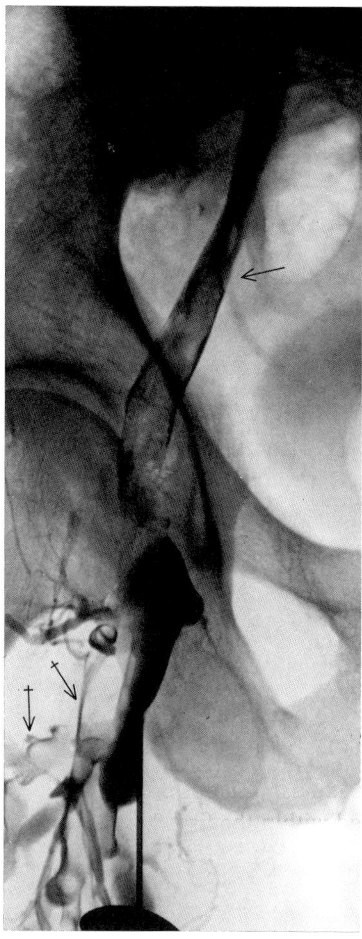

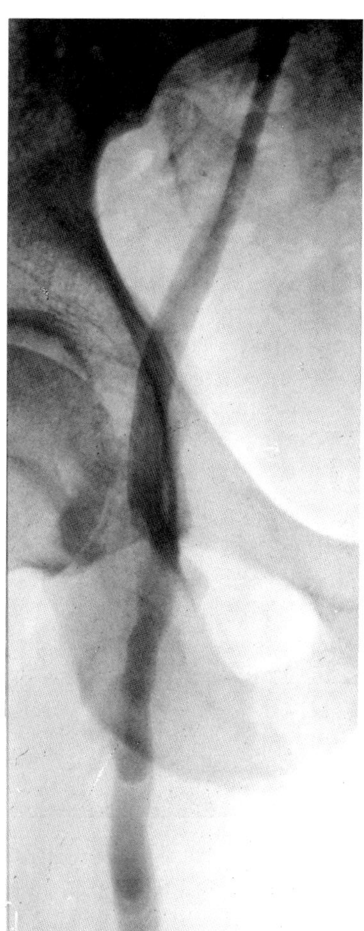

△

262. Ascending iliofemoral venous thrombosis with no apparent cause in a 73-year-old man. *Left,* ascending phlebography on the third day after symptom onset. → Dome sign; ↔ contour sign. *Right,* film 5 days after thrombectomy shows full restoration of patency with preservation of the venous valves

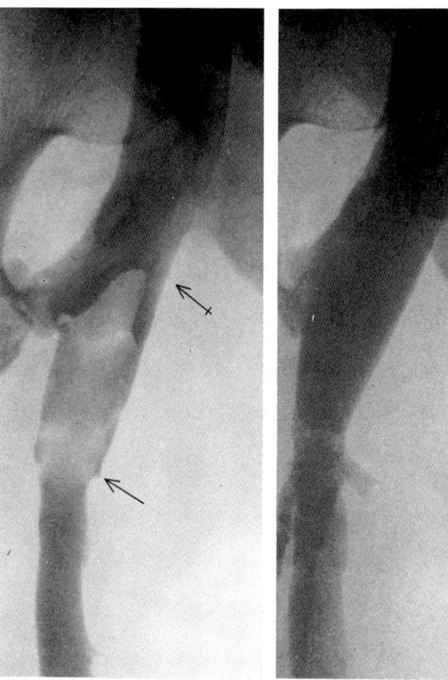

▷

263. Occluding thrombus in the common femoral vein of a 47-year-old man. *Left,* ascending phlebography on the third day after symptom onset. → Indistinct outline of the thrombus head; ↔ dome sign. *Right,* complete restoration of perfusion with preservation of venous valves after a 5-day course of streptokinase fibrinolysis

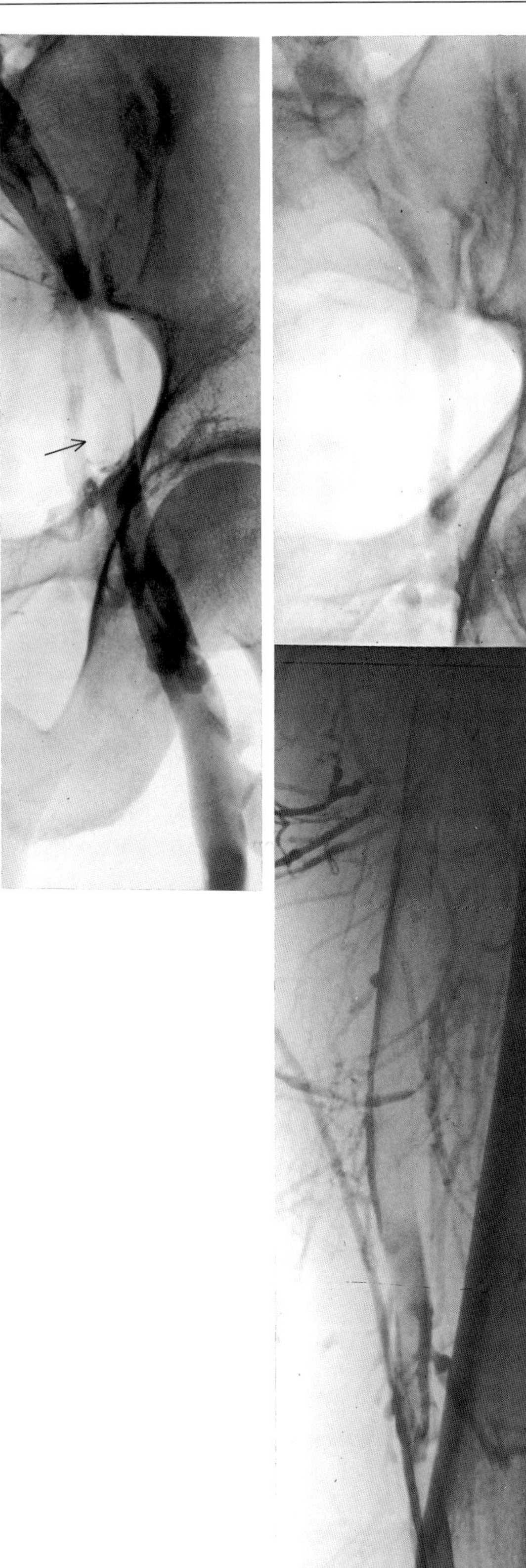

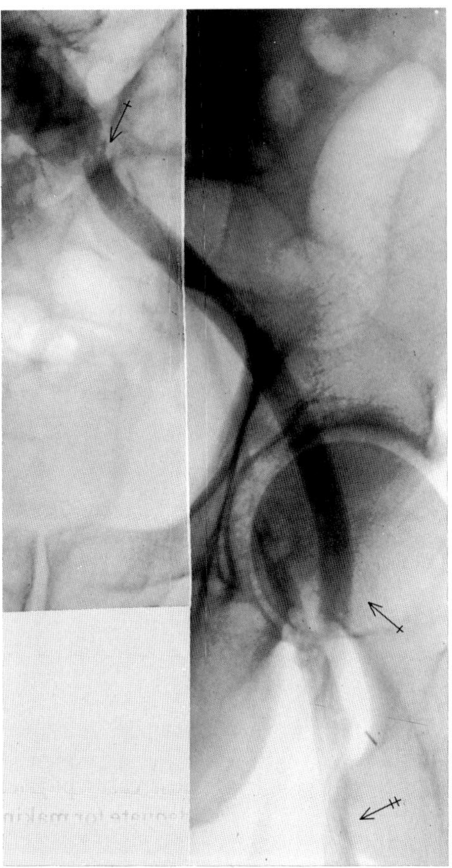

264. Descending iliofemoral venous thrombosis in a 57-year-old man. Acute compression of external iliac vein by indurated hematoma 6 weeks after diagnostic cardiac catheterization. Demonstrated by ascending phlebography. *Left,* subtotal constriction of the external iliac vein (→). *Middle,* next day, extensive descending thrombosis during heparin administration at therapeutic dosage. Surgery disclosed hard callosities with involvement of the vein wall; direct vascular reconstruction was not feasible. *Right,* status following thrombectomy and iliofemoral bypass with a polytetrafluoroethylene (PTFE) prosthesis; ↔ distal and proximal anastomoses. Contrast instilled through the thin intravascular catheter (⇸) for continuous local heparin therapy well-being. The benefits of fibrinolysis also extend to the peripheral stem veins and muscle veins with their important valvular apparatus. Operative treatment is probably the better option for pelvic vein thrombosis, though in this case facilities for *intraoperative phlebography* or *vascular endoscopy* should be available.

In descending iliofemoral venous thrombosis as
264 well, surgical revascularization is preferred over conservative therapy, as it is sometimes necessary to perform a *bypass operation*. In this case phlebographic delineation of the course of the affected veins can be decisive in terms of selecting the most appropriate procedure.

Circumscribed thromboses of the lower leg veins, nonoccluding thrombi, and recurrent and older thromboses are treated with *anticoagulants* at most centers. This creates a protective screen within which endogenous fibrinolytic activity can unfold. Anticoagulation is also used if there are contraindications to invasive treatment or if the patient refuses an invasive procedure. Under these conditions the need for follow-up phlebography or color-coded duplex scanning will depend on the individual situation. In most cases physical methods of measurement are adequate for making a hemodynamic assessment.

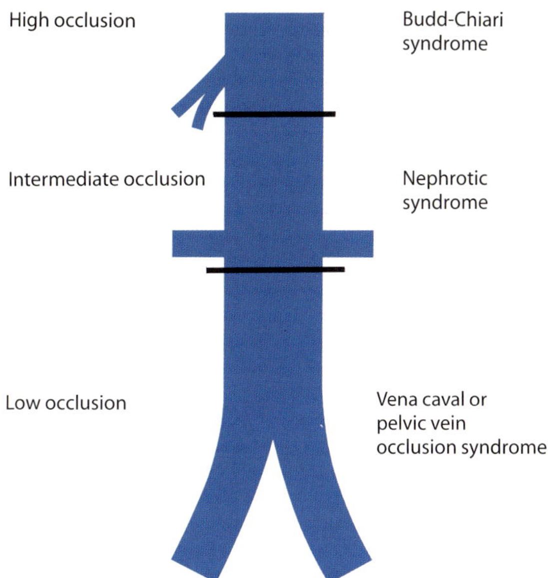

265. Levels of occlusion of the inferior vena cava

Etiology of obstruction of the pelvic veins and inferior vena cava
Thrombosis and post-thrombotic syndrome
Extravascular compression
Tumor infiltration
Surgery on the inferior vena cava
Spur formation in the left common iliac vein

Thrombosis of the Inferior Vena Cava

We devote a separate chapter to thrombosis of the inferior vena cava, because in some respects it is a unique disorder that differs from the peripheral thromboses. Its radiographic diagnosis must rely on conventional pelvic phlebography or digital subtraction angiography. Computed tomography and magnetic resonance imaging also furnish reliable information. These techniques, like color-coded duplex scanning, are advantageous in that they permit the assessment of surrounding tissue structures.

Occlusive Caval Thrombosis

Occlusive thrombosis of the inferior vena cava is rarely observed. Usually it signifies a *generalized disease process*. Caval thrombosis is a well-known complication of collagen disorders, and it occasionally results from a hypercoagulability state associated with a congenital coagulation defect or metastatic malignancy. Other causes of inferior vena caval obstruction are extravascular compression syndrome and tumor infiltration of the vessel wall.

In *low thrombotic occlusions* the cranial border of the thrombus extends to the level of the renal
veins. Involvement of the renal veins (*intermedi-* 265
ate occlusion) or the Budd-Chiari syndrome (*high occlusion*) are syndromes with organ-related symptoms and fall within the purview of internal medicine (Hach 1973).

The *clinical presentation* of an occluding infrarenal caval thrombosis corresponds to that of extensive bilateral pelvic vein thrombosis. Persistent, diffuse back pain is accompanied by marked swelling of both lower limbs with pale livid discoloration. Additionally there is prominence of the superficial veins of the abdominal wall. Because of the underlying disease alone, patients are seriously ill and have subfebrile to febrile temperatures.

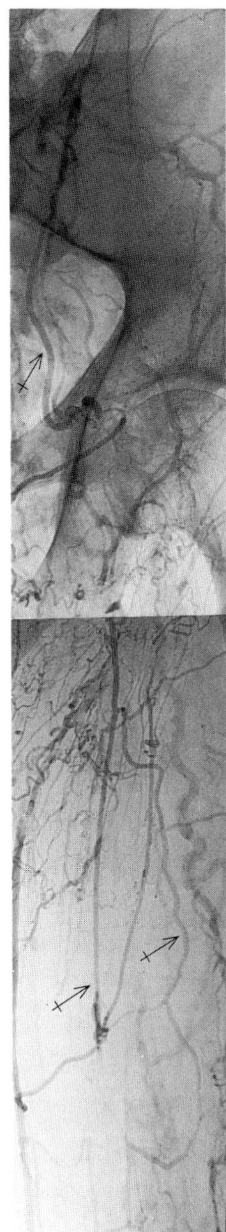

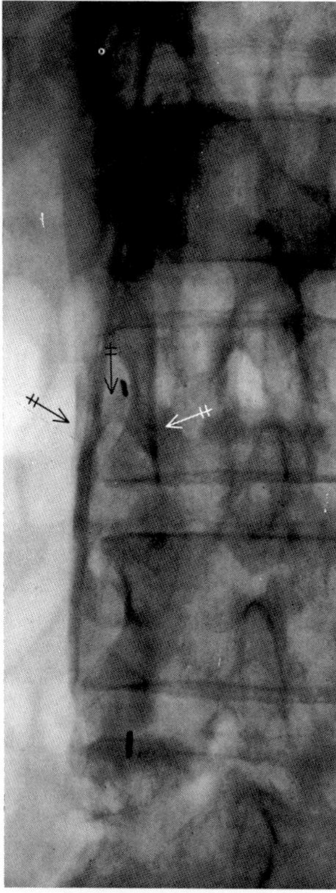

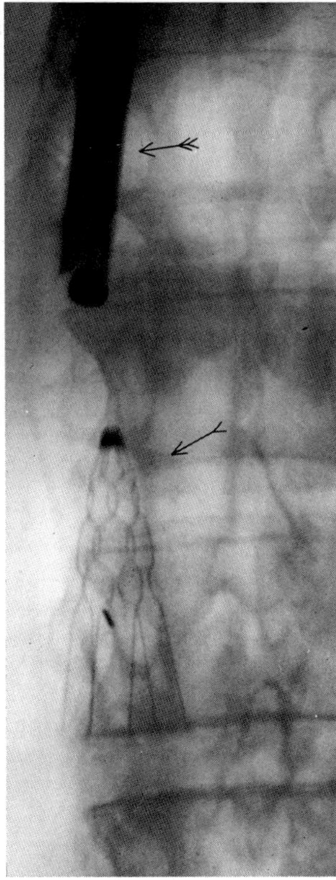

266. Extensive thrombosis of the leg and pelvic veins and inferior vena cava in a 67-year-old man with acute renal failure; right leg had been previously amputated. *Left,* ascending phlebography of the left leg and pelvic veins demonstrates muscle collaterals (→) and fine superficial veins (↔). *Top right,* transbrachial phlebogram demonstrates the tail of the thrombus in the inferior vena cava (⇸). *Bottom right,* film during insertion of a Greenfield filter (↣) to prevent pulmonary embolism during transport to the dialysis unit. ↠ Carrying instrument for filter
◁

Direct *phlebographic visualization* of the occluding caval thrombus can be accomplished from the 266
periphery only when the digital subtraction technique is employed. The film demonstrates an abundance of small and minute collateral veins. If there is a retroperitoneal venous occlusion associated with a marked paucity of collateral pathways, Ormond's fibrosis should be suspected.

Nonocclusive Caval Thrombosis

Occasionally a thrombus in the common iliac vein can enter the inferior vena cava by propagating in the direction of blood flow. The clinical symptoms are like those of unilateral pelvic vein thrombosis: unremitting lumbar pain, edematous swelling and slight livid discoloration of the affected extremity. Symptoms may be mild or absent during bed rest. Generally, involvement of the inferior vena cava by pelvic thrombosis can be detected only by digital subtraction angiography or by a routine contrast examination from the healthy opposite side.
The thrombus exhibits the typical dome and con- 267
tour signs. The less common mural thrombus is 268
easily mistaken for a compression effect.

A nonocclusive thrombus may also form on the inside of the vessel wall as an isolated lesion at sites where the intima has been disrupted by a primary tumor or by a malignancy infiltrating the wall from nearby tissues, inciting the release of thrombogenic substances. Detection of the mural thrombus is generally fortuitous. Clinical manifestations relate to a possible pulmonary embolism or to the underlying disease. The therapeutic approach depends on the individual situation.

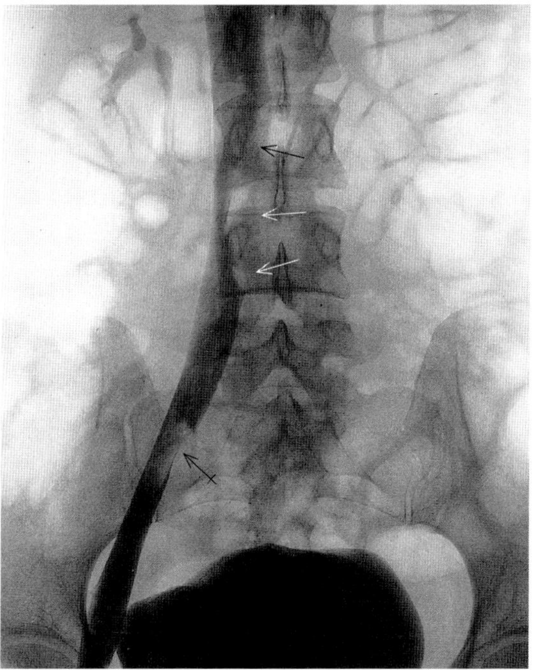

267. Descending and ascending iliofemoral venous thrombosis in a 31-year-old woman 7 days after symptom onset with severe back pain. Patient had been confined to bed for an influenzal infection with high fever. Operation disclosed an extravascular compression syndrome caused by perivascular callosities. There was thrombotic occlusion of the left pelvic veins merging with a mural thrombus of the inferior vena cava (→). Descending thrombosis in the right external iliac vein (↦) (see also Fig. 254)

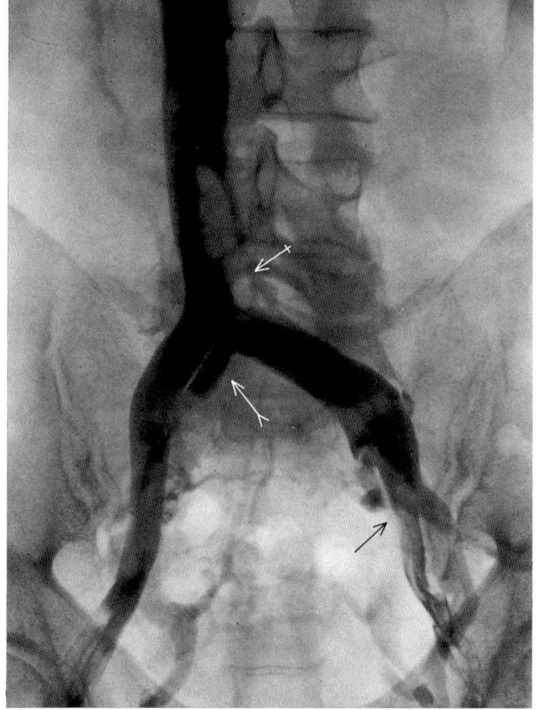

268. Ascending leg and pelvic vein thrombosis with no apparent cause in a 66-year-old man. Pelvic phlebography on day 12 after onset shows thrombi in the left external iliac vein (→) with suspicion of older postthrombotic changes. Floating thrombus in the inferior vena cava (↦), probably originating from a pelvic venous spur. Anomalous termination of the right internal iliac vein at the left common iliac vein (↣)

Role of Adjunctive Studies to Phlebography

Thrombosis of the inferior vena cava is a severe and often life-threatening disease that requires a comprehensive diagnostic assessment. *Real-time* and *color-coded duplex sonography* have a definite role to play in this setting. With a total occlusion, the inferior vena cava is distended and presents a circular cross-section. The typical double-beat phenomenon is no longer detected. In thin patients, intravascular reflections and vessel wall thickening become apparent within a few days. The compression test should be withheld due to the risk of pulmonary embolism. Evaluation of the perivascular tissues and organs is of major importance. Invasive tumors, aortic aneurysms, and other pathologic processes must be excluded or identified. This points to the potential value of
269 computed tomography and *magnetic resonance imaging* in selected cases.

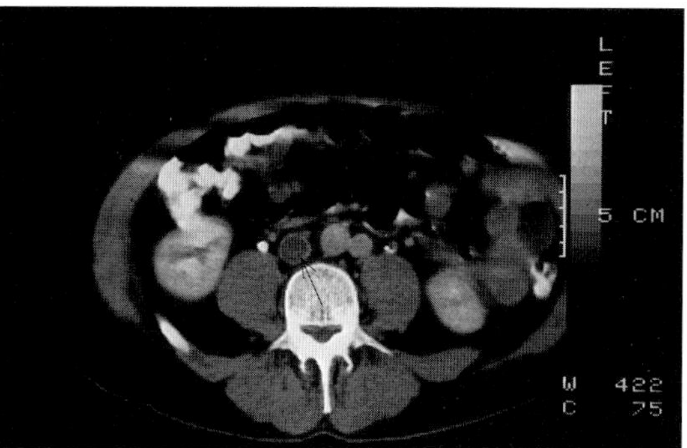

269. Computed tomogram of thrombotic occlusion of the infrarenal inferior vena cava (→). Ventral aorta of the vertebral body clearly shown by contrast medium. Additional finding of horseshoe kidney

References

Bartels D (1979) Therapie der tiefen Beinvenenthrombose und Lungenembolie. Fortschr Med 97: 1293

Benecke G (1976) Thrombogenese in Venen. In: Breddin K, Gross D (Hrsg) Moderne Thromboseprophylaxe. Schattauer, Stuttgart

Bollinger, A (1977) Doppler-Ultraschall zur Diagnose der tiefen Becken- und Beinvenenthrombose. In: Ehringer H (Hrsg) Akute tiefe Becken- und Beinvenenthrombosen. Huber, Bern

Dienstl E (1989) Isotopenuntersuchungen zur Diagnose venöser Thrombosen und Lungenembolien. Wiener Med Wschr 139: 551

Fridrich R (1977) Radio-Fibrinogen in der Diagnose der akuten tiefen Venenthrombosen. In: Ehringer H (Hrsg) Akute tiefe Bein- und Beckenvenenthrombosen. Huber, Bern

Grosser S, Kreymann G, Guthoff A, Taube C, Raedler A, Tilsner V, Greten H (1990) Farbcodierte Duplex-Sonographie bei Phlebothrombosen. Dtsch Med Wschr 115: 1939

Hach W (1973) Die Phlebographie beim Beckenvenen- und Vena-cava-inferior-Verschlußsyndrom. Phlebol Proktol 2: 143

Hach W (1981) Nicht-invasive instrumentelle Diagnostik venöser Thrombosen. In: Vinazzer H (Hrsg) Thrombose und Embolie. Springer, Berlin Heidelberg New York

Hach W (1982) Phlebologie in der täglichen Praxis. pmi-Verlag, Frankfurt

Hach W (1989) Beurteilung und Therapie des postthrombotischen Syndroms. Herz 14: 287

Hach W, Salzmann G, Radovic HW (1983) Die operative Behandlung der deszendierenden Thrombose und des akuten Kompressionssyndroms der Ileofemoralvenen durch Bypass mit wandverstärkter PTFE-Prothese. Vasa 12: 249

Hach W, Sternkopf M, Ott H (1989) Apparative und phlebographische Diagnostik der tiefen Bein- und Beckenvenenthrombose. Wiener Med Wschr 139: 543

Hach-Wunderle V (1990) Hämostaseologisches Risikoprofil bei venöser Thrombose. Habilitationsschrift. Johann Wolfgang Goethe-Universität, Frankfurt

Hartsuck JM, Greenfield LJ (1973) Postoperative thromboembolism. Arch Surg 107: 733

Jacobssen H (1983) Standardised leg temperature profiles in the diagnostic of acute deep venous thrombosis. Vasc Diagn 8: 3

Kakkar VV (1976) The 125J-labelled fibrinogen test and phlebography in the diagnosis of deep vein thrombosis. In: Breddin K, Gross D (Hrsg) Moderne Thromboseprophylaxe. Schattauer, Stuttgart

Martin M, Fiebach BJO (1985) Die Streptokinase-Behandlung peripherer Arterien- und Venenverschlüsse unter besonderer Berücksichtigung der ultrahohen Dosierung. Huber, Bern

Mostbach, A (1977) Diskussionsbemerkung. In: Ehringer H (Hrsg) Akute tiefe Becken- und Beinvenenthrombosen. Huber, Bern

Mostbeck A (1981) Isotopenmethoden in der Diagnostik venöser Thrombosen. In: Vinnazer H (Hrsg) Thrombose und Embolie. Springer, Berlin Heidelberg New York

Rotter W, Röttger P (1976) Über die Häufigkeit der Venenthrombose im Frankfurter Sektionsgut. In: Breddin K, Gross D (Hrsg) Moderne Thromboseprophylaxe. Schattauer, Stuttgart

Schmitt HE (1977) Aszendierende Phlebographie bei tiefer Venenthrombose. Huber, Bern

Vinazzer H (Hrsg) (1981) Thrombose und Embolie. Springer, Berlin Heidelberg New York

Wuppermann T (1986) Varizen, Ulcus cruris und Thrombose. Springer, Berlin Heidelberg New York Tokyo

Post-thrombotic Syndrome

The term "post-thrombotic syndrome," coined by Halse in 1954, is a collective term for numerous symptoms that persist in the wake of deep venous thrombosis or develop over a period of years. The diverse features of this syndrome range from mild recurrent swelling to very severe trophic disturbances associated with arthrogenic stasis syndrome (Hach et al. 1983) and with chronic fascial compression syndrome (Hach and Hach-Wunderle 1994). It is common for this condition to cause debilitating occupational and social problems for the patient. It has been estimated that more than 5 million people in the Federal Republic of Germany suffer from post-thrombotic disease. Contrast phlebography can aid in determining the optimum mode of treatment and help prevent long-term complications.

Post-thrombotic Syndrome in the Pelvic and Leg Veins

Post-thrombotic changes in the leg veins and ipsilateral pelvic veins fall within the same symptom complex, so it is appropriate to discuss them under one heading. Today it no longer appears justified to regard unilateral post-thrombotic pelvic venous syndrome as a separate entity. Consequently, terms such as "chronic pelvic venous block" (Wanke and Gumrich 1950) or "pelvic stenotic syndrome with siderosclerosis" (Schneider 1976) are considered to be obsolete.

Post-thrombotic disease of the pelvic venous system and inferior vena cava presents unique features owing to the specific patterns of collateral circulation that arise.

Pathophysiology

Reparative and compensatory processes are initiated within just days or weeks after the onset of

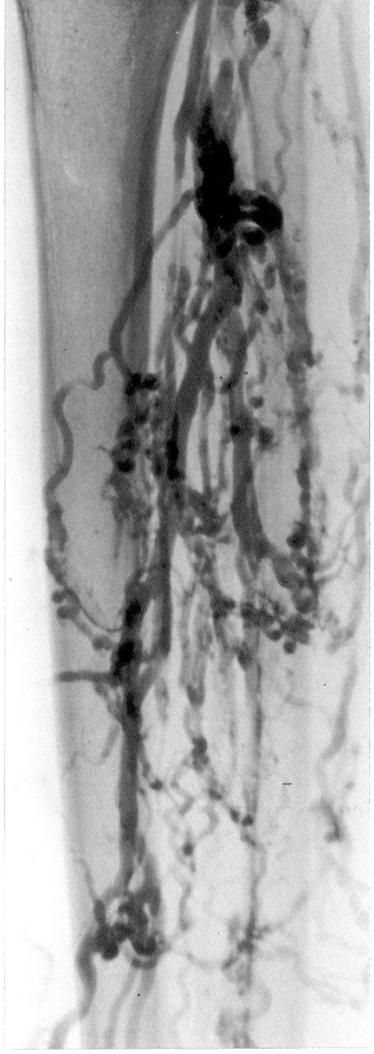
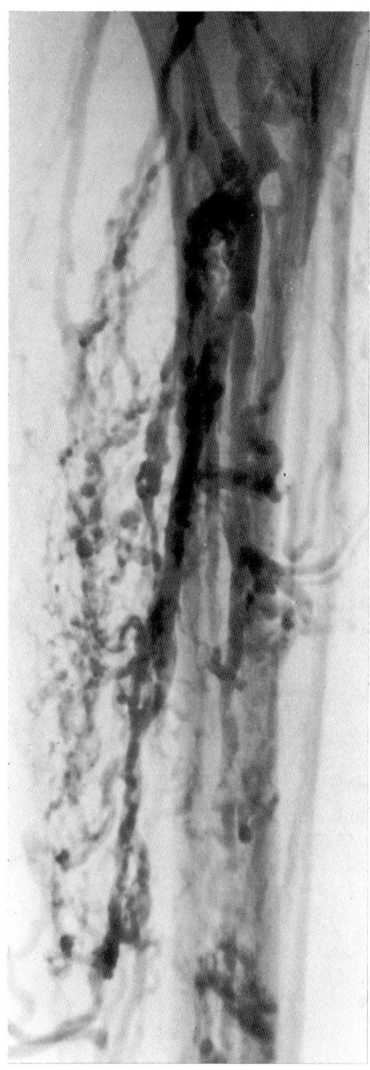

270. Post-thrombotic syndrome in a 54-year-old woman 4 months after the acute stage of the disease. There are marked signs of recanalization with islets and webs separated by the soft, rounded contours of persistent thrombi. Demonstrated by ascending pressure phlebography in the left leg, internal rotation (*left*) and lateral view (*right*)

an acute deep vein thrombosis. These processes are concerned mainly with handling the blood volume that has pooled in the lower limb due to the proximal outflow obstruction. Two physiologic mechanisms are available for this: recanalization and collateralization. Both processes are accessible to phlebographic investigation.

270 *Recanalization* begins with the formation of small voids within the thrombus due to spontaneous fibrinolysis. This is followed within 2 weeks by a gradual connective-tissue transformation and retraction of the thrombus away from the vessel wall. As this occurs, the crevices and cavities enlarge, coalesce, and acquire an endothelial lining. This recanalization process can take up to 12 months to complete.

The extent of recanalization can be assessed on phlebograms. In 35.5% of cases there is *complete*
restoration of a patent channel. Most common in 275
children and adolescents, complete recanalization is probably based on a high fibrinolytic activity of the vessel wall. In 53.4% of cases recanalization is
incomplete, and in 11.1% it is *absent* (Netzer 278, 279
1968).

Collateralization also serves to reestablish an adequate venous return when there is occlusion of the

277 main deep veins. When the proximal channels are obstructed, the peripheral venous pressure rises and serves as a stimulus for the development of bypass channels. Recanalization and collateralization are mutually antagonistic rather than synergistic in their effect.

274 Post-thrombotic *valve destruction* in the lower leg veins distorts the normal function of the calf muscle pump, the most important of the peripheral venous pumps, leading to retrograde flow in the axial vessels. The blood seeks new pathways through incompetent perforating veins to the superficial vessels, which in time adapt to the increased flow volume and become dilated.

A *loss of valvular function,* then, has adverse consequences in several respects: There is decreased blood flow toward the heart in the femoroiliac venous system, accompanied by retrograde flow toward the periphery with an inversion of normal intravascular pressure relationships. Because the peripheral muscle pumps in the lower leg are so critical for venous return, extensive post-thrombotic destruction of the crural venous valves has a particularly deleterious effect and is invariably associated with pronounced clinical symptoms.

The severe post-thrombotic *structural changes in the vessel wall*, involving a replacement of differentiated anatomic structures by contractile scar tissue, causes sacculations and dilatations to form at sites subjected to pressure and volume overloads. Turbulence and flow stasis in these areas give rise to dead spaces in the cutaneous and subcutaneous plexuses, which are thought to contribute to the dermatologic complications of chronic venous insufficiency.

Pathophysiologic factors in post-thrombotic syndrome
Elevation of dynamic venous pressure
Failure of the peripheral venous pumps
Retrograde blood flow
Pathologic secondary disturbances
Formation of hemodynamic dead spaces

Characteristics of acute thrombosis and the stages of post-thrombotic syndrome				
Duration	Peripheral edema	Vascular occlusions	Recanalization	Collateral circulations
Acute thrombosis (<4 weeks)	+++	+++	0	(+)
Early post-thrombotic syndrome (4 weeks–1 year)	++	++	+	+
Post-thrombotic syndrome proper (1–20 years)	+	+	++(+)	+++
Late post-thrombotic syndrome (1–20 years or more)	+++	+	++(+)	Decompensated

Clinical Symptoms

The progression from acute thrombosis to post-thrombotic syndrome should occur during the third to fourth week after disease onset in cases that take a spontaneous course. It is characterized by persistent edema due to continued venous outflow impairment that is most pronounced during exercise. *Early post-thrombotic syndrome* corresponds to the pathophysiologic processes of recanalization and collateralization. The duration of this stage is approximately 12 months. With increasing *adaptation* of the venous circulation, the clinical symptoms gradually subside.

Post-thrombotic syndrome in the strict sense is characterized by stable hemodynamic conditions. Through *compensation*, the venous system has achieved a maximum degree of adaptation to the pathomorphologic circumstances. The patient must learn to live with his complaints, peripheral stasis, and gradually progressive varicose veins.

With passage of time, the superficial collateral veins become overloaded by the excessive blood volume. They distend until their valves can no longer close, and varicose veins develop. *Secondary saphenous varicosity* has a particularly ad- 286
verse effect on venous hemodynamics. Blood can no longer be tapped from the smaller tributaries of the great saphenous vein, and contraction of the calf muscles produces ram effects over the sites of emergence of incompetent perforators. *Microcirculatory disturbances* lead to sites of brawny induration and finally incite the dermatologic complications of chronic venous insufficiency. *Decompensation* of the adaptive processes, es-

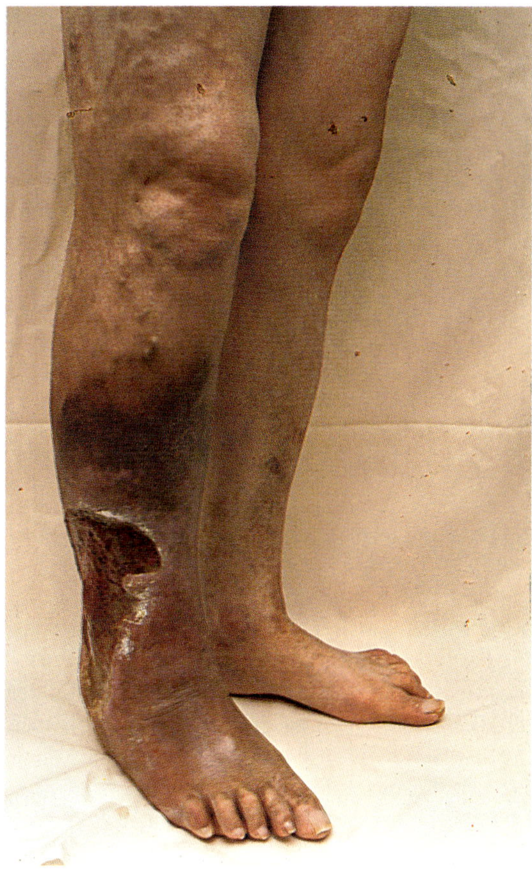

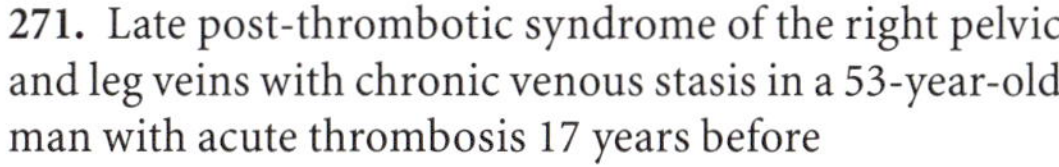

271. Late post-thrombotic syndrome of the right pelvic and leg veins with chronic venous stasis in a 53-year-old man with acute thrombosis 17 years before

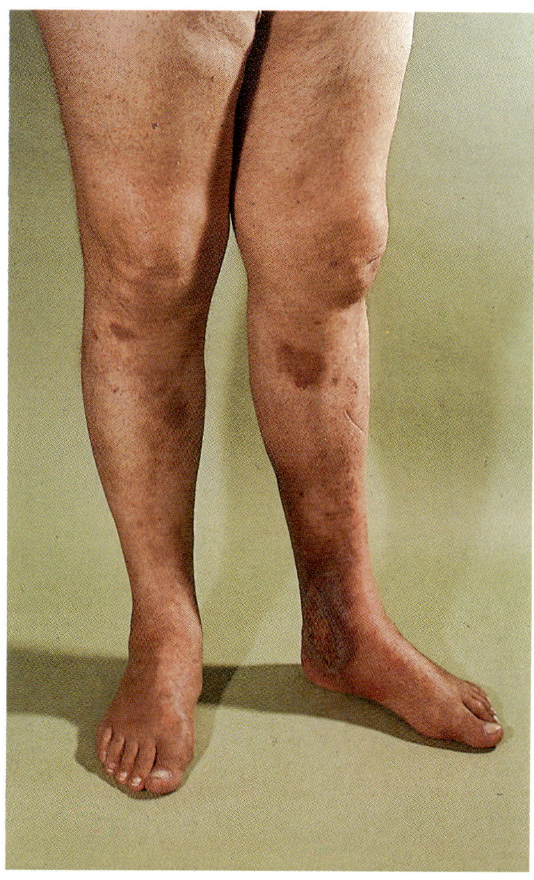

272. Arthrogenic stasis syndrome in a 44-year-old man with a 13-year history of post-thrombotic disease and a 4-year history of arthrogenic stasis syndrome in the left leg. Fixed equinus deformity, recurvatum at the knee, persistent crural ulcer

pecially varicose degeneration of the superficial collaterals, sets the stage for *late post-thrombotic*
271 *syndrome.*

The *rate of progression* of post-thrombotic disease is variable, depending on various factors such as preexisting anatomic and functional status, patient age, and previous therapeutic and prophylactic measures. Generally a period of 5–10 or 20 years is required for the development of late post-thrombotic syndrome.

The *clinical presentation of chronic venous insufficiency in* post-thrombotic states is marked by edema and induration of the skin and subcutaneous tissues in the supramalleolar area. Stasis eczema,
282 white atrophy, and ulceration are associated features. This symptom complex is by no means pathognomonic for post-thrombotic disease, however, and is also seen with the decompensated reflux circuits of saphenous varicosity, primary femoral valvular incompetence, or venous malformations. For this reason terms such as *chronic venous insufficiency* or *chronic venous stasis syndrome* should always be used to describe symptoms and should never be offered as a diagnosis.

The most severe complication is arthrogenic stasis 272
syndrome (Hach et al. 1983), which occurs when the chronic inflammatory process spreads to involve the ligaments of the ankle and subtalar joints. The patient favors this region by holding the foot in plantar flexion, which culminates in a fixed equinus deformity.

The two main peripheral *venous pumps* – the ankle and calf muscle pumps – rely on a freely mobile ankle joint in order to function. Ankylosis of that joint disables the major pumps and removes the principal motor for the centripetal transport of blood. As a result, the peripher-

Underlying diseases in chronic venous insufficiency
Saphenous varicosity with decompensated reflux circuit
Post-thrombotic syndrome
Arthrogenic stasis syndrome
Primary and secondary femoral vein insufficiency
Acquired arteriovenous fistula
Malformations

al venous pressure no longer falls during exercise but tends to equal the hydrostatic load.

The *fixed equinus deformity* can seriously handicap the patient in his ability to stand and walk. The supramalleolar ulcers respond well to strict bed rest and elevation but tend to recur quickly with resumption of ambulation. This accounts for the frequent poor results following repeated skin grafts. By the time a vicious circle has been established and the ankle has become immobile with fixed equinus, the symptom complex has given
273 way to a true disease entity. The treatment of choice is paratibial fasciotomy with passive remobilization of the ankle and subtalar joints followed by therapeutic exercises (Hach 1989). The goal is to achieve 20° of dorsiflexion, or at the very least 10°, from the neutral-0 position.

The end stage of the disease is *chronic fascial compression syndrome* (Hach and Hach-Wunderle 1994). As a result of structural changes in the crural fascia during orthostatism, the interstitial tissue pressure seems to be increased in the dorsal compartments of the lower leg, which leads to incurable circular crural ulcer. The necrotic process also involves the fasciae and the tendons. As the disease persists for a long time, humoral changes of the chronic inflammation occur, as well as iron deficiency syndrome with secondary anemia and functionally severely diminished blood supply to the muscles with a muddy yellow discoloration and glycogen deficiency. Patients often become dependent on medication and drugs; they become depressed and lose their social standing. Chronic fascial compression syndrome can now be cured by crural fasciectomy.

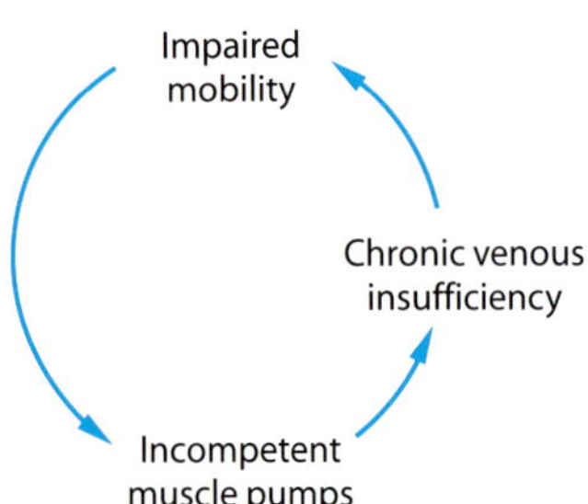

273. Development of arthrogenic stasis syndrome from disease symptoms to a nosologic entity

Phlebographic Diagnosis

The phlebographic evaluation of post-thrombotic syndrome requires biplane views of each vascular region in the leg and of the pelvic veins. The evaluation includes a description of the venous valves, the main deep veins and muscle veins, and the incompetent perforators. The collateral circulations and their hemodynamic efficacy are also assessed. Radiographic findings can be extremely diverse in post-thrombotic states. Small thrombi in the lower leg veins and nonocclusive clots generally leave

Clinical stages of post-thrombotic syndrome		
Stage	Tissue sclerosis	Clinical presentation
I	No tissue sclerosis	Reversible edema
II	Dermatoliposclerosis without involvement of the fasciae	Persistent edema
III	Regional dermatolipofasciosclerosis	Peripheral chronic venous insufficiency
IV	Circular dermatolipofasciosclerosis	Arthrogenic stasis syndrome

Phlebographic features of post-thrombotic syndrome
Venous valve destruction
Recanalization
Collateralization
Perivascular fibrosis
Hemodynamic abnormalities

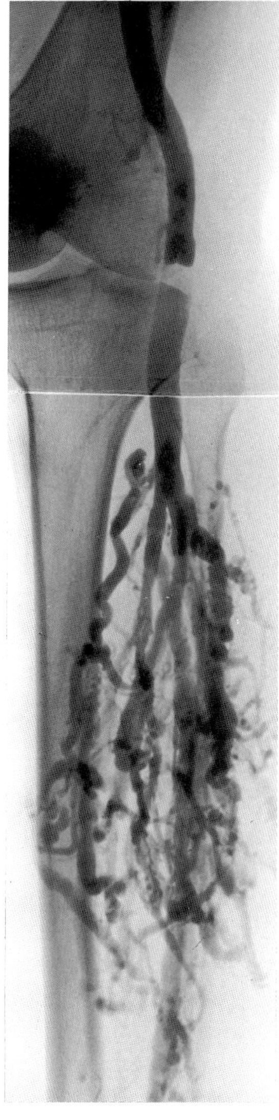

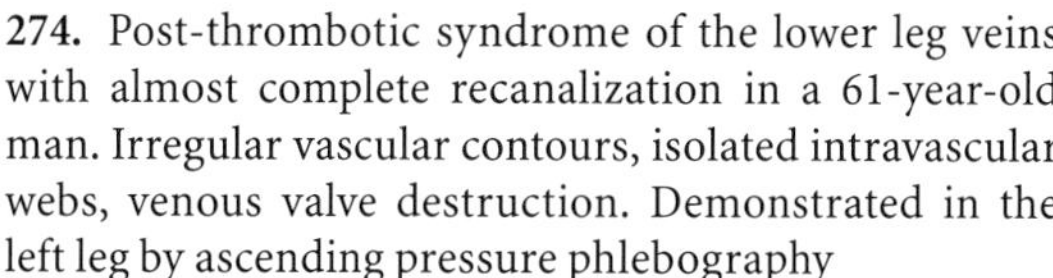

274. Post-thrombotic syndrome of the lower leg veins with almost complete recanalization in a 61-year-old man. Irregular vascular contours, isolated intravascular webs, venous valve destruction. Demonstrated in the left leg by ascending pressure phlebography

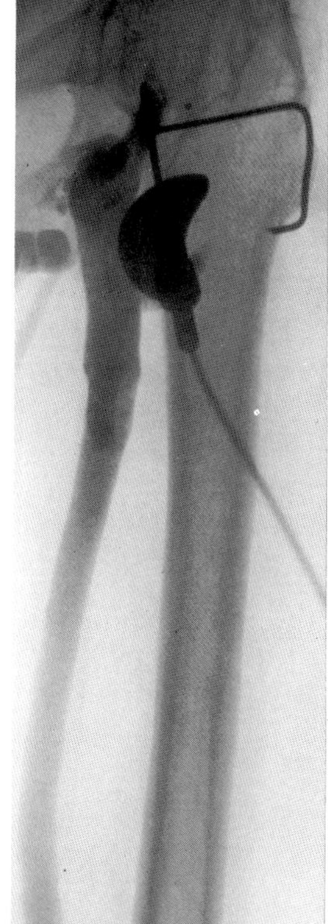

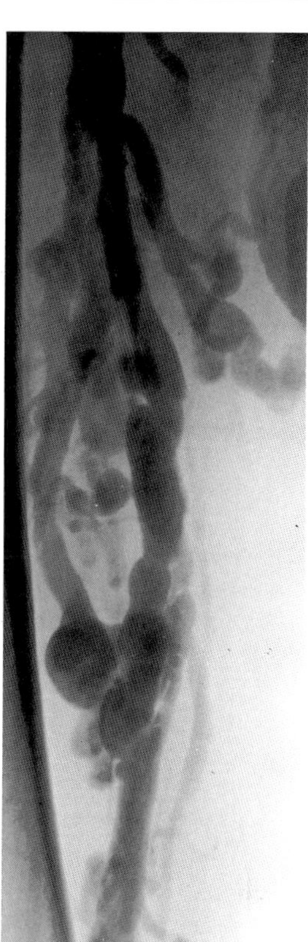

275 *(left).* Post-thrombotic changes in the superficial femoral vein with complete recanalization and valve destruction in a 35-year-old woman with a fused hip. Demonstrated by retrograde pressure phlebography

276 *(right).* Post-thrombotic syndrome with a multichanneled, partially recanalized superficial femoral vein. Demonstrated by ascending pressure phlebography

no residual signs, while in other cases there may be very obstrusive vascular changes following the deep thrombosis.
274 The degree of post-thrombotic vascular damage
275 depends above all on the severity and extent of the
276 original deep vein thrombosis. ***Recanalization*** is
also greatly influenced by previous therapeutic procedures that affect venous patency, such as fibrinolysis or thrombectomy. Thrombosis in children generally resolves with complete recanalization, so that post-thrombotic syndrome is difficult to appreciate during subsequent phlebography. The high fibrinolytic activity of the vein wall probably plays a major role in the breakdown of thrombi in young patients; with aging, these adaptive processes become much less efficient. Recurrent bouts of thrombosis also darken the prospects for successful compensation.

The visible *alteration of venous hemodynamics* on the video monitor is sufficient for diagnosing a post-thrombotic outflow obstruction. The transport capacity of the main deep veins is diminished, and outflow times are markedly prolonged. In response to brief manual calf compression, the contrast medium will surge a short distance through the affected vascular segments and then stop abruptly, with fading opacity, due to the central outflow delay (antegrade flow insufficiency).

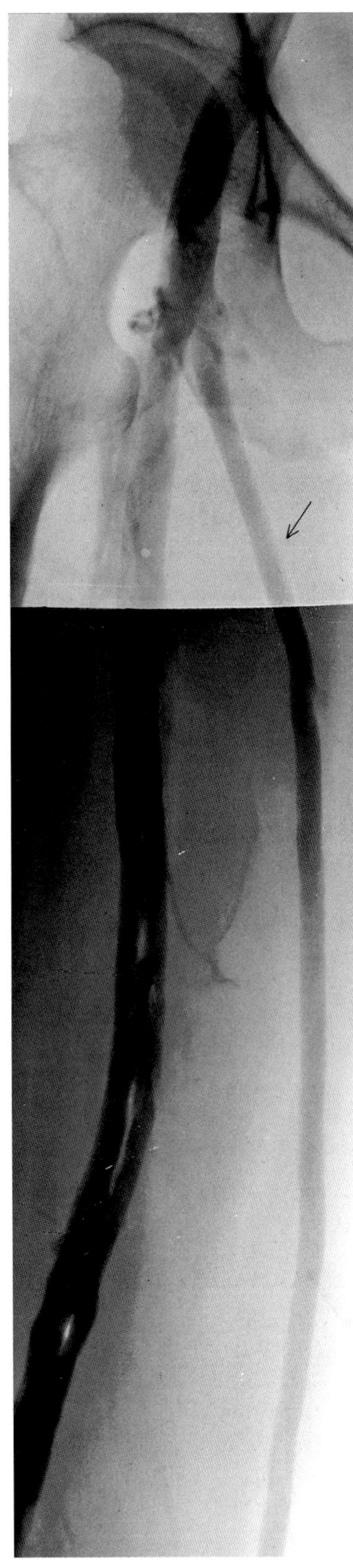

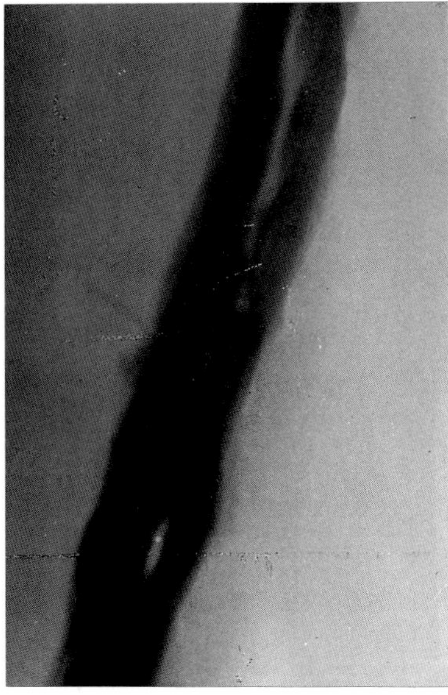

277. Partially recanalized superficial femoral vein in a 36-year-old woman with post-thrombotic syndrome. Irregular vessel contours, internal webs, collateral flow through the ectatic great saphenous vein (→). *Left,* ascending pressure phlebography. *Right,* close-up view of superficial femoral vein

Even with *complete recanalization,* thrombosis leads to valve destruction. An absence of valves or a decrease in their number is an important radiographic sign of post-thrombotic syndrome. This underscores the importance of examining the patient with a sharp table tilt to obtain optimum delineation of the anatomic valve structures through sedimentation of the contrast medium. 274

Ascending phlebography does not always provide a clear picture of the venous valves in the thigh. In these cases more reliable information is provided by retrograde pressure phlebography; the reflux of contrast medium down to and past the knee suggests the correct diagnosis (retrograde flow insufficiency). 275

A *partially recanalized deep vein* presents a typical phlebographic profile. The vessel is irregular in contour, and its lumen is subdivided by islets and lamellae. Segments narrowed by scarring alternate with circumscribed dilatations caused by turbulent and vortical flow. The vein has a tortuous, "unquiet" appearance. Hard, angular outlines imply a more recent process, while rounded contours are more suggestive of long-term disease. The blood seeks a new drainage route among the organized intravascular thrombus remnants and through bypass channels into parallel veins. 276 277, 278

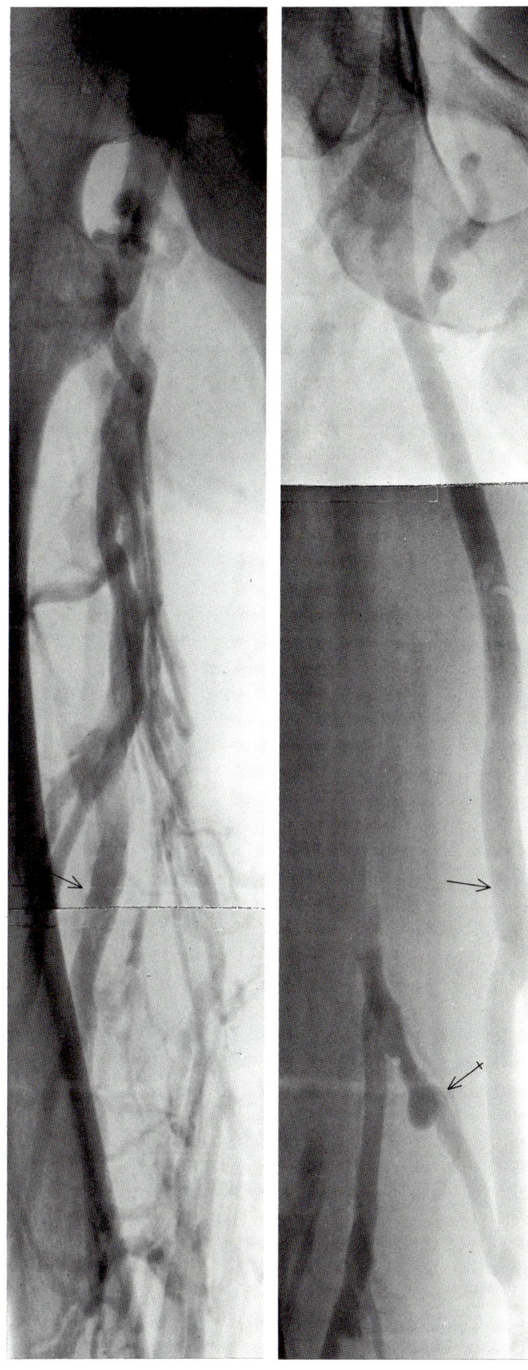

278 *(left).* Incomplete post-thrombotic recanalization of the superficial femoral vein. Pronounced intrafascial collateral flow through muscle veins and the profunda femoral vein (→)

279 *(right).* Absence of post-thrombotic recanalization in the superficial femoral vein with copious collateral flow through the ectatic great saphenous vein (→). Incompetent Dodd's perforator (↔)

Radiographic signs of recanalization
Rigid venous walls
Irregular wall contours
Luminal irregularities
Internal webs (septation)
Vascular islets
Bizarre course of vessel

With *absence of recanalization,* the affected venous segment is not opacified by phlebography, although obvious signs of prior thrombosis are 279
seen at the ends of the obliterated segment. The vessel contours appear sharp and irregular at the cutoff points.

With an extensive occlusion of the superficial femoral vein or with multilevel disease, the proximal vascular segments often are not well defined by the ascending techniques because of contrast dilution. If there is profuse collateral flow through the great saphenous trunk, the thigh veins can sometimes be visualized by retrograde filling from the saphenous termination during a Valsalva maneuver; otherwise retrograde phlebography is required.

Persistent obliteration of the stem veins in the lower leg combined with the development of collateral circulations through recanalized vessels and small intramuscular collaterals leads to the
characteristic picture of *chaotic collateralization* 280
on phlebograms, i.e., innumerable small veins and venules, showing varying degrees of opacification, in chaotic disarray. This phenomenon is the expression of inadequate adaptation to adverse hemodynamic conditions. Clinical symptoms are usually severe.

The ***collateral circulations*** are of major importance in the compensation of post-thrombotic syndrome with incomplete or absent recanalization. These circulations may develop at the extra- or intrafascial level.

Especially important is the *extrafascial collateral circulation,* whose development is explained by the function of the calf muscle pump. In a normal limb the pump propels blood in the main deep veins and muscle veins toward the heart with considerable force. Incompetent venous valves or an intrafascial outflow obstruction distorts the function of the pump, causing it to raise the peripheral venous pressure and propel the blood in a retro-

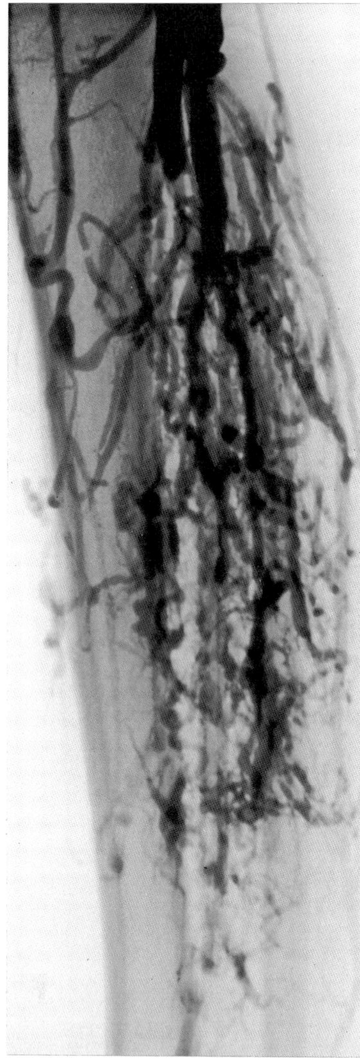

280. Post-thrombotic syndrome of the left lower leg veins with "chaotic recanalization" in a 39-year-old woman. Demonstrated by ascending pressure phlebography, internal rotation view

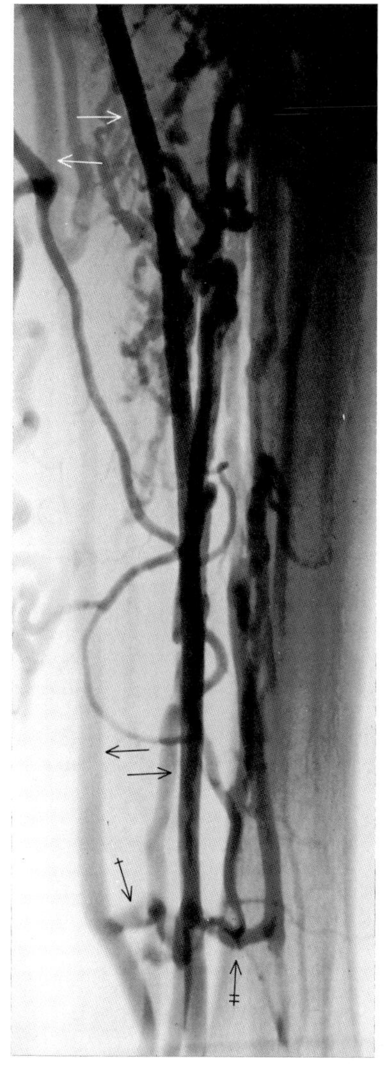

281. Post-thrombotic syndrome in the leg veins with partial recanalization. Incompetent middle Cockett's perforator (+→). Contrast medium drains through the trunks of a duplicated great saphenous vein (→), which is densely opacified peripherally and shows marked compensatory ectasia. ++→ Bridging vein functioning as a collateral. Lateral view of the left leg

281 grade direction. This causes the perforating veins to become dilated until their valves are rendered incompetent. This *perforator incompetence* allows the accumulating blood to drain from the intrafascial space into the extrafascial vessels. In the supramalleolar region, this leads to the clinical
285 symptoms of chronic venous insufficiency, eczema, induration, and ulceration.

The complex arborizations of the superficial venous system provide ample raw material for the development of collateral pathways, all draining into the great saphenous vein. This vessel is of central importance, therefore. Alternate pathways become functional only if the great saphenous becomes unavailable as a collateral. The following veins play a role in extrafascial collateral circula- 283
tions:

Great Saphenous Vein. Under normal conditions this vessel handles approximately 10% of the ve-

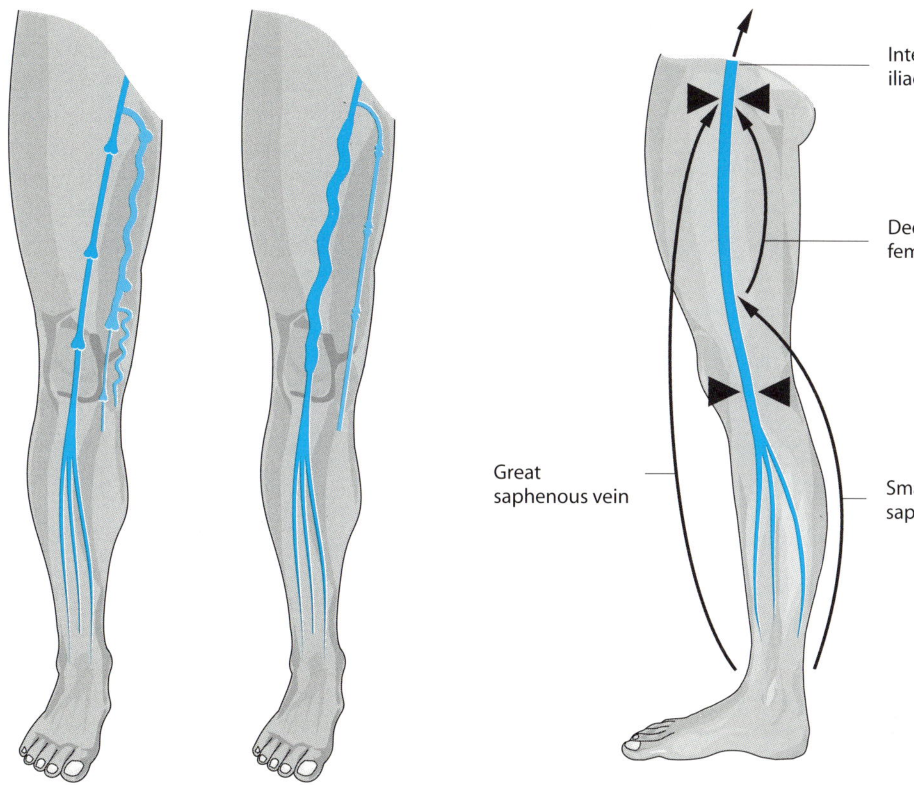

282. Main radiographic signs of primary saphenous varicosity (*left*) and compensatory ectasia (*right*) of the great saphenous vein. See table for explanation

283. Collateral circulations associated with obstructed popliteal and femoral venous outflow

nous return from the leg. When it becomes part of
a collateral circulation, it may conduct several
times that volume. The vein adapts to the altered
250 hemodynamics by ***compensatory ectasia,*** a phys-
282 iologic process of adaptation to an unaccustomed
284 volume load. This compensatory dilatation is
most pronounced in the periphery. The physiologic telescope sign in the terminal portion of the
241 vein is lost. The valves remain functionally sound
and, with a sharp table tilt, are well defined by
contrast sedimentation. Apparently the general
dilatation initially spares the valve rings, which
appear as circular constrictions on phlebograms –
282 the *girdle sign.*

The abnormal hemodynamics are immediately apparent on the video monitor. Opacification of the deep vessels is delayed or absent, and there is an immediate, profuse contrast runoff through the great saphenous vein.

As the volume overload increases, the lumen of the great saphenous vein expands until the venous valve cusps can no longer coapt, permitting retro-

Differences between compensatory ectasia and varicosity of the great saphenous trunk		
Roentgen sign	Saphenous varicosity	Phlebectasia
Visualization	Retrograde	Antegrade
Contrast density	Low	High
Venous valves	Incompetent	Competent
Telescope sign	Absent	Present or absent
Infravalvular dilatations	Typical	Absent
Aneurysms	Typical	Absent
Point of incompetence	Typical	Absent
Branch varix	Present	Absent
Girdle sign	Absent	Typical
Vessel wall	Morphologic transformation	Hypertrophy
Interpretation	Varicose vein	Collateral

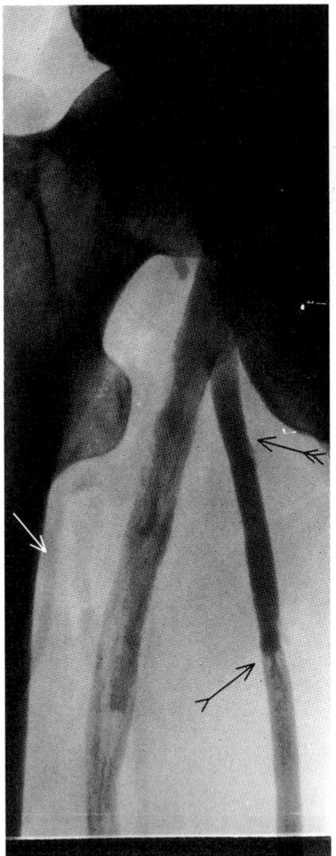

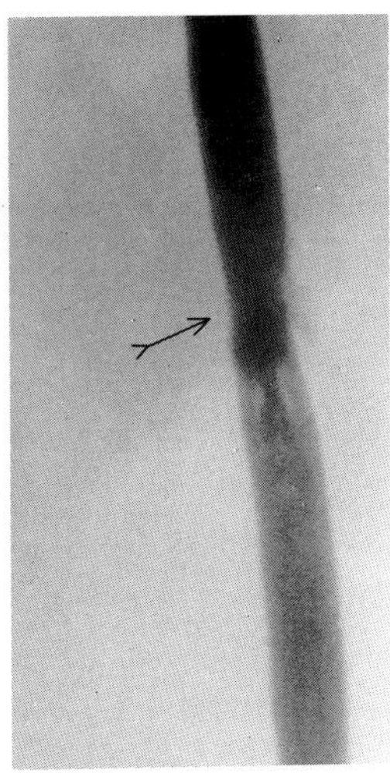

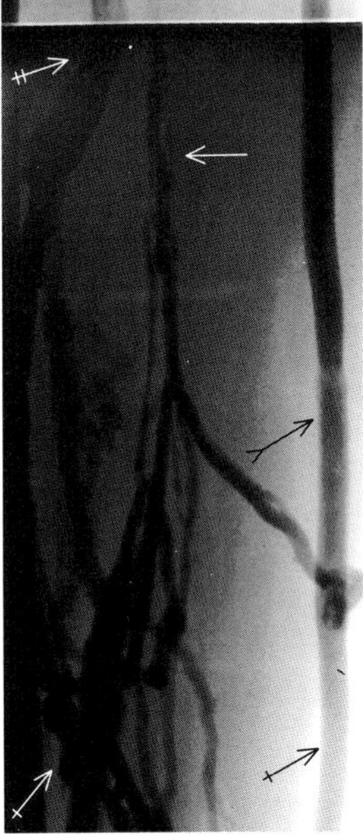

284. Post-thrombotic syndrome in a 50-year-old male. Slight recanalization of the superficial femoral vein (→). Collateral circulation through the distal femoral anastomosis (↔), the profunda femoris (⇸), and the ectatic great saphenous vein; ↣ girdle sign; »→ absence of telescope sign. *Left,* demonstrated by ascending pressure phlebography. *Right,* close-up view of the ectatic great saphenous vein with girdle sign. Circumferential constriction at the level of the valve plane; sedimentation effect of contrast medium signifies at least partial retention of valvular function. Effacement of valve sinuses; no infravalvular dilatation

grade flow. With progressive damage to the vessel wall, varicose degeneration and *secondary saphenous varicosity* ensue. 286  The phlebographic features of the compensatory ectasia are accompanied by the signs of saphenous varicosity, infravalvular dilatations, and venous aneurysms, so it is no longer possible to distinguish between ectasia and varicosity. The collateral circulation ceases to function. The vessel, initially perfused strictly by antegrade flow, can now permit a general hemodynamic reversal. Clinically, decompensation of the collateral circulation initiates the stage of late post-thrombotic syndrome. The pathophysiologic findings at this stage correspond to a *type IV decompensated reflux circuit.* Late post-thrombotic syndrome differs from primary saphenous varicosity in that it involves a *secondary reflux circuit* with less favorable hemodynamic conditions. The patient can derive significant benefit from surgical ablation of the extrafascial venous system.

The *reticular varices* that develop in post-thrombotic syndrome also fall under the heading of secondary varicosities. They can become quite extensive and hamper the conduct of the phlebographic examination. Today it appears unlikely that they are induced by volume overload alone, and the primary and secondary varicosities may be based on the same structural defects at the microscopic (Beneck 1973) or ultramicroscopic level (Staubesand 1977). The degree to which the saphenous veins are affected by these defects remains to be determined.

Small Saphenous Vein. The small saphenous vein plays only a minor role in the collateralization of post-thrombotic states. With functional loss of the 238
great saphenous vein, however, the small saphenous vein and femoropopliteal vein can form an 242
important collateral pathway to the internal iliac system. Giacomini's anastomosis and the medial accessory saphenous vein form another potential collateral route from the femoropopliteal vein to the saphenous hiatus.

Intrafascial Collateral Circulations. Little attention has been given to the intrafascial collateral circulations in previous studies. Some collateral channels are entirely adequate to compensate for circumscribed vascular occlusions, while others have a more theoretical than hemodynamic importance.

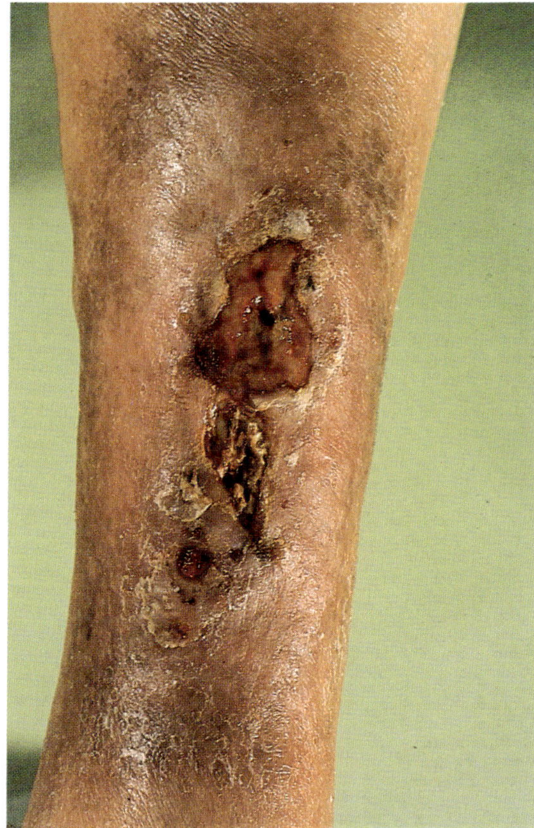

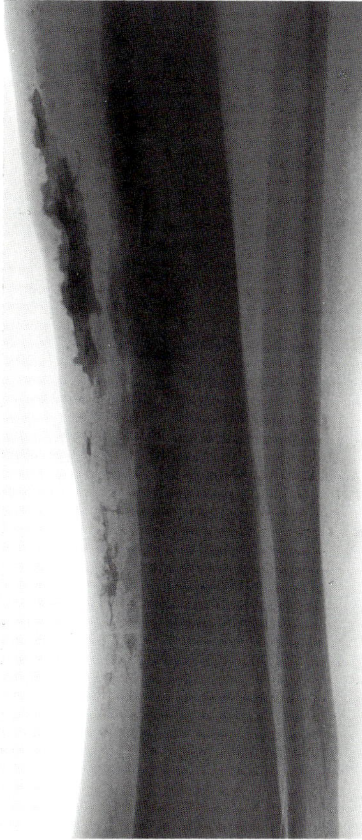

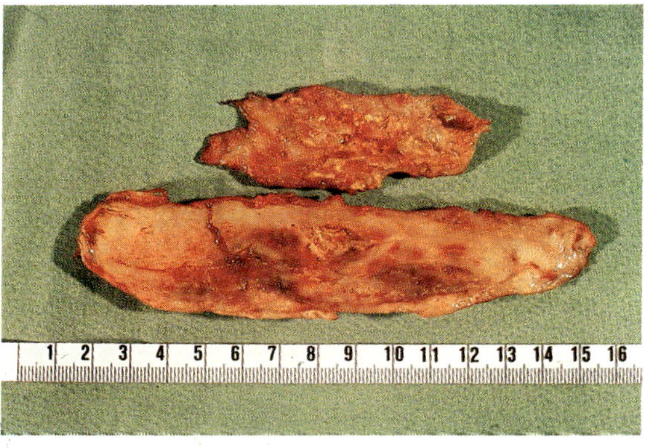

285. Post-thrombotic syndrome in an 86-year-old man with a 26-year history of persistent left crural ulcer. Extensive subcutaneous ossification. The ulcer healed at once following surgical removal of the ossified plates. *Left,* clinical appearance before operation. *Top right,* soft-tissue film of the bony plates. *Bottom,* surgical specimens

In post-thrombotic syndrome with partial or absent recanalization, the following vessels can function as collaterals:

43 – *Distal femoral anastomosis.* The connection between
287 the superficial femoral vein and profunda femoris
288 vein at the level of the adductor canal is the most important intrafascial communication. It can fully compensate for a superficial femoral vein occlusion when the inflow and outflow tracts are patent. Studies by our group (Hrivula-Pfeuffer 1976; Hach 1982) indicate that the distal femoral anastomosis can be demonstrated phlebographically in 18 % of cases.

– *One vessel of a reduplicated popliteal vein or superficial femoral vein.* Blood flow through duplicated stem veins has demonstrable hemodynamic significance in 4.7 % of patients with post-thrombotic syndrome (Hach 1982). This flow cannot be called collateral in

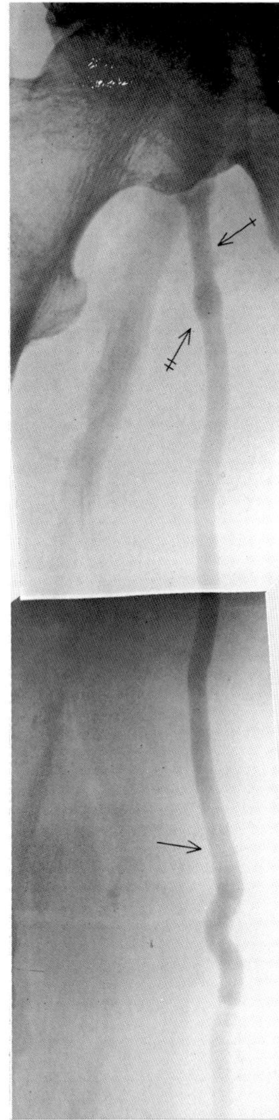

286. Secondary great saphenous varicosity in post-thrombotic syndrome with a very severe impairment of venous hemodynamics in a 47-year-old man who sustained a femoral fracture 15 years before. Ascending pressure phlebography shows little of the deep veins but densely opacifies the great saphenous trunk, which carries antegrade and retrograde flow. Vessel shows dilatation and tortuosity (→), no telescope sign (⇸), incipient infravalvular dilatation (⇻)

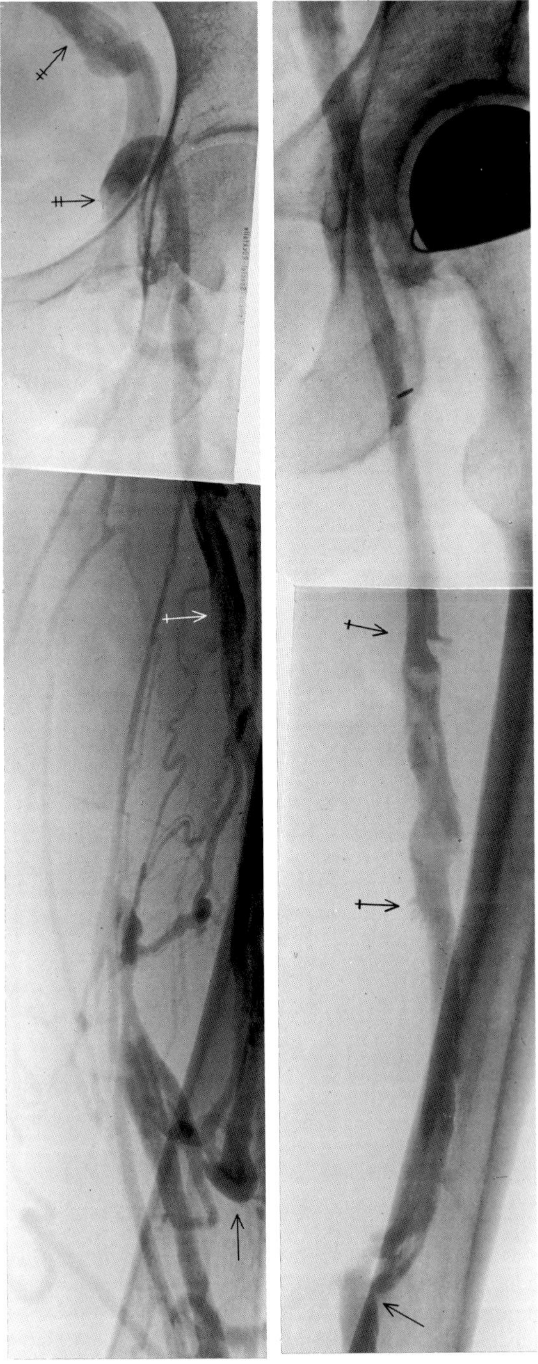

▷

287 *(left).* Well-compensated post-thrombotic syndrome of the left pelvic and leg veins in a 42-year-old woman. No recanalization of the superficial femoral vein or external iliac vein. Collateral flow through the distal femoral anastomosis (→) and profunda femoris (⇸) directly to the mouth of the external iliac vein (⇻). Demonstrated by ascending pressure phlebography

288 *(right).* Well-compensated post-thrombotic syndrome of the leg veins in a 53-year-old man. Persistent occlusion of the superficial femoral vein. Adequate collateral circulation through the distal femoral anastomosis (→) and profunda femoris (⇸). Demonstrated by ascending pressure phlebography the true sense of the word because it is not conveyed by a newly recruited vessel.

- *Muscle veins.* Numerous collaterals invariably form
280 within the muscles when there is persistent occlusion of the stem veins and no effective means of extrafascial diversion, usually due to secondary varicose degeneration or after surgical removal or sclerosing injection of the great saphenous vein. Muscle collaterals are always the expression of a profound hemodynamic impairment. They clearly have minimal importance as transport vessels. Combined with post-thrombotic changes, they contribute to the typical appearance of "chaotic collateralization."
38 - *Bridging veins.* The small connecting veins linking
281 the venae comitantes in the lower leg are integrated into the collateral circulation in 23.3% of patients but lack significant hemodynamic effect (Hach 1982; Hrivula-Pfeuffer 1976).
35 - *Rung veins ("ladder phenomenon").* These delicate
240 vessels are of some significance in compensating for partial occlusions of the posterior tibial veins, the blood perfusing the rung veins in a zig-zag pattern from one venous trunk to the other. The relative prevalence of these collaterals is 1.9%. They are though to have minor hemodynamic significance (Hach 1982; Hrivula-Pfeuffer 1976).

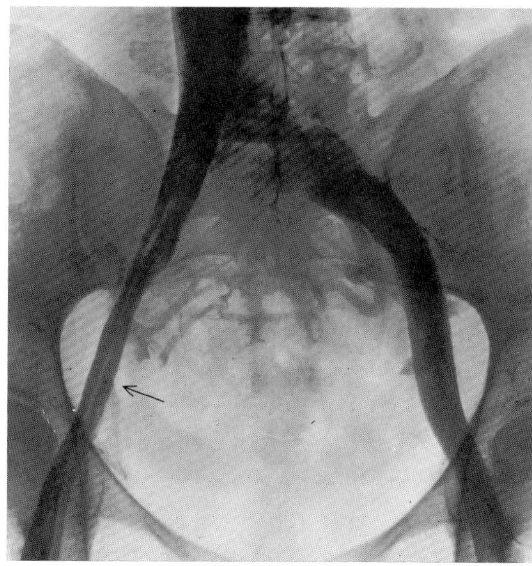

289. Post-thrombotic syndrome of the right leg veins in a 47-year-old woman. Constriction of the right external and common iliac veins by perivascular callosities (→); internal webs. Demonstrated by pelvic phlebography

Post-thrombotic syndrome commonly affects the *deep veins of the pelvis,* either alone or in conjunction with the leg veins. Post-thrombotic changes
289 in the external and common iliac veins are analogous to those affecting the major vessels of the
290 thigh. Partial recanalization is manifested by internal webs and islets within the vessel lumen. Another characteristic radiographic sign is *peri-*
289 *vascular fibrosis,* recognized by a concentric luminal narrowing. This process is not just a feature of post-thrombotic wall damage but also of Ormond's disease, radiation fibrosis, and post-traumatic or postinflammatory connective-tissue induration.

The arrangement of the collateral circulations that develop in response to a persistent occlusion of the main pelvic veins depends basically on the outflow conditions in the common femoral vein, which represents the proximal narrows in the pelvic venous system. The following vessels may function as preformed collaterals in the inguinal and pelvic region:

- *Gluteal veins and pudendal veins.* The femoropopliteal vein connects the terminal intrafascial portion of the small saphenous vein with the pudendal and gluteal veins, which are tributaries of the internal iliac.

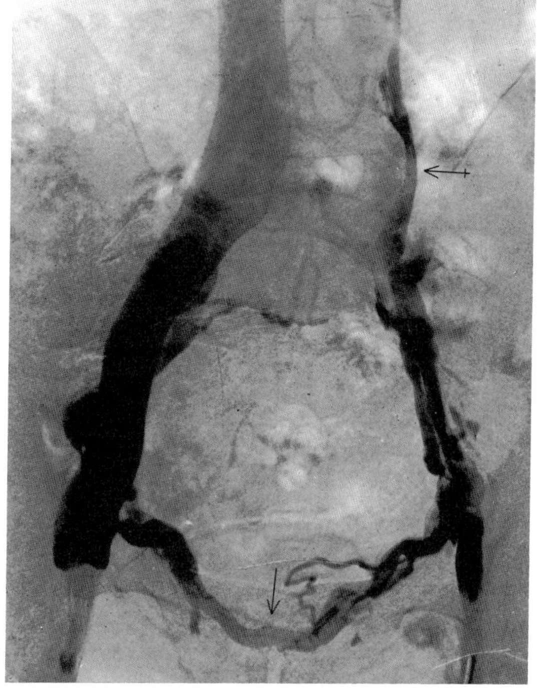

290. Post-thrombotic syndrome of the left external iliac vein with partial recanalization and obliteration of the left common iliac vein. Collateral circulation through suprapubic vessels toward the opposite side (→) and through the ascending lumbar vein (↔) to vertebral and paravertebral plexuses. Demonstrated by pelvic phlebography with photographic subtraction

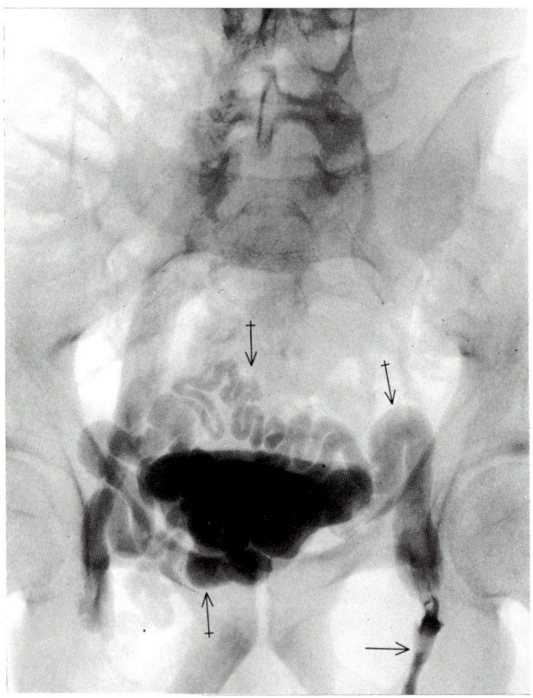

291. Post-thrombotic syndrome of the left pelvic and leg veins in a 25-year-old man with adequate clinical compensation. Persistent occlusions of the main deep veins of the thigh and pelvis. Collateral circulation from the ectatic great saphenous vein (→) directly through suprapubic vessels (↔) toward the opposite side. Demonstrated by pelvic phlebography

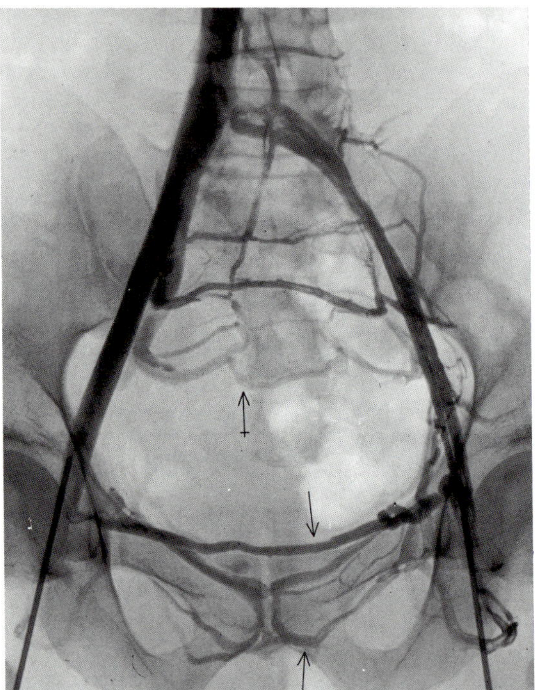

293. Post-thrombotic syndrome of the left external and common iliac veins with partial recanalization in a 43-year-old man. Collateral flow through suprapubic vessels (→) and presacral collaterals toward the opposite side. Demonstrated by pelvic phlebography

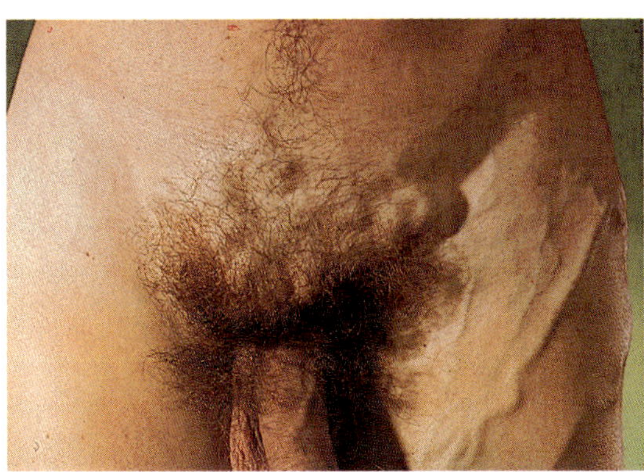

292. Post-thrombotic syndrome of the left pelvic and leg veins in a 25-year-old man who had acute deep vein thrombosis 5 years before. Note the development of suprapubic varices and superficial collaterals in the left hip region

- *Suprapubic collaterals.* Usually there is one
large vessel 3–5 mm in diameter or sometimes 290
two smaller veins passing along the superior margin of the pubic bone to the crosse on the opposite side. Occasionally the collateral arises from a great saphenous vein with compensatory ectasia, bridging the distance from that site 291
to the femoroiliac system. The suprapubic vessels are valveless. Later in the disease the vessels
undergo varicose degeneration with irregular 292
dilatation and tortuosity.
- *Presacral vessels.* The collateral pathways in front of the sacrum are anatomically preformed and are part the internal iliac system. They can
develop into very effective collaterals. From two 293
to five vessels are available following occlusion of the common iliac vein.
- *Pelvic venous plexuses.* The rich venous plexus- 294
es in the lesser pelvis of both men and women can largely compensate for post-thrombotic pelvic venous syndrome. The pudendal plexus or the gluteal veins with their connections in

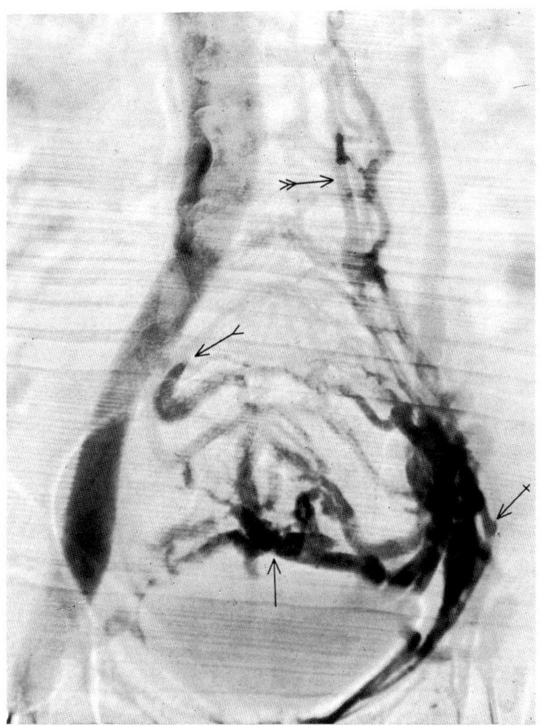

294. Post-thrombotic syndrome of the left pelvic veins with persistent occlusion in a 29-year-old woman with adequate clinical compensation. Collateral circulation through the rich venous plexuses of the uterus (→) and left ovary (+→) to the opposite internal iliac vein (≻→) and to the vertebral and prevertebral plexuses (≫→). Demonstrated by pelvic phlebography with photographic subtraction

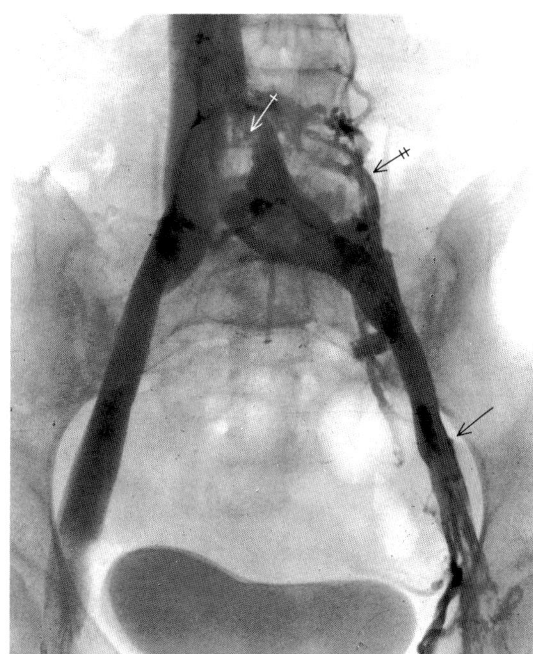

295. Post-thrombotic syndrome of the left pelvic veins with almost complete recanalization in a 47-year-old woman with deficient clinical compensation. Perivascular callosities and webs involving the external iliac vein (→); occlusion of the common iliac vein by a large central venous spur (+→). Collateral flow through the ascending lumbar vein (++→) to the vertebral and paravertebral plexuses

the inguinal region are available for bypassing an obliterated external iliac vein. This collateral route via the internal iliac veins is nearly always available when there is an isolated occlusion of the common iliac vein.

- *Ascending lumbar vein.* With obliteration of the common iliac vein, the ascending lumbar vein can channel venous return into the vertebral
295 and paravertebral venous systems, which have numerous connections with the inferior and superior vena cava.
- *External pudendal vein.* This vessel has anasto-
296 moses with the internal pudendal vein, which belongs to the territory of the internal iliac vein. With occlusion of the external iliac vein, this collateral pathway can acquire hemodynamic significance.
- *Veins of the abdominal wall.* These vessels, which carry blood in a caudal-to-cranial direction, do not function effectively as collaterals. They sometimes appear as large varices on 297
phlebograms.

Phlebographic Follow-Up

The progression from acute thrombosis to post-thrombotic syndrome is continuous and depends on the extent of the disease, individual factors, and applied therapeutic measures. Prompt fibrinolysis or thrombectomy can restore complete venous patency within a few days or earlier, whereas spontaneous recanalization and collateralization can take several months. In patients treated symptomatically, a stable, definitive state generally is not reached for about a year, and the term ***post-thrombotic syndrome*** (in the strict sense) is applicable. ***Early post-thrombotic syndrome*** refers to the interval between the acute phase of disease and hemodynamic stabilization at 2–12 months.

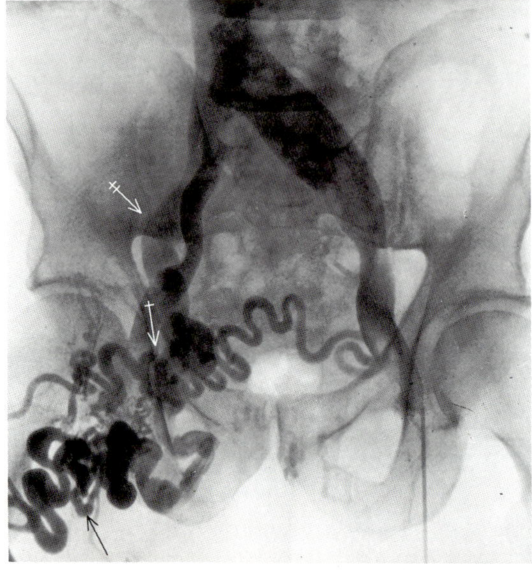

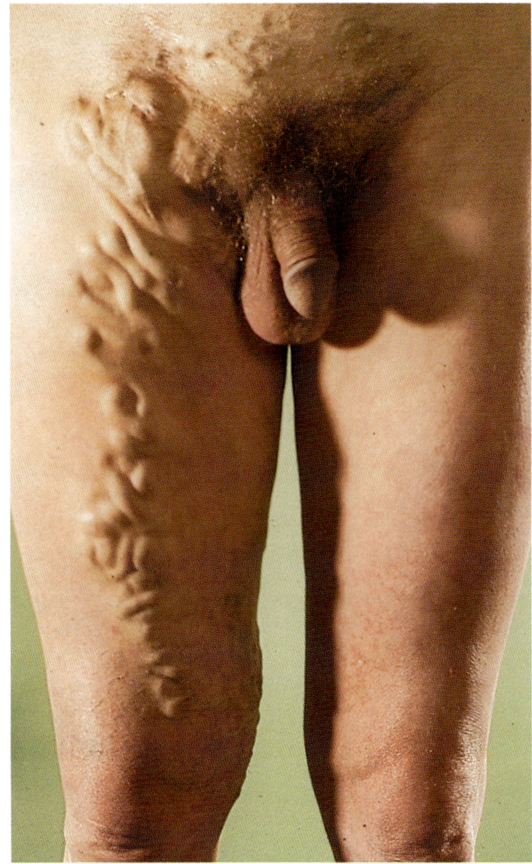

296. Occlusion of the right common femoral vein and external iliac vein by a war injury in a 58-year-old man. Marked collateral flow through the external (→) and internal pudendal veins (↔) to the internal iliac vein (⇸). *Top,* clinical appearance. *Bottom,* pelvic phlebogram

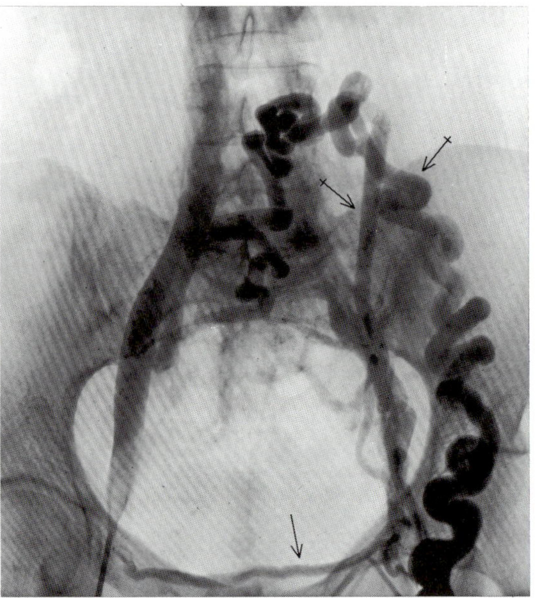

297. Post-thrombotic syndrome of the left pelvic and leg veins in a 44-year-old woman with poor clinical compensation. Inadequate recanalization of the external iliac vein and perivascular callosities; persistent occlusion of the common iliac vein. Suprapubic collaterals (→); extensive varicose collateral vessels in the anterior abdominal wall (↔). Demonstrated by pelvic phlebography

During this time the venous system has not yet completed its adaptation to the altered outflow conditions, and it is too early to assess the true impact of the occlusion. Early post-thrombotic syndrome, then, differs from post-thrombotic syndrome in that the vascular obliterations are more extensive while recanalization and collateralization are less advanced. Thus, in cases where acute thrombosis has been managed conservatively, a phlebographic follow-up examination should be scheduled for 1 year at the earliest so that a definitive assessment can be made as to the most appropriate plan of treatment.

In post-thrombotic syndrome proper, the hemodynamic conditions remain constant for years or decades. Decompensation of the collateral circuits marks the transition to ***late post-thrombotic syndrome,*** when a modification of treatment methods must be considered. Surgical treatment may be warranted, necessitating *follow-up phlebograms.*

Thus, only one or two radiographic examinations of the venous system are necessary during the lifelong course of post-thrombotic disease. All other information on disease compensation can be furnished by noninvasive diagnostic techniques.

Prior morphologic damage to the vein wall, pathologic flow conditions, and the continued presence of systemic risk factors are the essential causes of *recurrent thrombosis*. This condition can be very
298 difficult to diagnose phlebographically if no old films are available for comparison. The irregular lumina of the damaged post-thrombotic veins contain ill-defined filling defects that do not fit into the post-thrombotic architecture. Somewhat later the recurrent thrombus presents sharper, more angular contours with respect to its surroundings. Besides radiographic findings, the evaluating physician should assess the clinical presentation, the laboratory parameters of an inflammatory process, and also the efficacy of a therapeutic trial.

The age of a post-thrombotic syndrome cannot be determined from phlebographic findings beyond distinguishing between an early and late type of syndrome.

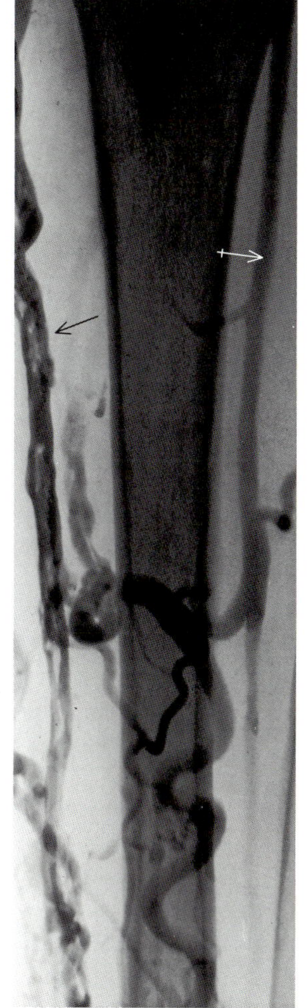

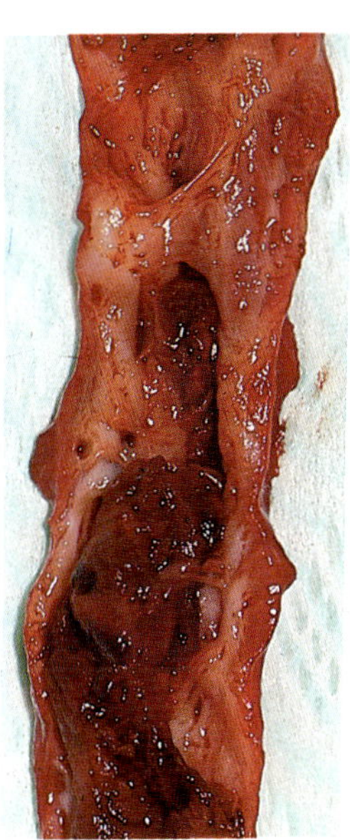

298. Recurrent thrombophlebitis of the ectatic great saphenous vein in post-thrombotic syndrome of the left leg. A 50-year-old man with repeated bouts of inflammation of unknown cause. *Left,* ascending pressure phlebography shows virtual nonfilling of the deep veins with contrast drainage through the ectatic great saphenous trunk (→). Old post-thrombotic changes and fresh thrombi in the vessel. ↔ Small saphenous vein. *Right,* surgical specimen of the great saphenous vein with thrombi

Formulating the Diagnosis

It is not very useful to classify phlebographic post-thrombotic syndromes by stages, mainly because there is no meaningful correlation with clinical symptoms. The most severe phlebographic changes may be well compensated, leading, for example, to an inadequate or erroneous disability assessment. A *descriptive diagnosis* conveys the most reliable information. Statements on the loca-
299 tion and extent of post-thrombotic changes, the degree of recanalization, and the functional adequacy of the collateral circulation are of immediate practical concern to the clinician. These points should be covered when the radiographic diagnosis is formulated.

Examples include the following:

- Post-thrombotic syndrome of the popliteal vein with complete recanalization
- Post-thrombotic syndrome of the deep lower leg veins and popliteal vein with partial recanalization and adequate collateral circulation through the great saphenous vein
- Post-thrombotic syndrome of the deep pelvic and lower limb veins with inadequate recanalization and deficient collateral circulation through the great saphenous vein

Essential diagnostic points in post-thrombotic syndrome
Location and extent
Degree of recanalization
Adequacy of collateral circulations

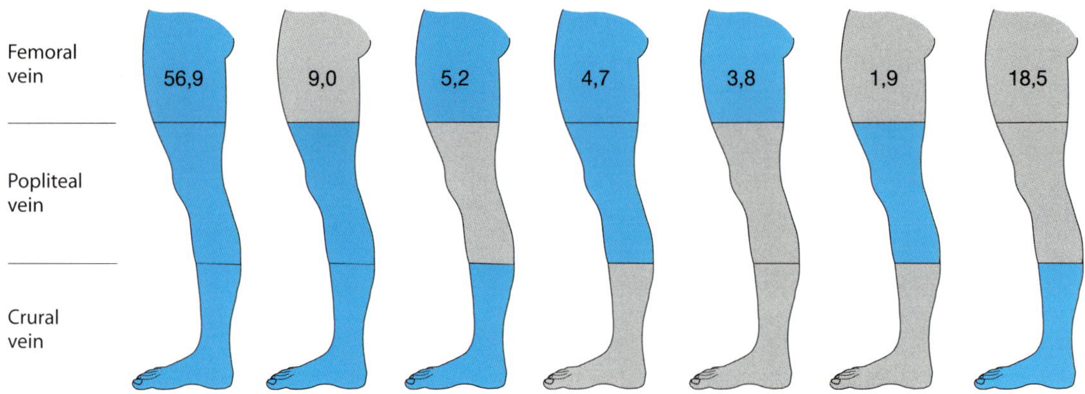

299. Frequency, location, and combination of post-thrombotic changes in the deep veins

Special Problems and Pitfalls

A major source of error in the interpretation of phlebograms is confusing internal webs and septa with flow phenomena, and mistaking vascular islets or mural structures for inflow effects. Doubts are quickly resolved by obtaining a second projection or delayed films.

101 The diagnostic difficulties relating to *nonopacification* of a vascular segment due to faulty technique were discussed earlier (see p. 65). Generally the affected segment can be visualized by administering a larger dose of contrast medium, injecting the medium under higher manual pressure, obtaining delayed films, or using the overflow effect. The selection of the injection site on the foot also plays a role, especially for visualization of the anterior tibial veins.

The diagnosis of post-thrombotic syndrome can be particularly challenging in patients who had *thrombosis in early childhood.* Radiographs demonstrate minimal alteration of venous morphology or hemodynamics. The only obvious abnormality is an absence of venous valves, which may be referred to a congenital anomaly.

Diagnosis is also difficult following an *optimum therapeutic response,* especially in younger patients. The purpose of thrombectomy and fibrinolysis, after all, is to forestall the development of post-thrombotic syndrome. Disordered, atypical muscle veins in the lower leg often provide the only radiographic clue to the original disease.

A strict distinction should be drawn between ***ectasia of the great saphenous vein*** in the setting of collateralization and *primary saphenous varicos-*
282 *ity.* The former condition represents a physiologic adaptive process to an increased volume load, whereas saphenous varicosity is based on pathologic structural changes in the vessel wall with incompetence of the venous valves. These conditions can be differentiated by their phlebographic features.

Primary varicosity of the great saphenous vein develops in a proximal-to-distal direction, whereas compensatory ectasia progresses from distal to proximal. Accordingly, the varicose saphenous
vein shows its greatest caliber increase proximally 143
with a gradual narrowing of the vessel in the peripheral direction. Compensatory ectasia, on the other hand, is characterized by a straight, uniform
expansion of the saphenous trunk from ankle to 241
groin. There are no retrograde flow signs such as infravalvular dilatations or aneurysms and meandering curves.

The characteristic flow patterns can be observed on the monitor and used as needed for differential diagnostic assessment. With compensatory ectasia there is immediate contrast filling of the great saphenous trunk, which shows an unusually intense degree of opacification. The varicose saphenous vein opacifies weakly in a later phase of the examination, when the contrast medium has already become diluted in the blood stream.

Technical errors in the phlebography of post-thrombotic syndrome
Overlapping superficial veins
Incomplete filling of the deep veins
Single-plane view
Nonvisualization of the pelvic veins

A combination of these findings points to *secon-*
286 *dary varicose degeneration* of the great saphenous vein and heralds the transition to late post-thrombotic syndrome.

In patients with severe chronic venous insufficiency, the contrast medium sometimes drains at once through incompetent perforators into large superficial varices. These superimposed opacities make assessment of the deep veins quite difficult. A clearer picture can be obtained by taking early films, but a successful examination may require occluding the superficial varices with a tight compression bandage.

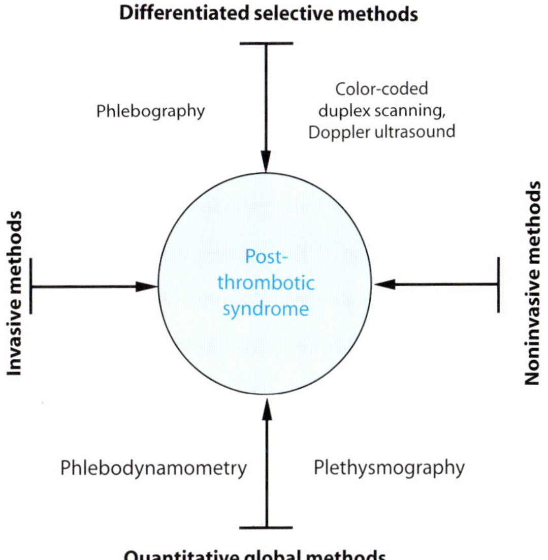

300. Instrumental techniques of venous diagnosis in post-thrombotic syndrome

Comparison of Phlebography with Other Diagnostic Methods

In most cases a *prior history* of thrombosis will direct suspicion toward post-thrombotic syndrome, but occasionally the diagnosis must be made in a patient with no prior history who is presenting for evaluation of local edema. These patients often report a tendency for swelling to persist in the lower extremity following an injury or operation. In other patients the dermatologic complications of chronic venous insufficiency are predominant. For a comprehensive assessment of the phlebologic status, it is necessary to combine phlebography with the measurement of various parameters of venous function. Each individual method provides particular information; in post-thrombotic syndrome, in contrast to other vascular diseases, imaging techniques and other methods are equally important. Thus in post-thrombotic disease the invasive and noninvasive and the selective and global measurements are combined, constituting the tetard of the instru-
300 mental diagnostic workup.

Real-time and *color-coded duplex scanning* allows for effective imaging of post-thrombotic changes in the veins. The patient is first examined in the supine position. The vessel lumen is filled with echogenic structures having the characteristics of
301 islets and webs. Calcium deposits are marked by acoustic shadows. The vein wall appears irregular-
302 ly thickened and also echogenic. The flow profile is permeated by turbulent zones. A major disadvantage of this method is it us not useful for evalu-
303 ating the extent of collateralization.

304 The destruction of the venous valves permits regurgitant blood flow in the main deep veins (*ret-rograde insufficiency*) during standing, coughing, and straining. This flow can be detected by *directional or unidirectional Doppler ultrasound*
measurement during a Valsalva maneuver in the 305
supine patient or by the calf decompression test in the standing patient. The *more severe* the changes are, the longer the apparent period of reverse flow. In the calf compression test, the flow amplitude of the directional Doppler curve also provides diagnostic clues. An intravascular obstacle in front of 305
or behind the transducer causes the amplitude to become smaller and wider according to the acoustic weakening of the A sound; in the frequency analysis profile, the fenestration is lost and the flow assumes a turbulent character.

Doppler ultrasound demonstrates a respiration-dependent flow pattern over the deep stem veins only if there is unobstructed proximal outflow. Spontaneous Doppler signals normally are not recorded from the great saphenous trunk. But if the vessel is part of a competent collateral system resulting from deep venous occlusion, at least the proximal segments will show definite respiratory
modulation of flow within the thigh. 306

The question of whether the great saphenous vein has retained its ***compensatory phlebectasia*** or whether there has already been a transition to secondary saphenous varicosity is significant in terms of selecting patients for operative treatment. Ascending pressure phlebography can pro-

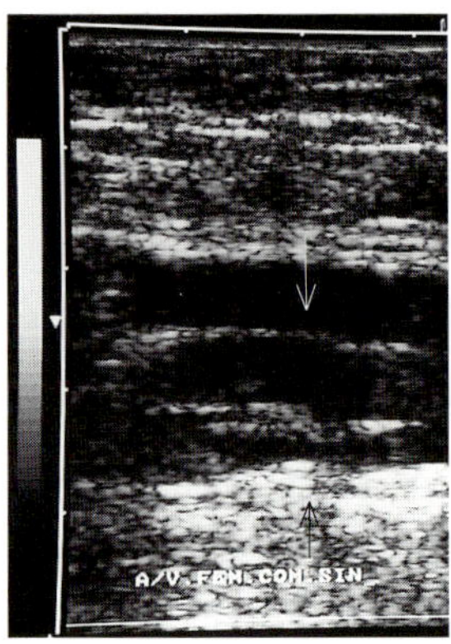

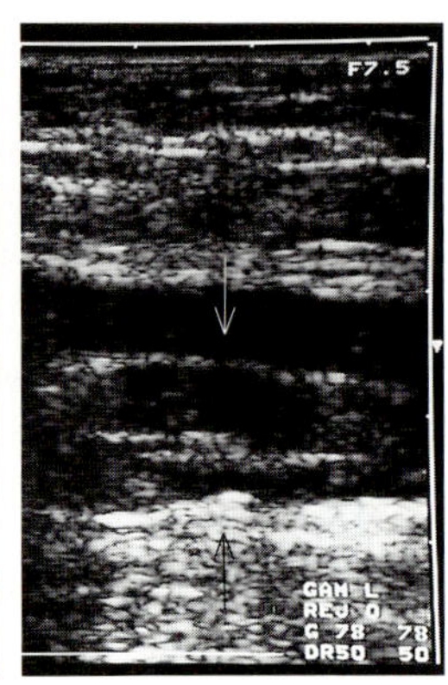

302. Post-thrombotic syndrome (in the narrow sense) in the superficial femoral vein. A 55-year-old woman with thrombosis of the leg and pelvic veins 29 years previously. Irregular vascular borders (→) with strong reflections from the lumen and septa. Increase in thickness of the vascular wall (*left*). Incompressibility (*right*) as evidence of the occluded lumen. Demonstrated by real-time sonography. (Acuson, 7-MHz transducer)

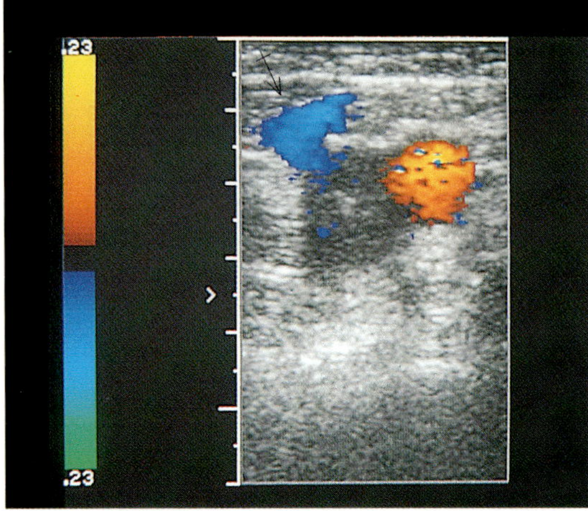

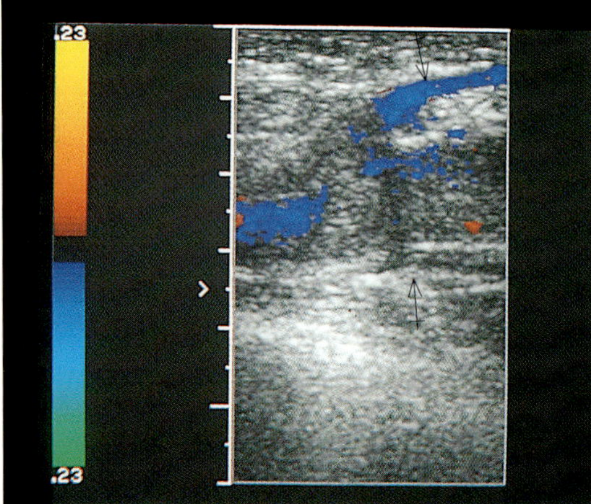

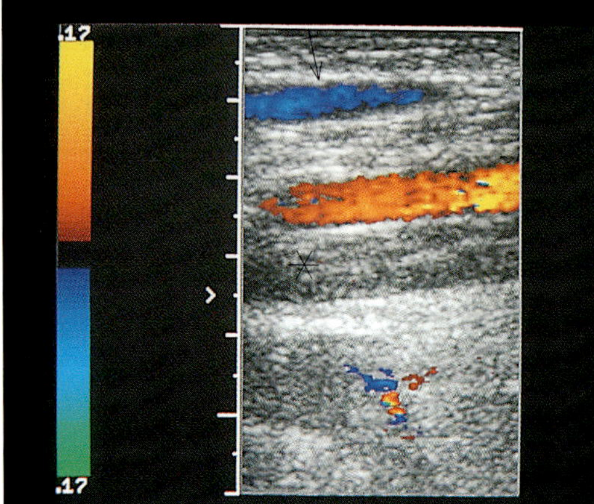

◁

301. Recurrent thrombosis in the superficial femoral vein 4 weeks previously (immediate syndrome) in post-thrombotic disease of long duration with phlebectasia of the great saphenous vein. A 50-year-old man with systemic disease. The occlusive thrombus reaches as far as the junction of the enlarged great saphenous vein (→); clearly demonstrated by sonography, particularly in the center of the lumen. Demonstrated by color-coded duplex sonography in the groin; *top,* cross-section; *middle,* longitudinal section. Clear increase in thickness of the dorsal vascular wall (↔). Occlusion of the superficial femoral vein (*) in the midthigh (*bottom*); enlarged great saphenous vein with spontaneous blood flow. Arteries coded *red.* (Acuson, 7-MHz transducer)

vide a clear *morphologic differentiation* of these conditions. Loss of the girdle sign as a criterion of compensatory ectasia and the detection of infravalvular dilatations or venous aneurysms justifies a diagnosis of secondary saphenous varicosity.
306 Doppler flowmetry permits *a functional assessment,* with absence of reflux after calf *de*compression in the standing patient indicating compensatory phlebectasia, and brief or limited reflux signifying delayed valve closure due to vascular dilatation corresponding to the radiographic girdle sign. Prolonged, inexhaustible reflux confirms 306

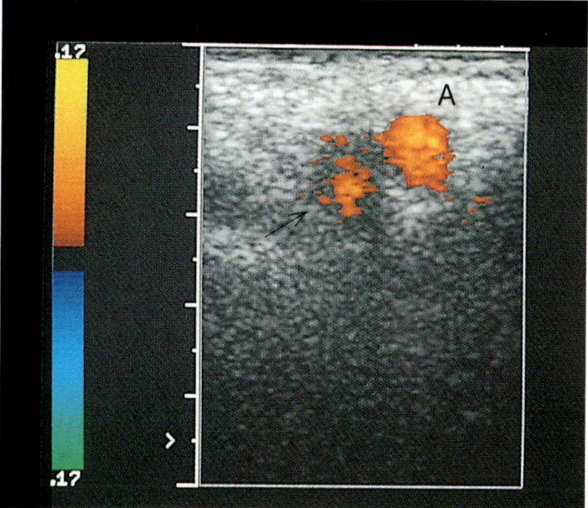

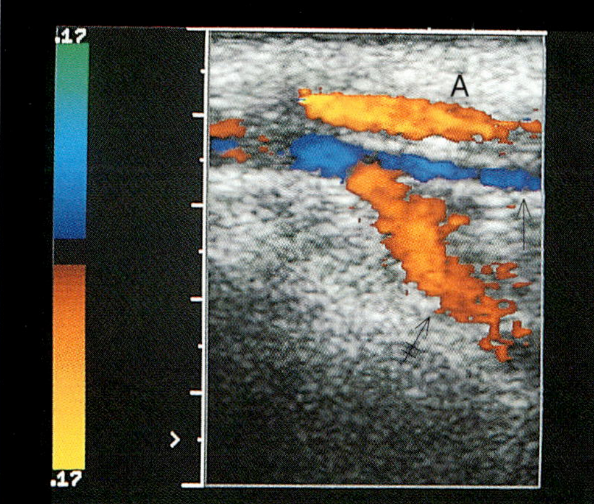

303. Post-thrombotic syndrome in the leg and pelvic veins on the left side in a 60-year-old woman. Ablation of the thrombus 8 years previously. *Top,* demonstrated by color-coded duplex sonography (cross-section). Partial reopening of the common femoral vein with retrograde flow direction during inspiration and Valsalva maneuver (→). *Bottom,* longitudinal section showing considerable narrowing of the superficial femoral vein with collateral enlargement of the deep femoral vein (⇸). Reversed flow direction with destroyed venous valves. Femoral artery (*A*) coded *red.* (Acuson, 7-MHz transducer)

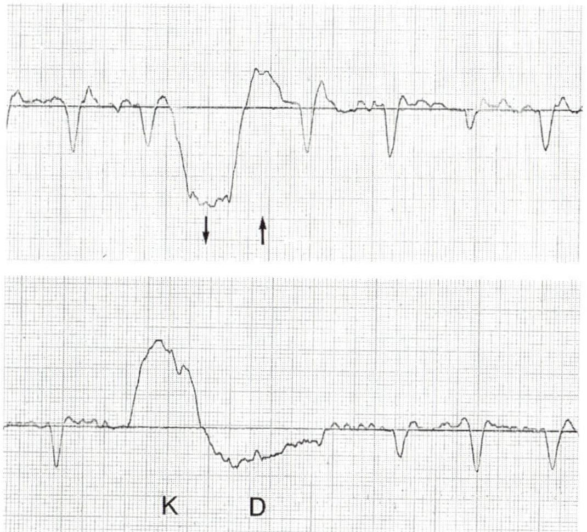

304. Directional Doppler hemodynamics in post-thrombotic syndrome with recanalization and loss of valve function. Taken over the superficial femoral vein with a 4-MHz transducer and paper speed of 20 cm/s; patient standing. *Top,* retrograde flow during the Valsalva maneuver (↓); brief overshoot effect following the Valsalva maneuver (↑). *Bottom,* low, broad amplitude during calf compression test (*K*), brief reflux during calf *de*compression test (*D*)

▷

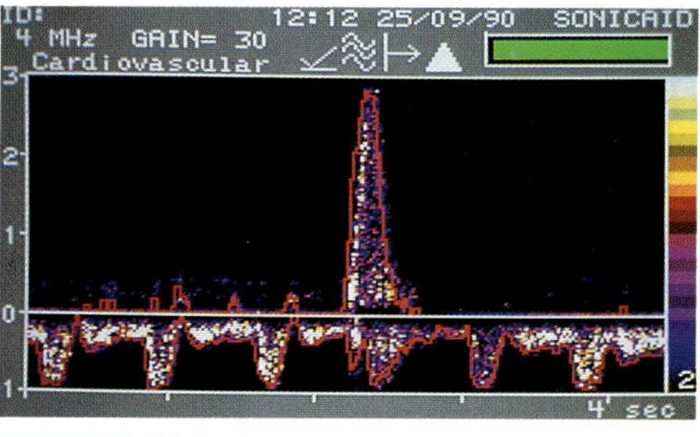

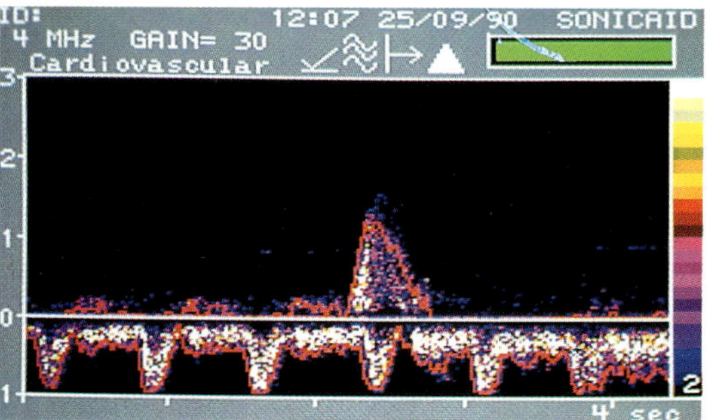

305. Doppler waveforms recorded over the superficial femoral vein using directional frequency analysis. Calf *com*pression and *de*compression test in the standing patient. Sonicaid unit, 4-MHz probe. *Top,* normal waveform shows high amplitude and spectral broadening on calf compression, minimal reflux due to valve closure on decompression. *Bottom,* amplitude decrease caused by outflow obstruction. Turbulent waveforms with no spectral broadening. Prolonged reflux effect on calf decompression

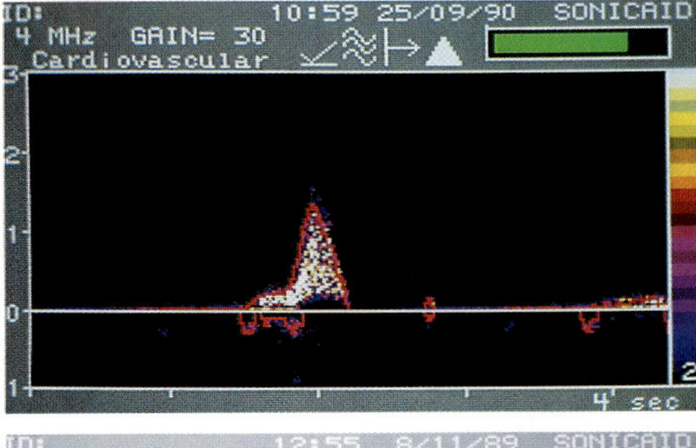

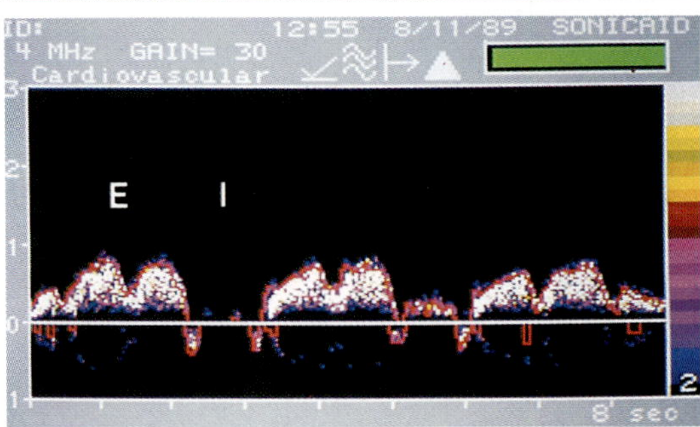

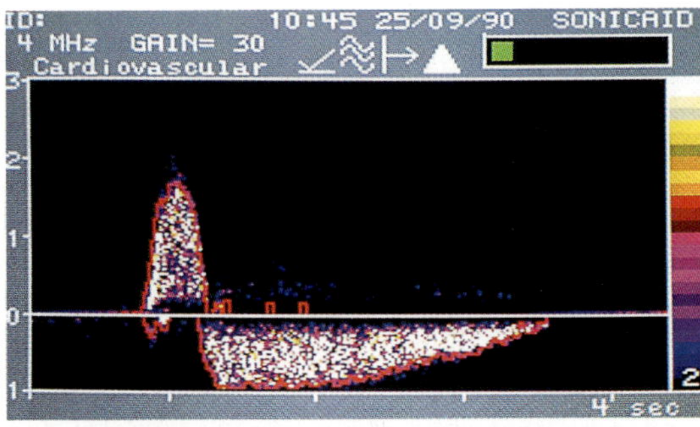

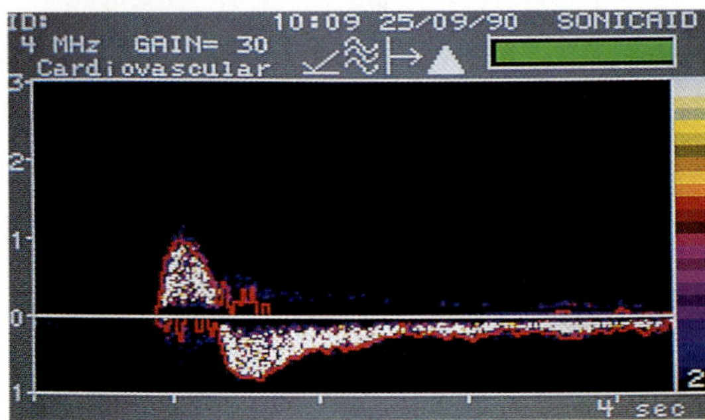

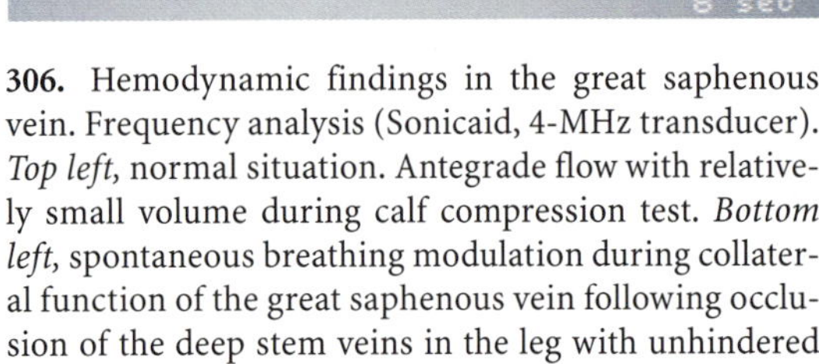

306. Hemodynamic findings in the great saphenous vein. Frequency analysis (Sonicaid, 4-MHz transducer). *Top left,* normal situation. Antegrade flow with relatively small volume during calf compression test. *Bottom left,* spontaneous breathing modulation during collateral function of the great saphenous vein following occlusion of the deep stem veins in the leg with unhindered pelvic drainage. *E,* expiration; *I,* inspiration. Arterial pulsation recorded. *Top right,* compensatory phlebectasia with clearly delayed valve closure. Correlation with morphological findings of the girdle sign. Calf compression and decompression test with patient standing. *Bottom right,* secondary saphenous varicosity without venous valve closure. Inexhaustible return flow effect during calf decompression test

complete valvular incompetence relating to secondary saphenous varicosity. If X-ray findings conflict with the result of the Doppler ultrasound examination, then treatment planning should be directed by the phlebographic findings. In principle, morphologic criteria provide the basis for the decision to manage a case surgically.

While the various parameters of *global venous function* convey information on the degree of compensation of the post-thrombotic disease, the morphologic substrate of the disease must be defined by radiography before a general evaluation can be made. This requirement is especially important in disability assessment cases.

The *dynamic venous pressure* is an essential parameter of venous function. A decrease in the delta-P pressure drop and a shortening of the *t2* refill
time provide important evidence of venous circu-
307 latory impairment in the post-thrombotic state.
The *combined,* consecutive use of phlebography and phlebodynamometry, then, conveys decisive information on the status of the post-thrombotic syndrome (Weber and May 1990). A butterfly needle in the dorsal foot vein can help facilitate the combined study.

Photoplethysmography (light reflection rheography) yields a tracing that is reciprocal but otherwise similar to the dynamic venous pressure curve, but instead of pressure relationships it reflects shifts of blood volume in the subdermal venous plexuses of the lower leg. Despite the indirect 308
nature of the light-reflection measurements, this simple study appears useful for monitoring the course of post-thrombotic disease. The exercise program consists of foot dorsiflexions performed by the seated patient. The refill time correlates best with the severity of venous insufficiency.

Venous capacity and drainage also convey important information on the compensation of post-
thrombotic syndrome. They are determined by
venous occlusion plethysmography. Combined 309
with phlebography, this study also provides a means of quantifying the blood flow disturbance. A decrease in *venous capacity* signifies inadequate

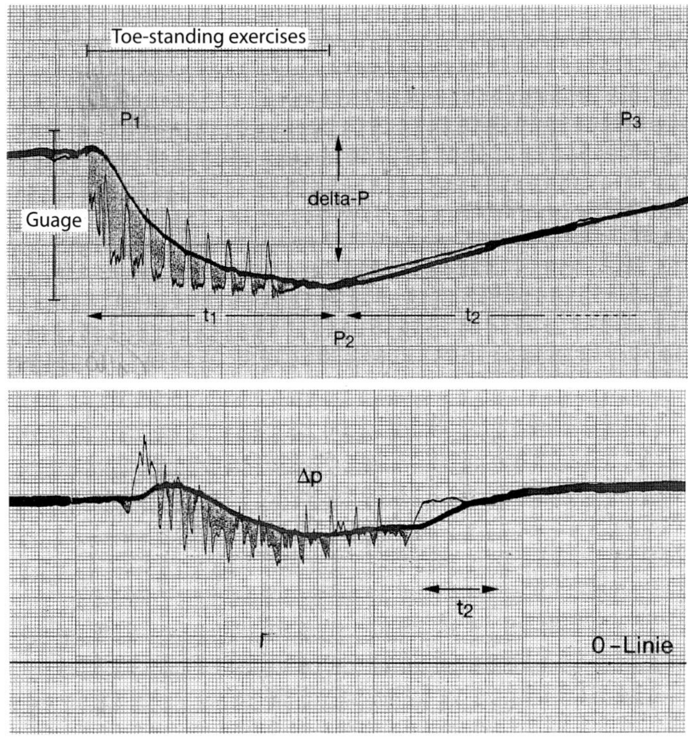

307. Dynamic venous pressure curve in post-thrombotic syndrome. *Top*, normal findings with the principle parameters *P1* (resting pressure), *delta-P* (pressure decrease during exercise), and *t2* (time until return to baseline pressure) (see also Fig. 125). *Bottom*, severe post-thrombotic syndrome. Pressure decrease delta-P 20 mmHg (normal>55 mmHg); *t2* decreased to 2 s (normal>25 s)

recanalization and is typical of post-thrombotic syndrome. An increase in venous capacity is seen with increasing secondary varicosity or may result from sacculations in decompensated collateral pathways of the deep venous system.

Venous drainage, an index of the outflow velocity of blood from the lower extremity, reflects the sum of recanalization and collateralization as an expression of compensatory conditions in the outflow tract. Drainage measurements are not affected by the function of the peripheral muscle pumps. Drainage remains at a markedly decreased level during the phase of early post-thrombotic syndrome but then gradually increases with adaptation.

Phlebography and the various physical measurements *supplement each other* in the evaluation of post-thrombotic syndrome. As in no other venous system disorder, the indication for specific operative procedures is based on an awareness and critical analysis of all findings. The noninvasive techniques are adequate for long-term follow-ups, however.

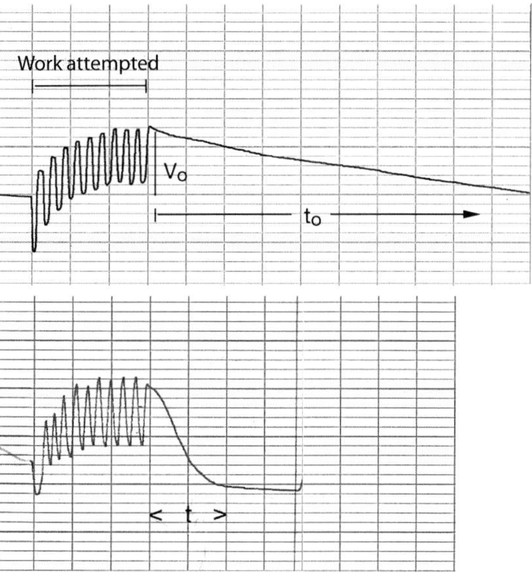

308. Photoplethysmograhpic results in post-thrombotic syndrome. *Top*, normal curve (see also Fig. 124). *Bottom*, refill time *t* decreased to 10 s (normal, 30 s)

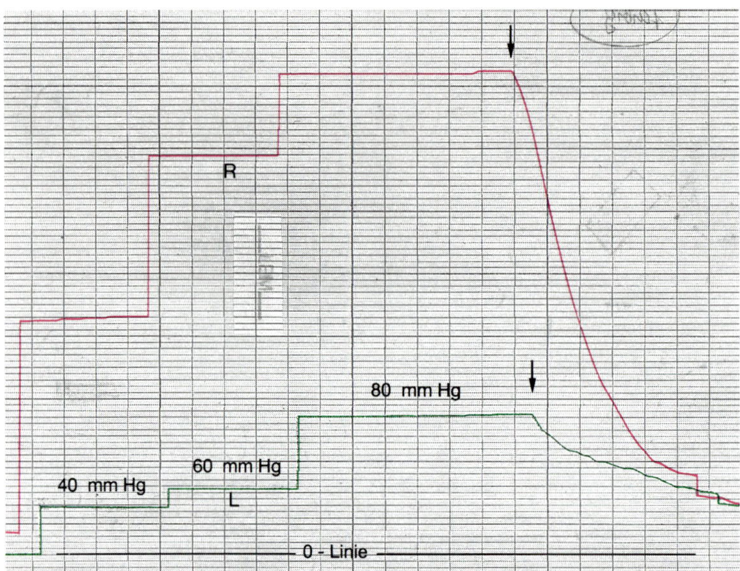

309. Plethysmographic curves in venous occlusion. *R*, normal curve for the right leg. Venous capacity 4.5 ml blood/100 ml tissue; drainage (↓) 68.3 ml blood/100 ml tissue per min. *L*, severe post-thrombotic syndrome on the left side. Capacity 1.4 ml; drainage (↓) 11.6 ml

In patients with a unilateral post-thrombotic syndrome of the pelvic veins, a special indication exists for venous pressure measurement when a bypass procedure is being considered. This can be done with the same needle used for selective pelvic phlebography, or with a separate needle inserted into the common femoral vein. The pressures are measured in the supine patient using a Statham element at rest and then during exercise consisting of 20 maximum ankle excursions. If the pressure rises by more than 30% relative to the resting value, a bypass procedure is indicated.

Therapeutic Implications

The therapeutic mainstay in post-thrombotic syndrome is *compression*. Clinical and phlebographic findings will determine whether compression therapy should be limited to the lower leg or encompass the whole limb. The prescribed class of compression stocking depends on the degree of compensation of the venous flow impairment.

Surgical *removal of the great saphenous vein* is advised when the vessel has ceased to function as a collateral and there has been a deterioration of peripheral hemodynamics in the setting of secondary saphenous varicosity. The surgeon must base patient selection on pertinent phlebographic findings, Doppler flow sampling, and especially on quantitative data from a comprehensive evaluation of venous hemodynamics. *Selective perforator dissection* or *operations at the crural fascia* can be of substantial benefit in improving chronic venous insufficiency.

With inadequate recanalization at the pelvic level and favorable hemodynamic conditions in the leg veins, the main surgical options to consider are *Palma's bypass operation,* the alloplastic crossover bypass, or Hach's inverse crossover procedure. The clinical information necessary for patient selection are derived from the phlebogram and from femoral venous pressure data. In special cases value reconstruction or transplantation is possible.

Bilateral Post-thrombotic Syndrome of the Pelvic Veins and Post-thrombotic Syndrome of the Inferior Vena Cava

It is useful to classify the level of occlusion of the inferior vena cava as low, intermediate, or high on the basis of clinical symptoms. Each type is a separate disease entity, and all are associated with 265
more or less pronounced venous congestion in the trunk and lower limb. Similar effects are associated with bilateral obstruction of the pelvic veins.

Besides digital subtraction imaging, studies that contribute to the diagnostic workup of inferior vena caval occlusion syndrome include computed tomography and magnetic resonance imaging, which are advantageous in that they also permit a differentiated assessment of surrounding tissue structures. Real-time sonographic imaging and duplex scanning also are used routinely. The ultrasound techniques convey reliable information on the condition of the inferior vena cava but not on the collateral pathways.

Low Caval Occlusion

Low (infrarenal) occlusion of the inferior vena cava and bilateral post-thrombotic pelvic venous syndrome cause lower limb edema, secondary varices, and in severe cases chronic venous insufficiency. The occlusion terminates below the entry of the renal veins, which inhibit further progression of the thrombosis owing to their high blood flow. Farther peripherally, the deep leg veins may be involved in the circulatory disturbance. *Etiologic considerations* should include a systemic disorder (e.g., a collagen disease), a disturbance of homeostasis, or an extravascular compression syndrome.

Recanalization processes are less effective in the large pelvic and retroperitoneal vessels than in the peripheral veins. Collateralization plays a far greater role owing to the numerous anatomically preformed vascular connections that exist in the retroperitoneal space. Digital subtraction phlebography is the technique most commonly used at present for the radiographic scrutiny of these vessels.

Five collateral pathways are available for bypas-
310 sing a low caval occlusion. A knowledge of these pathways is important for understanding the pathophysiology of the occlusion and interpreting the roentgenograms.

Collateral circulations associated with various types of inferior vena caval occlusion			
	Type of occlusion		
	Low	Intermediate	High
Central collateral circulation	+	+	+
Superficial collateral circulation	+	+	+
Parietal collateral circulation	+	+	0
Portal collateral circulation	+	+	0
Intermediate collateral circulation	+	0	0

Vertebral Plexuses and Paravertebral Trunks. This central collateral pathway constitutes a functional unit. It is closely related anatomically to the parietal vessels. Because the venous plexuses are valve- 311
less, they can carry blood in all directions and communicate with the inferior vena cava at any level. The anastomoses between the ascending lumbar veins and the azygos vein on the right side or the hemiazygos vein on the left establish direct connections with the superior vena cava.

The central collateral circulation has the greatest hemodynamic significance. It is best demonstrated by subtraction films.

Parietal Collateral Pathways. Collateral flow 312
through the deep circumflex iliac vein to the costal

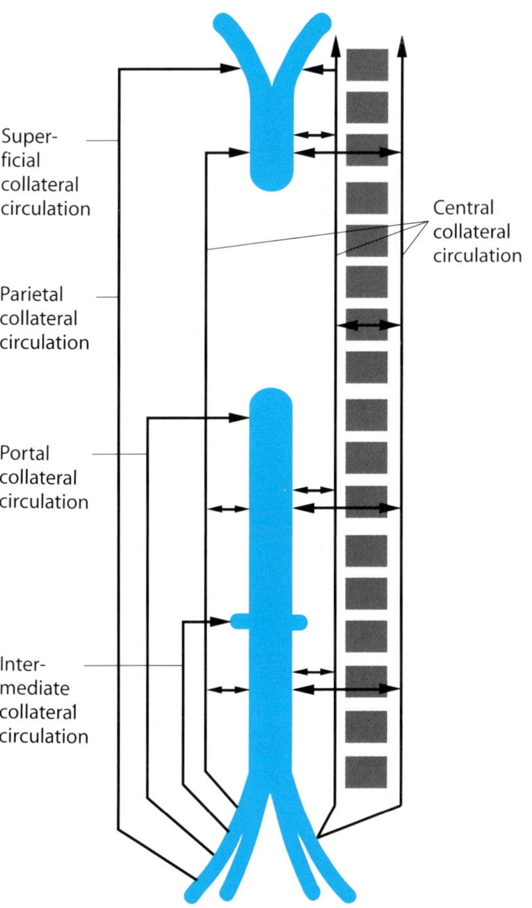

310. Collateral systems associated with a low occlusion of the inferior vena cava

Anastomoses between the inferior vena caval and portal systems
Primary anastomoses (anatomically preformed)
Inferior and medial rectal veins, Rectal venous plexus → Superior rectal vein → Inferior mesenteric vein
Paraumbilical veins → Vein of falciform ligament
Left ovarian vein or left spermatic vein → Inferior mesenteric vein → Left colic veins
Lumbar veins, Renal veins, Renal capsular veins, Suprarenal veins → Superior and inferior mesenteric veins
Secondary anastomoses (via peritoneal adhesions)
Pelvic venous plexus → Ileal veins →Superior mesenteric vein
Pelvic venous plexus, Inferior epigastric vein → Epiploic veins → Gastroepiploic veins

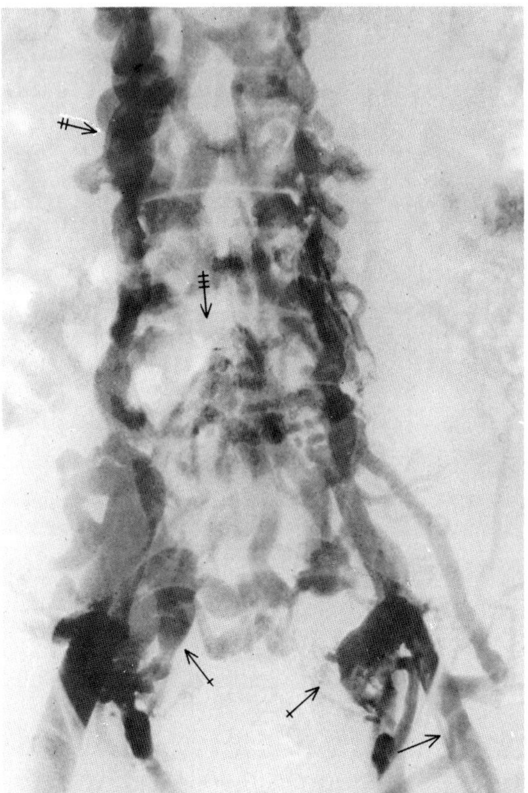

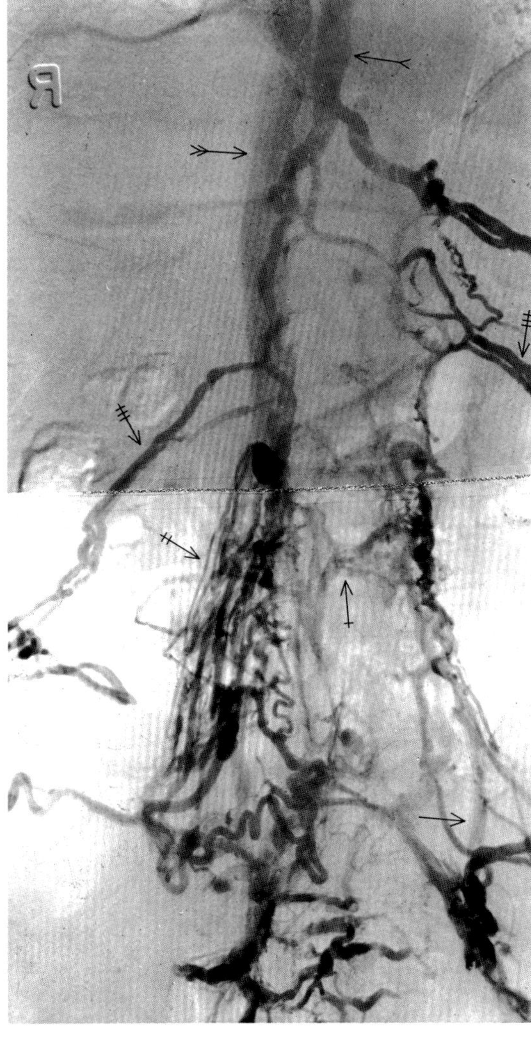

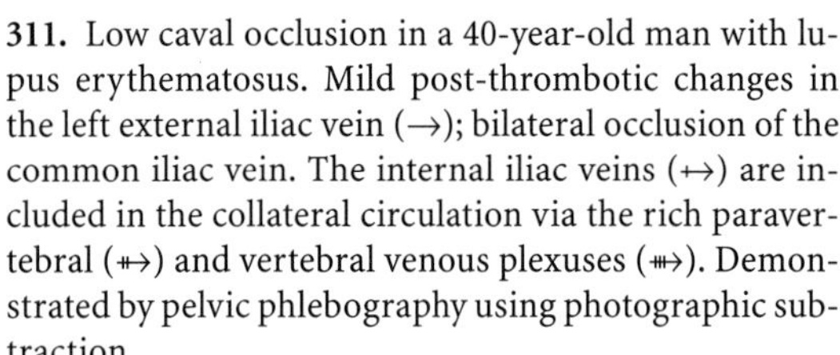

311. Low caval occlusion in a 40-year-old man with lupus erythematosus. Mild post-thrombotic changes in the left external iliac vein (→); bilateral occlusion of the common iliac vein. The internal iliac veins (↦) are included in the collateral circulation via the rich paravertebral (⇸) and vertebral venous plexuses (⇻). Demonstrated by pelvic phlebography using photographic subtraction

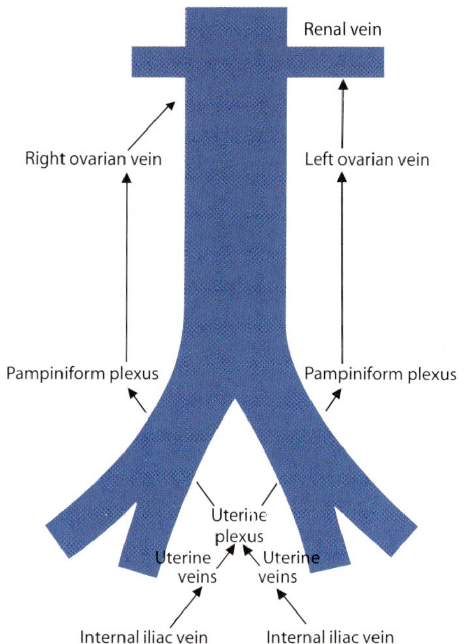

313. Intermediate collateral circulation through the ovarian veins

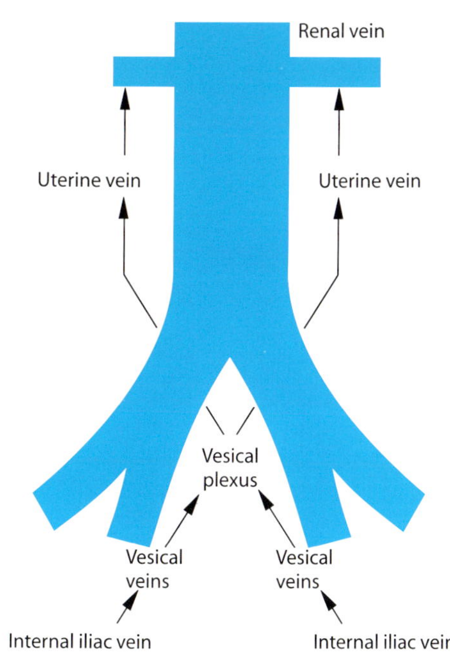

314. Intermediate collateral circulation through the uterine veins

◁ **312.** Low caval occlusion in a 45-year-old woman with lupus erythematosus. Parietal collateral circulations. → Ascending lumbar vein; +→ vertebral plexus; ++→ psoas veins; +++→ subcostal vein; ↣ azygos vein; ↣↣ inferior vena cava. Enhanced by photographic subtraction

▷

315. Occlusion of the left common iliac vein in a 29-year-old woman. Demonstrated by pelvic phlebography with photographic subtraction. Shown are the uterine plexus (→), the left ovarian plexus (+→) and ovarian veins (++→), and the vertebral and paravertebral plexuses (+++→)

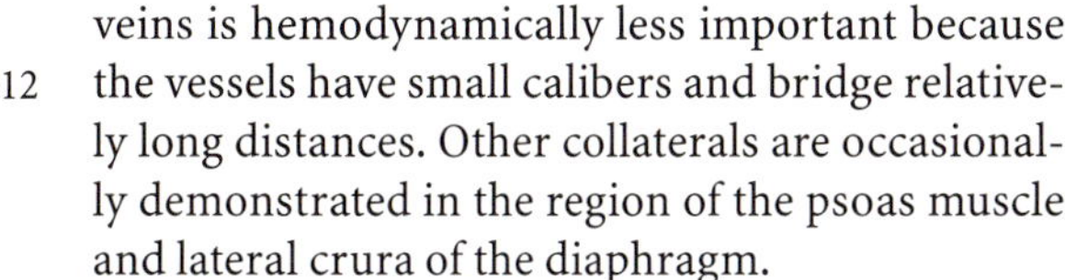

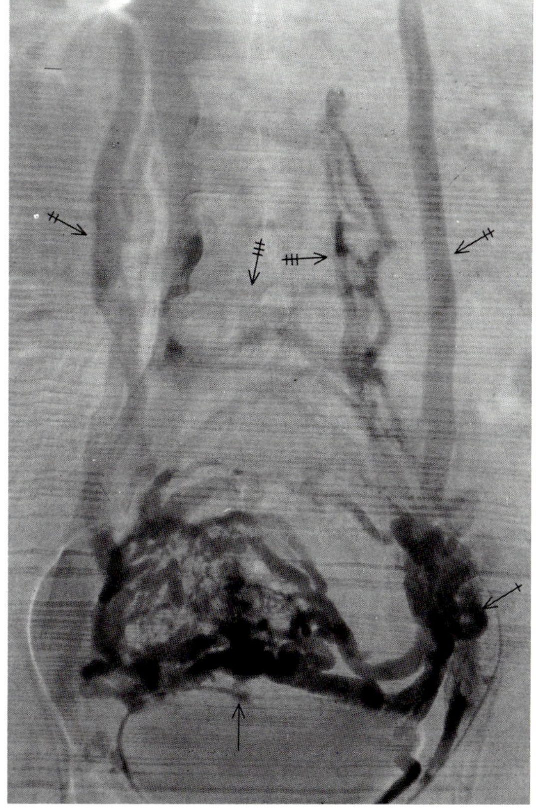

veins is hemodynamically less important because
312 the vessels have small calibers and bridge relatively long distances. Other collaterals are occasionally demonstrated in the region of the psoas muscle and lateral crura of the diaphragm.

Ovarian and Uterine Veins. Part of the intermedi-
313 ate collateral circulation, these vessels arise from
314 the pelvic plexuses and in women can attain thumb-size calibers. The uterine vessels have comparatively little hemodynamic significance.
315 They are recognized on phlebograms by their distinctive tortuosity.

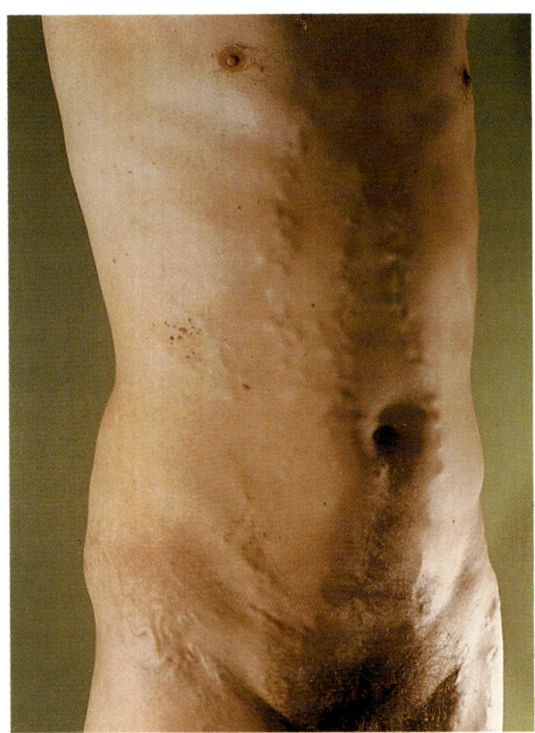

Primary and Secondary Anastomoses with the Portal Venous System. Venous drainage in the pel- 316
vic region and abdominal wall occurs through the same vessels as in portal hypertension, but in the opposite direction. The anatomically preformed anastomoses (primary anastomoses) have very little hemodynamic significance. Small veins in proximity to the umbilicus are important for the clinical differential diagnosis of portal hypertension, but all are not demonstrated on phlebograms. Secondary anatomoses that develop through peritoneal adhesions can assume major importance.

Collaterals of the Abdominal and Chest Wall. 317
These delicate vessels have very little importance as collaterals because of their small caliber, marked tortuosity, and their distance from the superior vena caval system. However, prominence

◁

316. Collateral vessels on the anterior abdominal wall associated with a low occlusion of the inferior vena cava

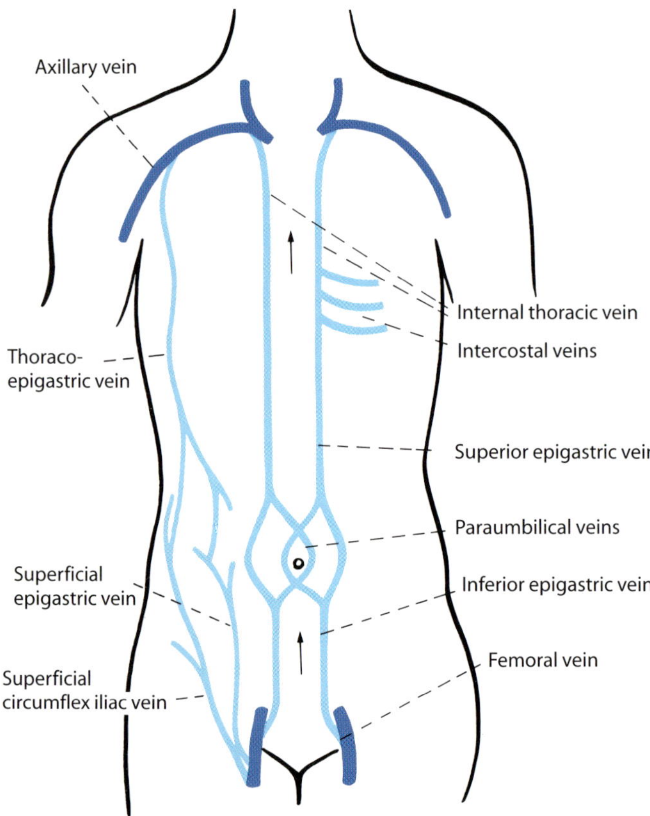

317. Superficial collateral circulation associated with a low occlusion of the inferior vena cava

of these vessels is a very useful clinical indicator that permits an immediate presumptive diagnosis to be made.

Intermediate Caval Occlusion

Intermediate occlusion of the inferior vena cava with involvement of the renal vessels is very rare. Usually there are associated occlusions in the pelvis and lower limbs. Intermediate caval occlusion should be suspected clinically whenever *venous inflow stasis* coexists with a *nephrotic syndrome*. Acute renal venous thrombosis causes excruciating, unremitting pain in the lumbar region, while post-thrombotic syndrome presents with less drastic symptoms.

The intermediate type of occlusion can result from systemic inflammatory vascular diseases and especially from neoplastic processes that infiltrate and compress the inferior vena cava from surrounding tissues.

The same systems can function as collaterals as in the low type of occlusion. Another important potential pathway, first described by Leja in 1888, is the *renolumbar anastomosis* between the renal veins and the paravertebral plexuses (Bücheler et al. 1968; Weber 1978).

High Caval Occlusion

High occlusion of the interior vena cava is a rare entity characterized by involvement of the hepatic veins. It may be caused by obliterative endophlebitis of the hepatic veins, congenital septa in the inferior vena cava, or tumor compression syndrome.

The clinical picture corresponds to the chronic form of *Budd-Chiari syndrome* combined with chronic venous insufficiency symptoms in the legs. The liver is greatly enlarged and tender to pressure. Because the collateral circulations of the portal system and of the pelvic venous congestion develop synergistically, there is very marked prominence of the superficial trunk veins. The central collateral pathway has the greatest hemodynamic importance.

References

Benecke G (1973) Pathologie der Venenerkrankungen. In: Haid-Fischer F, Haid H (Hrsg) Venenerkrankungen. Thieme, Stuttgart

Bücheler E, Düx A, Sobbe A (1968) Die renolumbale Anastomose im direkten retroperitonealen Veno- und selektiven Azygogramm. Fortschr Röntgenstr 109: 712

Fischer H, Widmer LK, Biland L (1982) Sozioepidemiologische Untersuchung der Venenkrankheiten. Phlebol Proktol 11: 94

Hach W (1982) Der venöse Kollateralkreislauf. In: Fischer H, Betz E (Hrsg) Restitutive Vorgänge in Gefäßwänden, Kollateralkreisläufe. Wissenschaftl Verlagsges, Stuttgart

Hach W (1989) Paratibiale Fasziotomie. In: Denck H, van Dongen RJAM (Hrsg) Therapie der Venenerkrankungen. TM-Verlag, Hameln

Hach W, Hach-Wunderle V (1994) Die Rezirkulationskreise der primären Varikose. Springer, Berlin Heidelberg New York Tokyo

Hach W, Langer C, Schirmers U (1983) Das arthrogene Stauungssyndrom. Vasa 12: 109

Halse T (1954) Das postthrombotische Syndrom. Steinkopff, Darmstadt

Hrivula-Pfeuffer A (1976) Phlebographische Untersuchungen über die Bedeutung des Kollateralkreislaufs im tiefen Venensystem für die Kompensation des postthrombotischen Syndroms. Inauguraldissertation, Universität Frankfurt

Netzer CO (1958) Die Strömungsverhältnisse beim postthrombotischen Syndrom. Zbl Chir 83: 1698

Netzer CO (1968) Die Strömungsverhältnisse beim postthrombotischen Zustandsbild. In: Kappert A, May R (Hrsg) Das postthrombotische Zustandsbild der Extremitäten. Huber, Bern

Schneider W (1976) Zur Pathophysiologie der venösen Insuffizienz unter Berücksichtigung der lymphovenösen Beziehungen. In: Klüken N, Schmutzler R (Hrsg) Fragivix. Ergebnisse d. Angiologie, Bd 11. Schattauer, Stuttgart

Staubesand J (1977) Matrix-Vesikel und Mediadysplasie. Med Welt 28: 1943

Wanke R, Gumrich H (1950) Chronische Beckenvenensperre. Zbl Chir 75: 130

Weber J (1978) Phlebographie und Venendruckmessung im Abdomen und Becken. Witzstrock, Baden-Baden

Weber J, May R (1990) Funktionelle Phlebographie. Thieme, Stuttgart

Venous Aneurysms

Few reports have been published to date on aneurysms of the venous system (Hartling and Hach 1973). Most venous aneurysms are detected fortuitously during surgery or radiographic examination.

The term "aneurysm" by definition refers to the arterial system due to the pathogenetic potential of the high intra-arterial pressure. Even in the veins, however, intravascular pressures can exceed 100 mmHg during

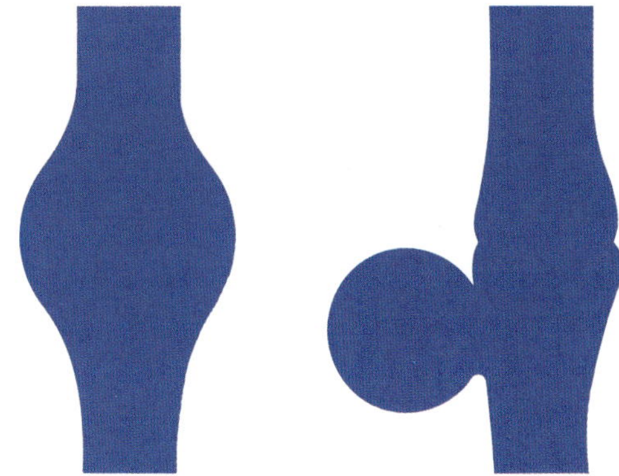

318. Fusiform and saccular venous aneurysms

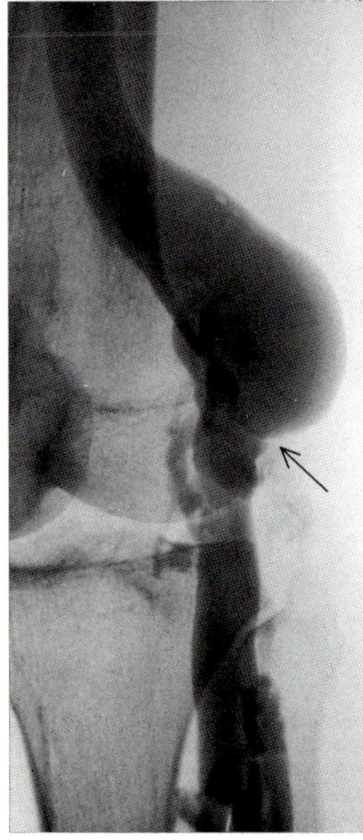
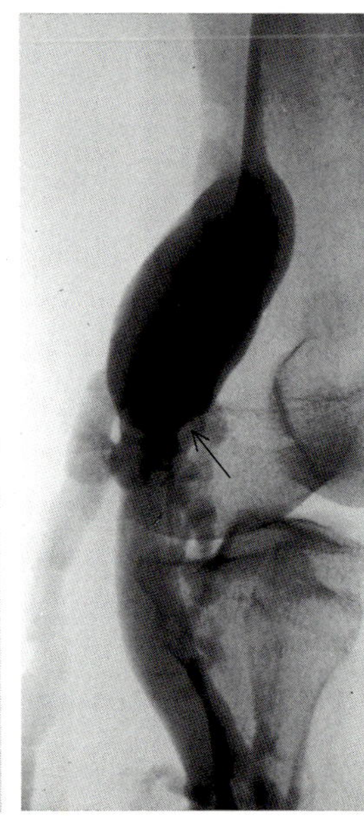

320. Regional ectasia of the popliteal vein due to a valvular anomaly (→); no aneurysm. Incidental finding during ascending pressure phlebography, internal rotation (*left*) and lateral view (*right*). Incidental finding

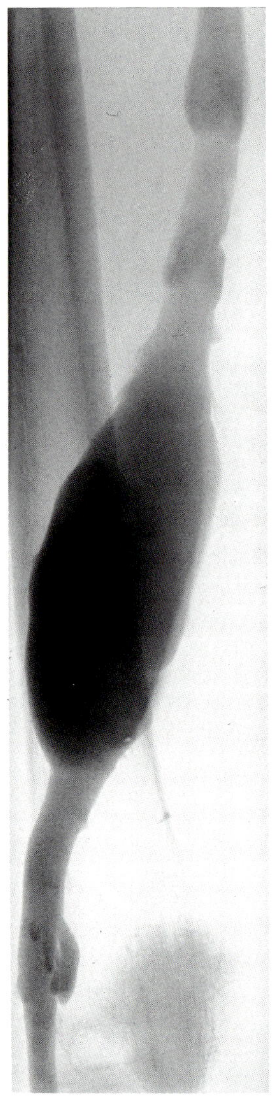

◁ **319.** Fusiform aneurysm of the superficial femoral vein. This lesion gave rise to a severe pulmonary embolism in a 47-year-old man with an otherwise negative history. (Phlebogram courtesy of Prof. Dr. H.E.Schmitt, Kantonspital Basel, Switzerland)

coughing or straining (Prerovski et al. 1960). In a vein with preexisting wall damage, this pressure is sufficient to produce a localized dilatation with all the symptoms of an aneurysm.

We know from arterial pathology that three main types of aneurysm can occur. A *true aneurysm* is one involving all layers of the vessel wall. A *false aneurysm* is caused by injury or disease of the middle and outer wall layers. A *dissecting aneurysm* involves a longitudinal splitting of the vessel wall by the dissection of blood between the wall layers. All of these types have been described within the venous system as well (Hartling and Hach 1973).

Venous aneurysms are either fusiform or saccular 318
in shape. The morphologic criteria for a *fusiform* 319
aneurysm on phlebograms are the localized involvement of a venous segment and an abrupt caliber increase relative to the adjacent, normal-size segment. Together, these features allow for positive differentiation from phlebectasia and varicos- 320
ity, which also may be confined to short venous segments.

Radiographic features of fusiform aneurysm
Segmental involvement Abrupt caliber increase Spindle shape

Radiographic features of saccular aneurysm
Segmental involvement Unilateral outpouching of the vessel wall Presence of a neck Tendency to occur below a venous valve

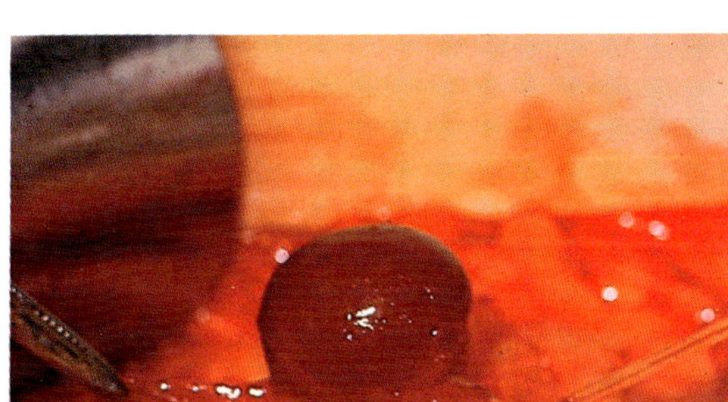

Fusiform aneurysms of the peripheral veins are rare. A typical site of occurrence, apparently, is at the femoropopliteal junction. We have personally observed three such cases. Weber and May (1990) reported on 19 cases in the literature. Fusiform aneurysms are seldom encountered in the large proximal venous trunks.

On the other hand, the *saccular aneurysm* typical
of great saphenous varicosity is a common find- 321
ing. It invariably forms below an incompetent venous valve. With an asymmetrical incompetence 136
of the valve cusps, the blood refluxes into the vein
during straining and impinges on one surface of
the wall at an oblique angle. With passage of time, 137
shear effects and turbulence produce an outpouching of the vessel at that location. By definition, an aneurysm is present as soon as there is a
discernible "neck" whose diameter is at least half 139
the maximum diameter of the sac. 323

Saphenous vein aneurysms tend to occur distal to 322
the second sluice valve, i.e., a hands width below
the entry of the saphenous trunk into the deep venous system. Apparently the strong flexure of the
crosse creates a site of predilection, although aneurysms can also occur about other venous valves. 326

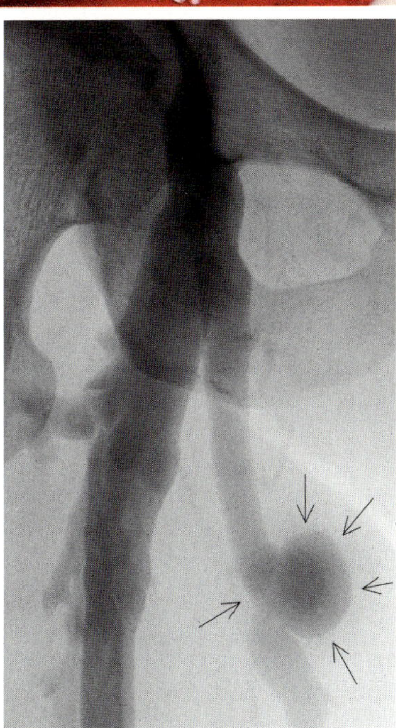

321. Saccular aneurysm in a varicose great saphenous vein. Typical site of occurrence below an incompetent venous valve. *Top*, surgical specimen. *Bottom*, ascending pressure phlebography

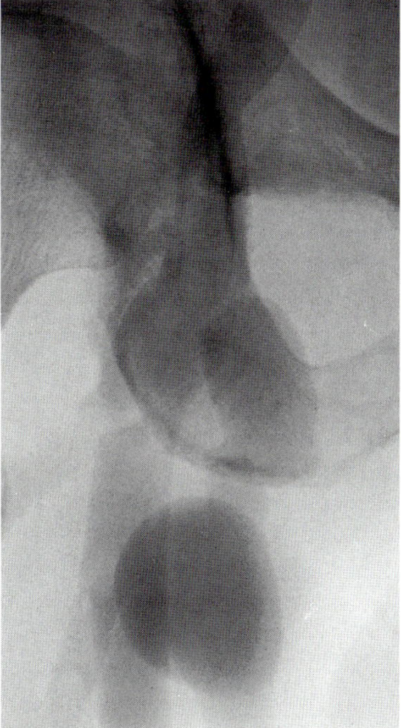

322. Saccular aneurysms of a great saphenous vein with severe stage IV varicosity. The lesions are located below the terminal valve and sluice valve

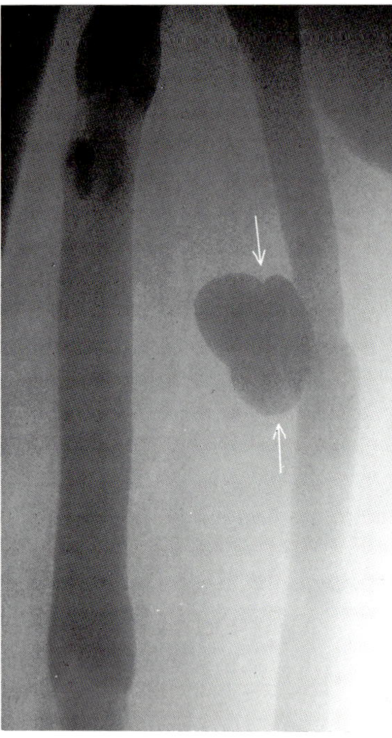

323. Infravalvular saccular aneurysm (→) of a varicose great saphenous vein in the midthigh

324. Infravalvular aneurysm of a varicose great saphenous vein. → Ball thrombus

They are very rarely observed in the small saphenous vein.

Hemodynamic factors are of prime importance in
the pathogenesis of saccular saphenous vein aneurysms. Congenital defects in the vein wall, inflam-
323 matory processes, and traumatic insults have less
causal significance. The prevalence of saccular aneurysms in varicose saphenous veins is 10.9%
(Hartling and Hach 1973).

324 Venous aneurysms can easily become thrombosed
325–327 and thus inaccessible to phlebographic inspection. Spherical ball thrombi are occasionally seen.
Saccular aneurysms are very rare in the deep venous system of the leg. Their pathogenesis relates to congenital defects and secondary wall damage in post-thrombotic syndrome. We have personally observed aneurysms of the popliteal vein, superficial femoral vein, and soleus veins.

Aneurysms of the deep axial veins are easily detected by *real-time ultrasound imaging* and *color-coded duplex scanning.* Intra-aneurysmatic thrombi can be identified by their relatively high echogenicity. Ultrasound has a special role in the search for an unknown embolus source; fusiform aneurysms of the femoropopliteal region can be particularly life-threatening in this regard. Most aneurysms are incidental findings, however.

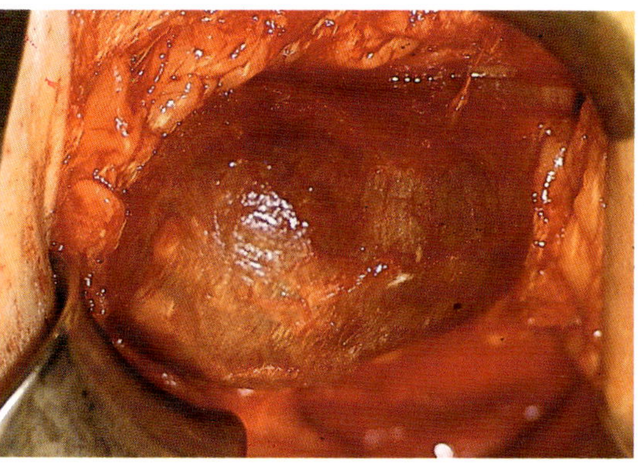

325. Plum-size thrombosed aneurysm of the great saphenous vein in the groin region. Appearance at operation

During *phlebography,* an effort is made to demonstrate the aneurysm in two planes. This is done by
attempting to rotate the neck into the lateral pro- 326
jection. Otherwise the lesion may be mistaken for
coiling of the vein due to regressive changes.

A large venous aneurysm is at risk for thrombosis and thus poses a hazard of potentially severe pulmonary embolism. It is prudent, therefore, to consider *surgical treatment* in addition to compression therapy and anticoagulation. In suitable cases the aneurysm can be ex-

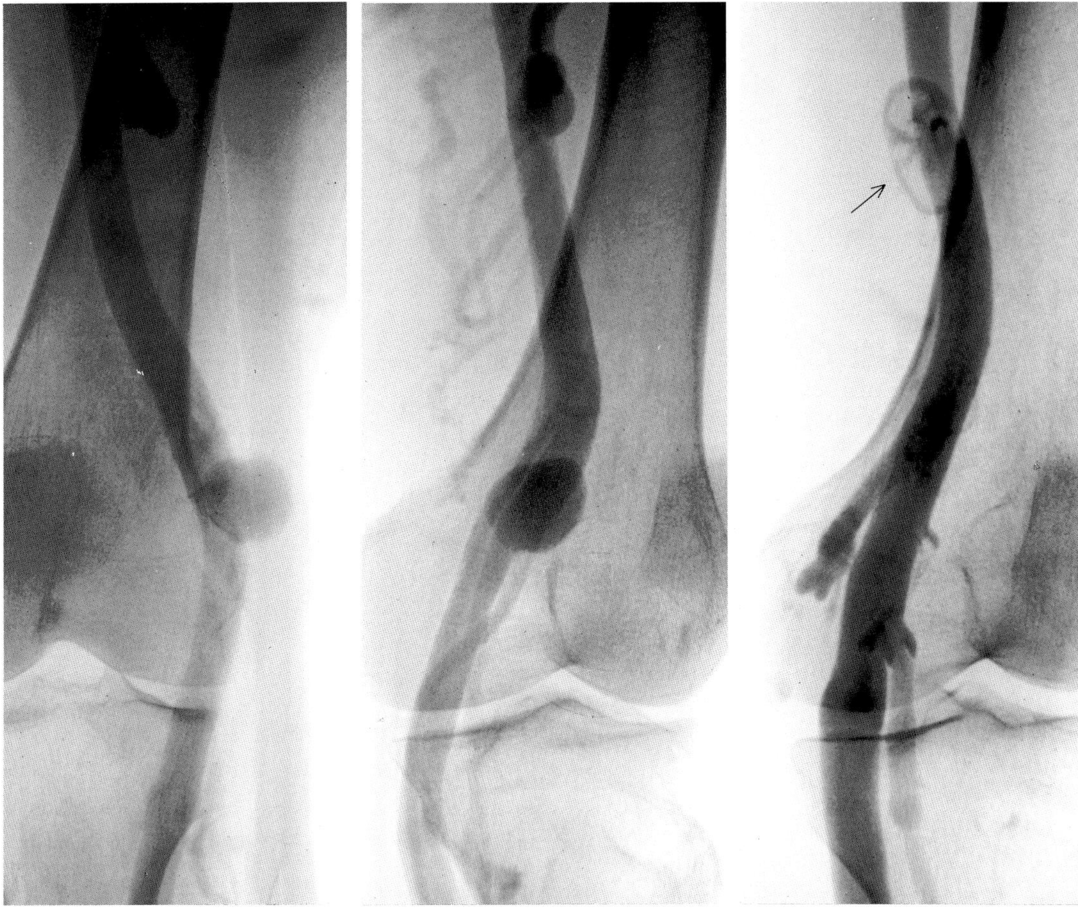

326 (*left, middle*). Aneurysms of the popliteal vein in post-thrombotic syndrome with complete recanalization. Ascending pressure phlebography, internal rotation (*left*) and lateral view (*middle*)

327. Aneurysms of the superficial femoral vein with old thrombi (→). Cause unknown. Incidental finding in a 72-year-old woman

cluded using a Husni-May type venous bypass and peripheral arteriovenous fistula. Saphenous aneurysms are removed as part of the standard surgical procedure for extrafascial varicose veins.

References

Hartling F, Hach W (1973) Das venöse Aneurysma. Phlebol Proktol 2: 159

Prerovski I, Linhardt J, Dejdar R (1960) Krankheiten der tiefen Venen und unteren Gliedmaßen. VEB Gustav Fischer, Jena

Weber J, May R (1990) Funktionelle Phlebographie. Thieme, Stuttgart

Congenital Venous and Mixed Dysplasias

Clinically relevant malformations of the pelvic and leg veins are encountered with some frequency. They can cause significant functional disability and cosmetic deformity in the affected limb. In severe cases the malformations exert secondary effects on the cardiovascular system and blood volume.

It is common for malformations to affect multiple vascular systems at one time, and many are associated with circumscribed skeletal growth disturbances and cutaneous nevi. The prevalence of these symptoms varies from case to case. Monosymptomatic disorders are seen less commonly on the venous side of the circulation. Various proposals have been made in the literature regarding the

Congenital angiodysplasias
Arterial dysplasias
Venous dysplasias
Arteriovenous fistulas
Lymphatic dysplasias
Combined forms

Classification of venous dysplasias
Anomalies of number, course, or termination
Persistence of embryonic structures
Hypoplasias, aplasias
Valvular anomalies
Ectasias
Angiomas

classification of congenital vascular dysplasias (Malan and Puglionisi 1965; Pratesi 1972). The author essentially follows the scheme of Schobinger (1977) and Vollmar (1974). Summaries on the subject can be found in Belov et al. (1985, 1989).

Anomalies of Number, Course or Termination, and Persistent Embryonic Structures

Numerous variations of the leg veins were described earlier in the chapter on normal phlebographic anatomy. Anomalous terminations and numerical anomalies are of limited clinical importance, though sometimes it is important for the venous surgeon to be aware of them.

Outflow obstructions exist in the proximal segment of the left common iliac vein in about 20% of the popula-

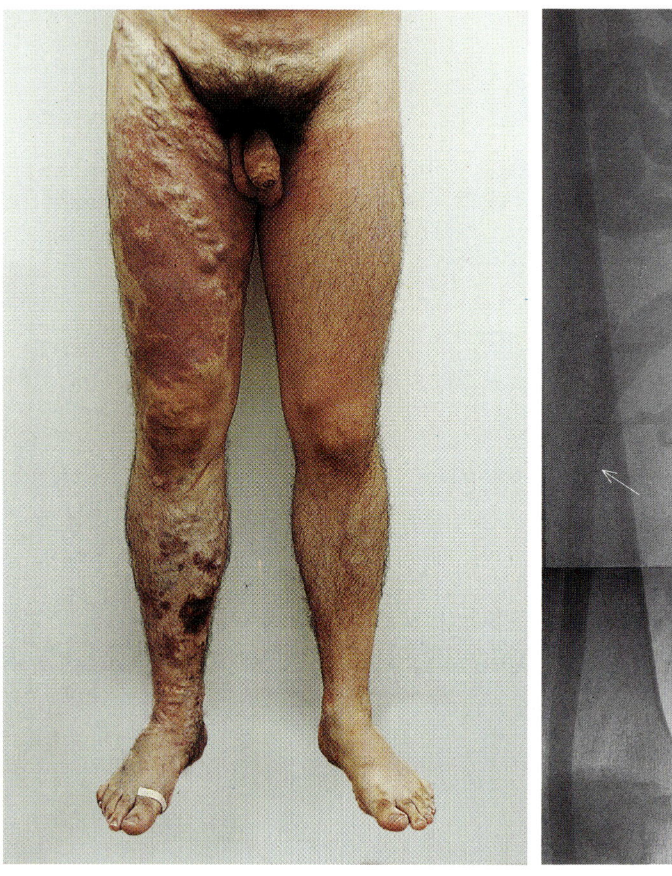

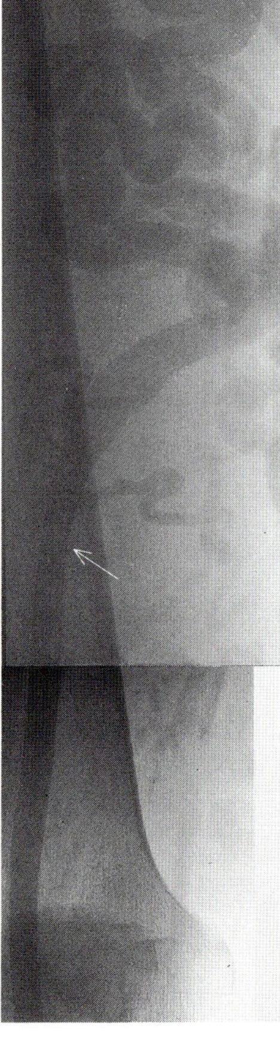

328. Aplasia of the superficial femoral vein in a 33-year-old man. The popliteal vein opens directly into extensive superficial varices (→). Great saphenous vein previously extirpated. *Left,* clinical appearance, with slight swelling of the right extremity; varices and naevi flammei. *Right,* femoropopliteal flow demonstrated by ascending pressure phlebography

tion (Sztankay and Szabo 1970). Called pelvic venous spurs by May and Thurner (1956), some of these lesions are congenital adhesions or occlusive membranes, while others are a response to chronic irritation of the vein wall by the crossing artery (see p. 233).
Anomalies of the inferior vena cava include duplication, left-sided vena cava, and a persistent supracardinal system; they are based on errors of embryologic development (Edwards 1951). Absence of the suprarenal caval segment or a membranous stenosis or occlusion between the hepatic veins and the right atrium can precipitate a Budd-Chiari syndrome (Hach 1973). Anomalies in the course of the inferior vena cava are described in detail by Weber and May (1990).
Digital subtraction angiography is useful for the investigation of anomalies in the retroperitoneal venous system. It may be supplemented by films in the semiupright or lateral position and by having the patient perform a Valsalva maneuver.

Anomalies of the major retroperitoneal veins are occasionally detected during routine abdominal sonography. Duplication of the inferior vena cava is most commonly encountered. Phlebography should follow the sonographic examination to provide a more detailed diagnosis.

Hypoplasias and Aplasias

Congenital hypoplasias and aplasias of the deep
328 pelvic and leg veins are rare as isolated anomalies but occasionally occur in association with other dysplastic conditions such as Klippel-Trenaunay syndrome. Aplasia of the inferior vena cava, especially its suprarenal segment, was mentioned above.

Valvular Anomalies

The venous valves are subject to various numerical and morphologic anomalies.

Avalvulosis

Agenesis of the venous valves may affect the whole venous system of an extremity or only part of it. It is frequently associated with other valvular malformations. Several members of the same family may exhibit avalvulosis, so genetic damage appears to be a factor (Lodin et al. 1961). Symptoms appear during the second decade of life with leg edema, mild varicosity, and acrocyanosis, sometimes accompanied by hypotensive circulatory problems.

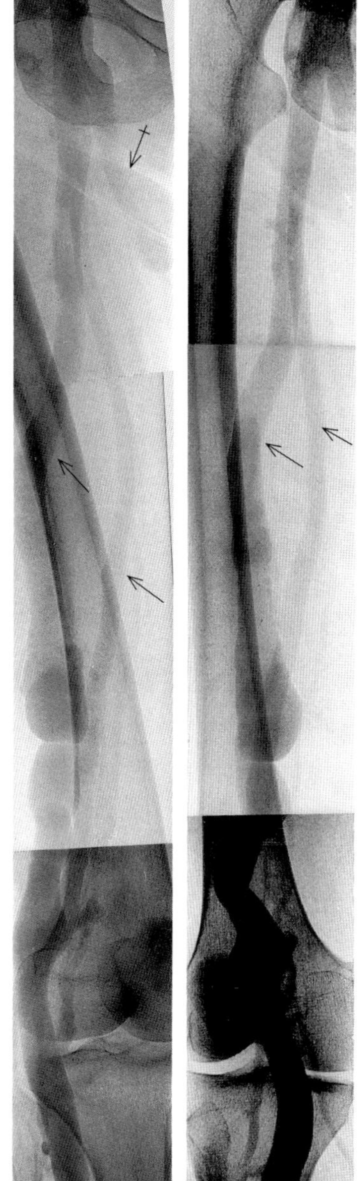

329. Probable congenital aplasia of the venous valves in a 41-year-old woman. Dysplastic dilatation and slight tortuosity of the deep stem veins; → Duplication of the superficial femoral vein; ↔ Stage III great saphenous varicosity. Demonstrated by ascending pressure phlebography. *Left,* internal rotation. *Right,* lateral view

This anomaly can be detected by ascending and
retrograde pressure phlebography. It is sometimes 329
difficult to differentiate from low-grade postthrombotic changes and, in patients with saphe-

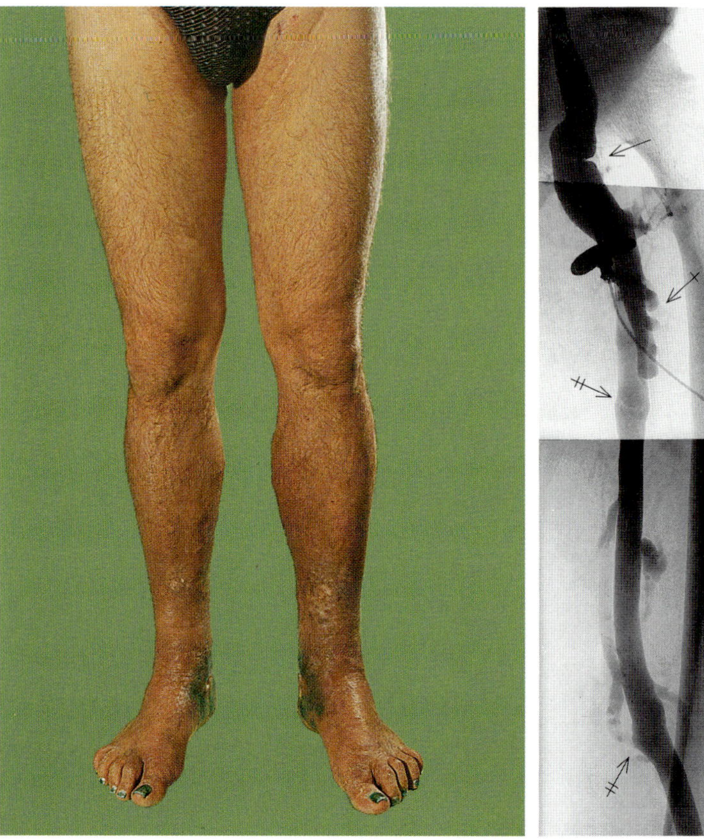

330. Primary femoral valvular incompetence in a 47-year-old man with recurrent swelling of both legs since early youth and a crural ulcer since age 17. *Left,* clinical appearance. *Right,* retrograde pressure phlebography. → Dysplastic venous valve; +→ profunda femoris vein; ++→ superficial femoral vein with dysplastic valves

nous varicosity, from secondary popliteal and femoral vein insufficiency. The patient's history figures prominently in the differential diagnosis, therefore.

Primary Femoral Valvular Incompetence

330 In young patients, primary femoral valvular incompetence must be considered as a potential cause of problems ranging from nonspecific leg discomfort to severe chronic venous insufficiency with bursting calf pain (Kistner 1978). The disease is probably based on a congenital defect of the valve cusps in the common and superficial femoral veins, and sometimes in the popliteal vein. The valves are located at the anatomically correct site, but one or both cusps are flabby and elongated and cannot coapt securely to prevent regurgitant flow.

The diagnosis is established by ascending and retrograde pressure phlebography, which demonstrate retrograde blood flow from the groin to the distal thigh and on to the calf. The morphologic changes in the valve cusps are well defined on high-contrast phlebograms.

In certain cases, according to Kistner (1978), primary femoral valvular incompetence is amenable to *microsurgical repair,* using extremely fine sutures to restore tension to the valve cusps. Another technique involves the transposition of the superficial femoral vein onto the produnda femoris vein. Thus, a detailed phlebographic study can have major practical implications, although the efficacy of these surgical techniques remains to be proven.

Secondary femoral valvular incompetence is ac- 157
quired during postnatal life. Hach et al. (1980) point to degenerative processes and especially to volume overload associated with decompensated reflux circuits in primary varicose disease as the

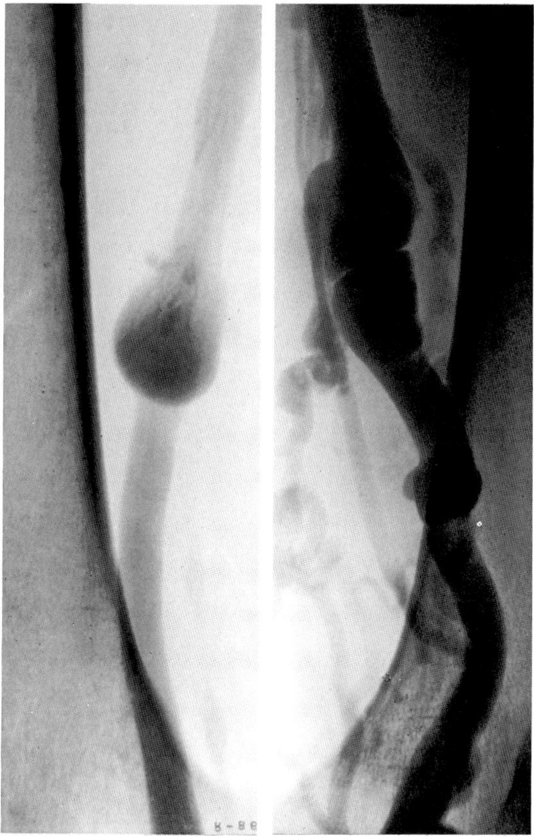

331 *(left).* Dysplastic, pear-shaped venous valve detected incidentally during ascending pressure phlebography

332 *(right).* Venous valve dysplasia. Infravalvular dilatation signifies valve incompetence in a 45-year-old woman with no clinical symptoms. Incidental finding during ascending pressure phlebography

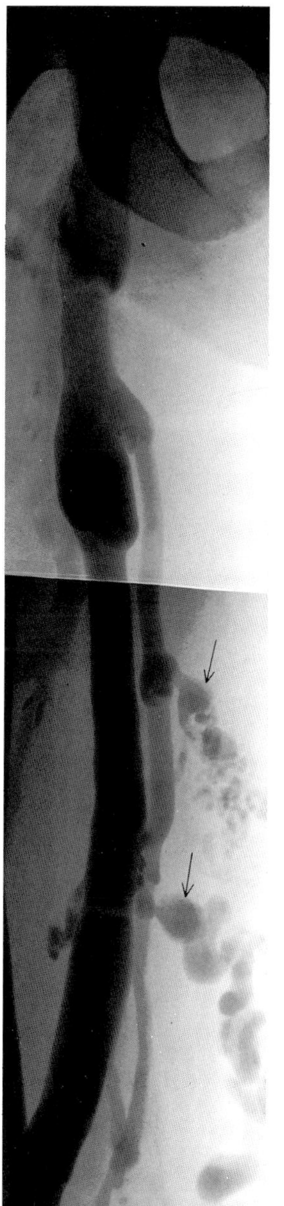

333. Ectasia of the superficial femoral vein and popliteal vein with grotesque-appearing venous valves. Incidental finding in a 27-year-old woman with mild recurrent swelling of the legs. Incompetent Dodd's perforators (→) with associated varices. Demonstrated by ascending pressure phlebography

principal causes. The valve cusps lose their ability to coapt due to dilatation of the valve ring. Secon-
158 dary femoral and popliteal vein insufficiency bears strongly on the prognosis of the disease in patients with great saphenous varicosity (Hach and Hach-Wunderle 1994).

Valvular Dysplasia

The valve cusps may be asymmetrically positioned or situated at an angle within the vein. The anomalous valve morphology is easily recognized on phlebograms. Valvular displasias are said to be relatively common in Rendu-Osler disease and Marfan's syndrome (Schobinger 1977).

A typical anomaly is frequently observed in a constant valve of the superficial femoral vein located 331
at the level of the adductor canal. The sinuses show a pear-shaped dilatation and are poorly delineated proximally with respect to the vessel lumen. Sometimes the valve exhibits an isolated in- 332

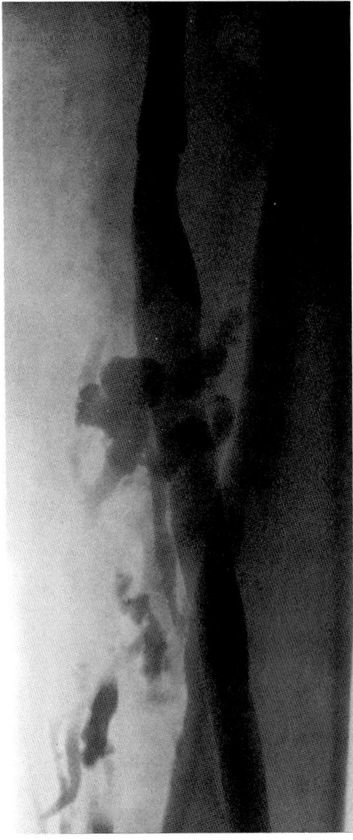

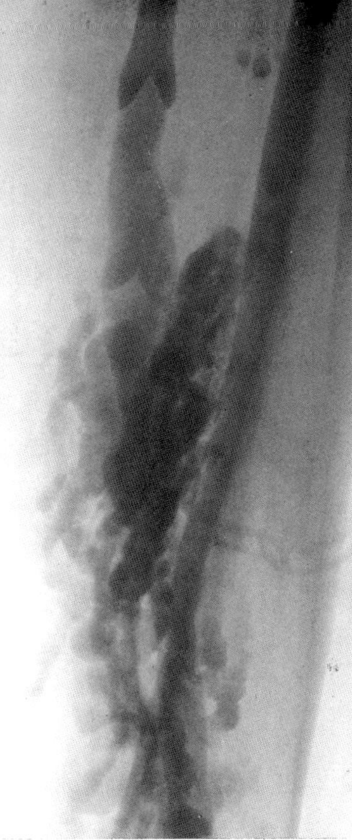

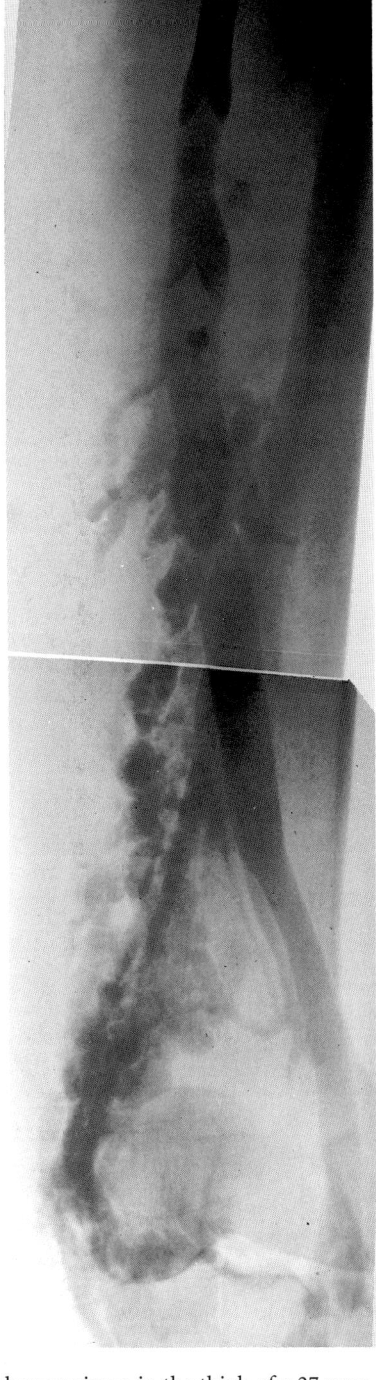

332 competence of its cusps. The cause of this anatomic variation is unknown but may relate to hemodynamic as well as congenital factors.

Dysplastic Ectasias

In contrast to the compensatory ectasia of the great saphenous vein seen in post-thrombotic syndrome as a physiologic adaptive response to increased volume flow, the dysplastic venous ectasias are regarded as pathologic malformations.

Localized Phlebectasia

This is a rare disease that is usually detected incidentally in younger individuals. It is associated with mild congestive complaints, slight varicosity, and sometimes edema. The affected venous segment appears markedly dilated on phlebograms.
333 The valves are grotesquely enlarged but apparently are competent. Post-thrombotic changes are absent. There are no surgical implications.

334. Cavernous hemangioma in the thigh of a 27-year-old woman with moderate recurrent leg swelling and significant congestive complaints. Ascending pressure phlebography. *Left,* early film demonstrates the vessels feeding the angioma. *Middle,* filling of the angioma. *Right,* extensive recurrence 1 year after skeletizing surgery

It is very unlikely that local ectasia of the fibular
37 vein represents a true malformation. Indeed, the dilatation is so common that it serves as a distinguishing feature of the vein.

Genuine Diffuse Phlebectasia

Diffuse phlebectasia, described by Bockenheimer in 1907, is extremely rare. It remains uncertain whether this condition is in fact a disease entity. The dilatations are distributed equally among the superficial and deep veins. Differentiation from systemic hemangiomatosis may be impossible (Schobinger 1977).

Venous Angiomas

Angiomas (hemangiomas) are tumor-like vascular malformations that are classified among the hamartomas, or congenital tumors of maldevelopmental origin.

Cavernous angioma consists of an irregular, tan-
334 gled mass of veins with a primitive tissue structure. It most commonly occurs in subcutaneous tissue, muscle, and bone. Subjective complaints arise from circumscribed thromboses and occasionally from effects on neighboring organs. Cavernous angioma occurring in the intrafascial compartment of the leg can cause pain and edema. The correct diagnosis is established, often incidentally, by ascending phlebography. Contrast medium from the deep veins drains into an atypical, irregular, very tortuous and valveless mass of blood vessels. Manual compression rapidly expels the contrast medium from the mass, which otherwise retains its opacity for some time and finally "fades" with the appearance of a large contrast pool devoid of internal detail. Arteriographic findings are negative.

The radiographic visualization of a cavernous hemangioma requires multiplane views to convey a spatial impression of the relations of the mass to surrounding structures. Particular attention is given to the early phase of the study, during which the large feeding vessels, which may be accessible to surgical treatment, fill with contrast medium. If the topographic relationships of the lesion are unclear, as is frequently the case, the examination is repeated by taking spot films immediately after elimination of the contrast medium.

Combined Dysplasias

Dysplasias of the arterial, venous, and lymphatic systems can combine in a variety of ways. It is most common for venous and lymphatic malformations to coexist. Arteriovenous shunts also have causal importance in some disorders. The diagnostic workup must be tailored to these individual variations. As a general rule, arteriography and ascending phlebography are indicated in younger patients. Physical and radioisotope studies also contribute to the diagnosis. The combined dysplasias include Klippel-Trenaunay syndrome, Servelle-Martorell syndrome, and F. P. Weber syndrome.

Klippel-Trenaunay Syndrome

In 1900 the French physicians N. Klippel and P. Trenaunay published their observations on a symptom complex characterized by *nevus flammeus,* 335
varices, and *limb hypertrophy.* The lower extremity is most commonly involved. Active arteriovenous shunts are not observed.

Klippel-Trenaunay syndrome is often combined with malformations of the lymphatic system and with dysplasias of the intrafascial veins, leading to a diverse range of clinical presentations. Not infrequently, ascending phlebography will demonstrate severe *deformities of the deep venous trunks.* Often entire venous segments are absent or incompletely formed. In other cases irregular dilatations alternate with grape-like or garland-like vessels that may contain calcified thrombi (phleboliths).

The typical finding is *a persistent lateral marginal
vein,* which is demonstrable in 14% of patients 336
with Klippel-Trenaunay syndrome (Vollmar and Voss 1979). The finger-thick, valveless vessel runs up the lateral side of the leg and unites with the
deep veins in the thigh or pelvic region. A residu- 337
um of early embronic development, the persistent marginal vein signifies a profound malformation
of the venous system. 338

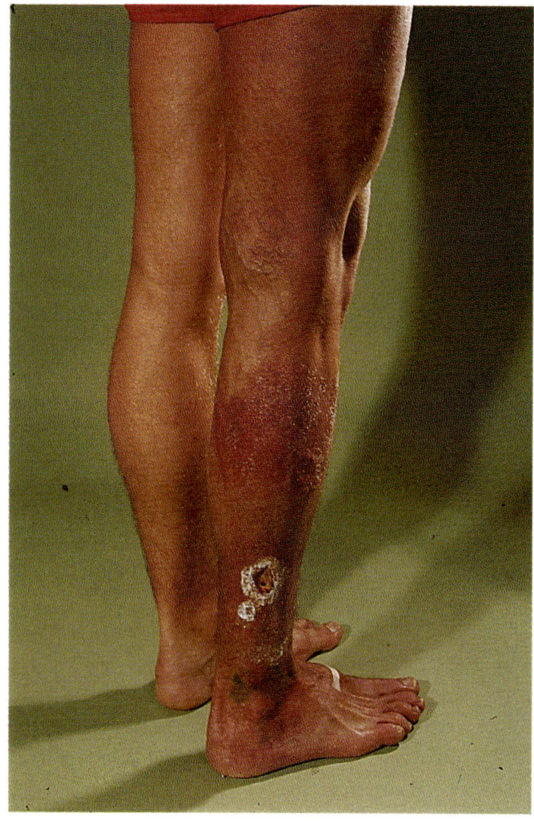

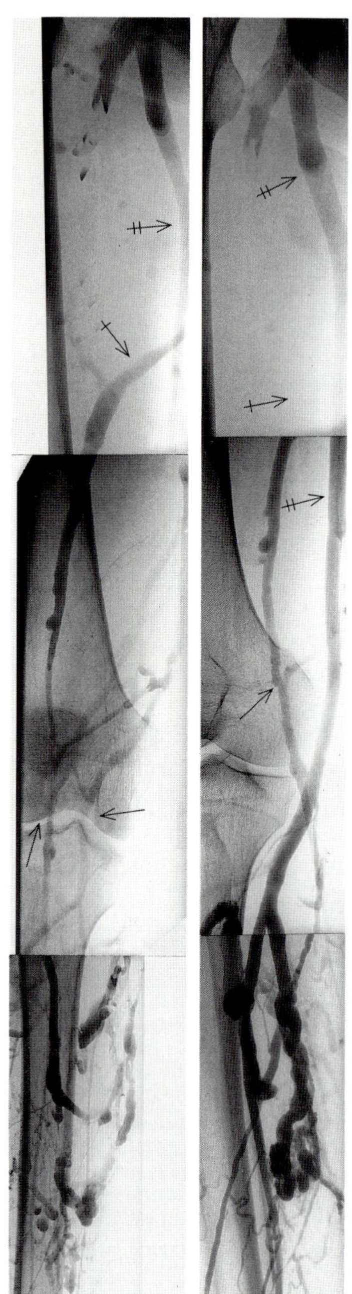

335. Klippel-Trenaunay syndrome in a 22-year-old man. *Left,* clinical appearance. Nevi flammei, varices, 2-cm lengthening of the right leg; 1-year history of crural ulcer. *Right,* ascending pressure phlebography, internal rotation and lateral view. Dysplastic dilatation of the popliteal vein (→) with development of a Giacomini anastomosis (⇸). The deep lower leg veins join directly with the ectatic great saphenous trunk (⇻)

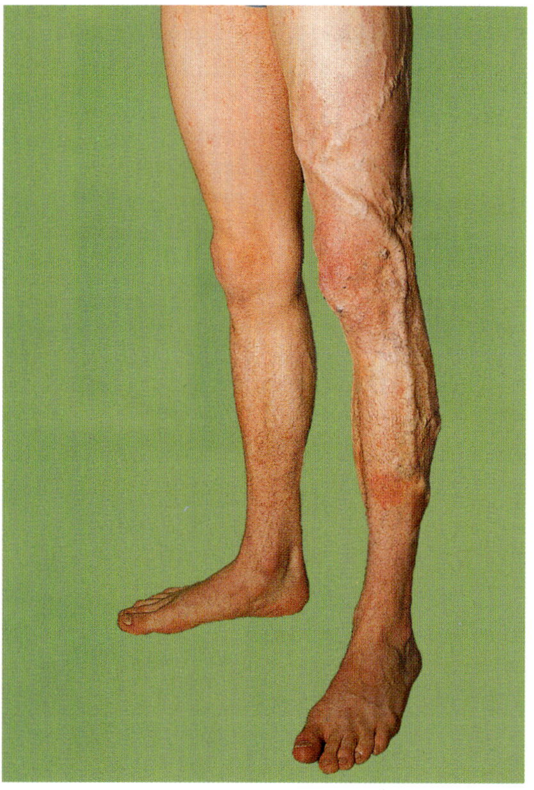

◁
336. Prominent lateral marginal vein in a 20-year-old man with Klippel-Trenaunay syndrome

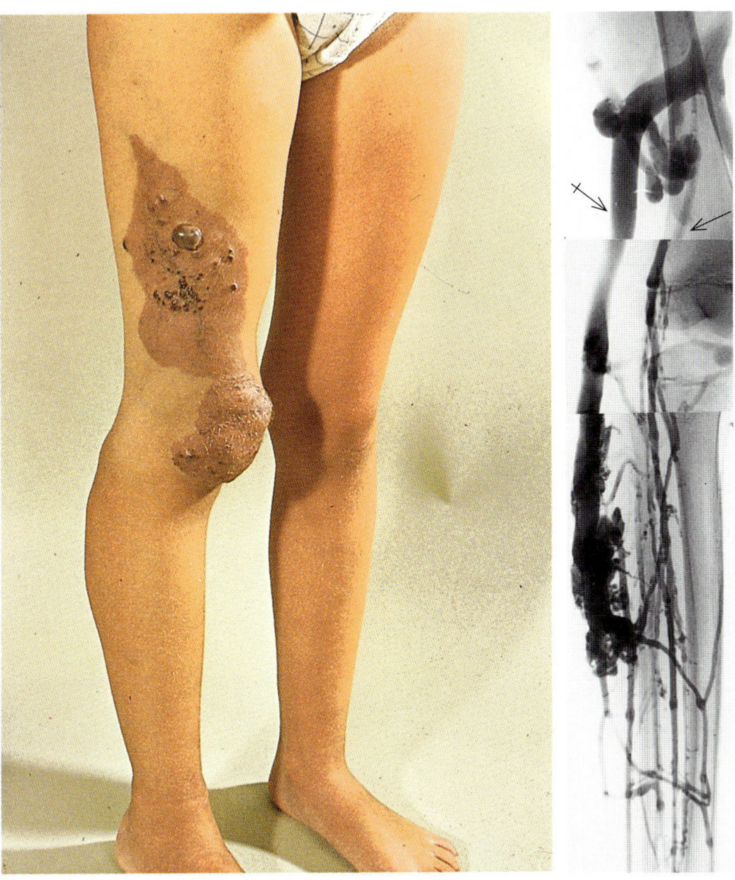

337. Klippel-Trenaunay syndrome in a 5-year-old girl. *Left,* clinical appearance. Pigmented nevus, cavernous hemangioma, varices, minimal lengthening of the right leg. *Right,* ascending pressure phlebography shows hypoplasia of the popliteal vein (→) and superficial femoral vein. Most of the contrast medium drains through a persistent lateral marginal vein (↔)

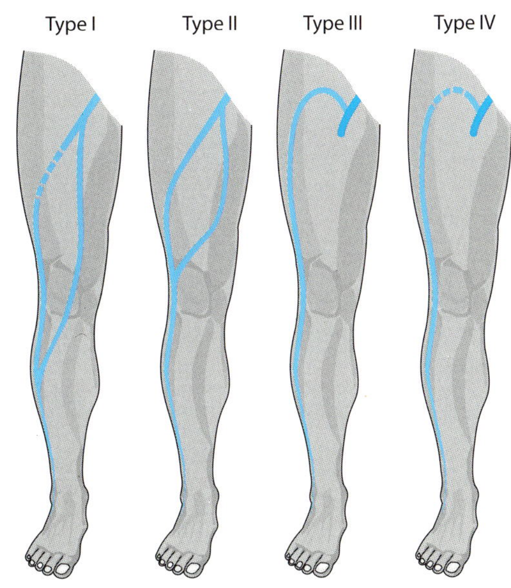

338. Types of persistent lateral marginal vein by course and extent. (After Vollmar and Voss 1979) ▷

Servelle-Martorell Syndrome

Servelle-Martorell syndrome is a congenital arteriovenous dysplasia (Servelle and Trinquecoste 1948; Martorell 1949) that more commonly affects the upper extremity. Its triad of features consist of *varicosity, systemic hemangiomatosis,* and *asymmetrical growth retardation,* based on structural changes in the bone caused by intraosseous hemangiomas. The disease is sometimes associated with dementia, neurofibromatosis, and other developmental defects.

The diagnosis is established by angiographic and phlebographic findings and by assessment of the skeletal deformity.

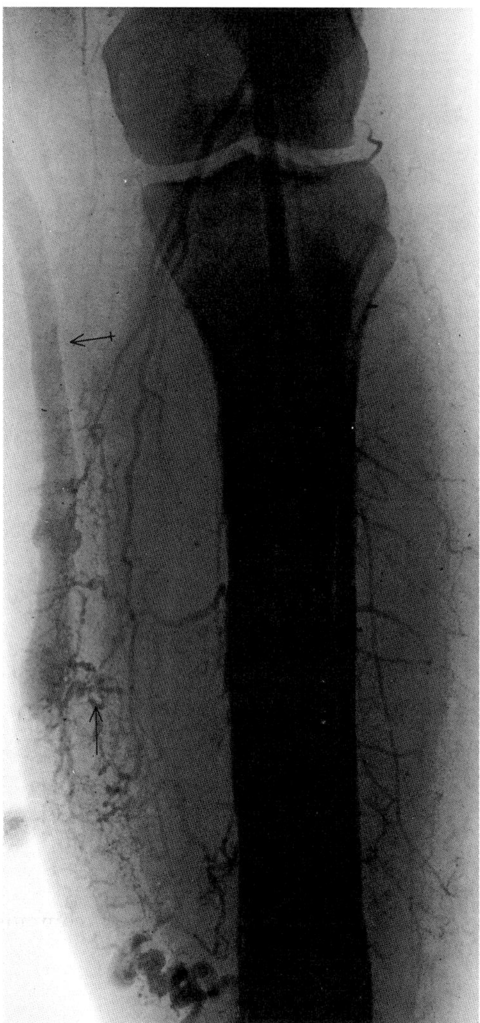

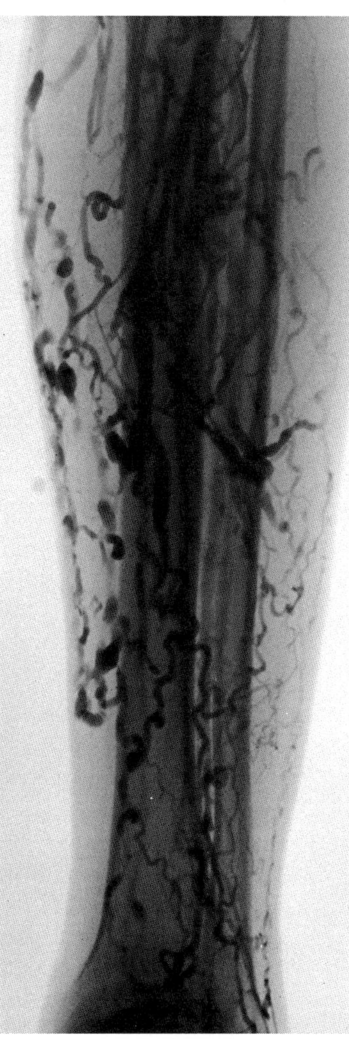

339. F. P. Weber syndrome in a 30-year-old man. *Left,* arteriogram demonstrates multiple transverse shunts (→); early venous phase (↔). *Right,* ascending phlebography with a Valsalva maneuver shows dysplasia of the deep and superficial venous systems with an absence of valves

As in Klippel-Trenaunay syndrome, a persistent lateral marginal vein is present in 17 % of Servelle-Martorell cases (Vollmar and Voss 1979). This vessel sometimes functions as a collateral for the dysplastic deep veins, in which case it should not be removed.

F.P. Weber Syndrome

The English internist F. P. Weber (1863–1962) de-
339 scribed in 1907 a syndrome characterized by *limb hypertrophy* and *angiodysplasia* based on the presence of congenital arteriovenous fistulas. The shunts correspond to the type II transverse shunt defined by Vollmar (1974). Hemangiomas, lymphangiomas, and cutaneous nevi are generally absent. The prognosis is guarded. Some cases are amenable to skeletizing surgery, but conservative treatment is advised in most patients.

The diagnosis is established by *arteriography.*
Films in the late arterial phase define the multiple 339
arteriovenous shunts, which open directly into varicose veins. *Ascending phlebography* occasionally shows dysplastic deep veins whose valves are absent or diminished in number.

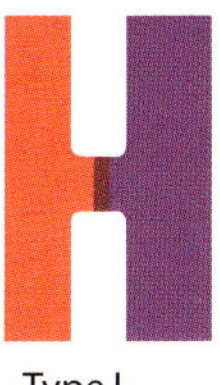

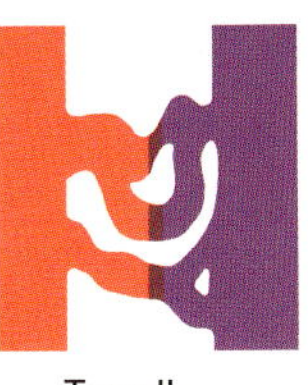

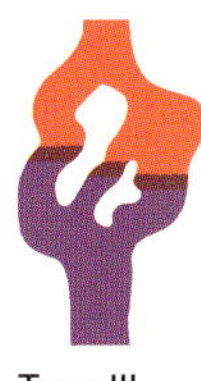

340. Types of congenital arteriovenous fistulas. See text for details. (After Vollmar 1963)

Differences between congenital and traumatic arteriovenous fistulas		
Feature	Congenital	Traumatic
Number of connections	Usually multiple	Single
Hemodynamic effect	Slight	Pronounced
Operative treatment	Problematic	Indicated
Prognosis of cases taking a spontaneous course	Doubtful	Unfavorable

Congenital Arteriovenous Fistulas

The vascular system develops from the embryonic capillary network. If there is a failure of arterial and venous differentiation of the primitive vessels, and multiple connections persist, the stage is set for the establishment of arteriovenous fistulas. Sometimes arteries and veins are separated only by a thin membrane, which tears at some point during postnatal life and leads to a *late manifestation* or sudden exacerbation of vascular disease (Lawton et al. 1975).

Vollmar (1974) has classified congenital arteriove-
340 nous fistulas into *3 different types* based on morphologic criteria. Only types I and II occur in the extremities and are of phlebologic interest. Every arteriovenous fistula should be evaluated for its activity or inactivity.

Active fistulas can be detected only by *arteriography*. The pathologic connections are directly visualized in a late phase of the examination, when the contrast medium enters the venous system rapidly and in relatively high concentration.

Solitary Transverse Shunts

Solitary congenital transverse shunts between major arteries and veins correspond to the ductus arteriosus type of fistula, or *type I* in the Vollmar classification. They rarely occur in the extremities. In shunts with high volume flow, the severe hemodynamic impairment can even be detected by phlebography, and the features are like those of a traumatic fistula.

Multiple Transverse Shunts in Smaller Vessels

It is more common to find multiple transverse shunts between arteries and veins of all calibers. The vessels communicate through an interposed angiomatous vascular network (*type II*). An inactive, clinically undetectable shunt can give rise to a cavernous hemangioma, Klippel-Trenaunay syndrome, or Servelle-Martorell syndrome, while the active form can lead to F. P. Weber syndrome.

Localized Tumor Shunts

This type of congenital arteriovenous fistula is characterized by the direct communication of small arteries with veins, without an interposed capillary network (*type III*). The prototype of this anomaly is the racemose aneurysm, which occurs chiefly on the head and in the brain.

Value of Adjunctive Studies to Phlebography

Every case involving a congenital dysplasia must be individually evaluated. Whenever there is the least suspicion of a systemic impairment of the peripheral circulation, a comprehensive diagnostic workup is indicated. It should be added that, in children, the use of invasive diagnostic procedures should be held to a minimum.

In addition to phlebography, diagnostic imaging of the *arterial vascular system* is frequently necessary to exclude pathologic arteriovenous connections. *Color-coded duplex scanning* is effective for this purpose in patients with clinically relevant findings. Angiomatous changes in the soft tissues of the affected extremities also are detected by this technique.

It is desirable for an experienced vascular surgeon to make a *synoptic interpretation* of the various diagnostic findings. While there are many cases in which causal treatment is not feasible, local surgical procedures can often effect a significant improvement of hemodynamic status.

References

Belov S, Loose DA, Müller E (1985) Angeborene Gefäßfehler. Einhorn, Reinbek

Belov S, Loose DA, Weber MD (1989) Vascular malformations. Einhorn, Reinbek

Bockenheimer P (1907) Über die genuine diffuse Phlebektasie der oberen Extremität. Festschrift für G.E. von Rindfleisch. Universität Leipzig

Edwards EA (1951) Clinical anatomy of lesser variations of the inferior vena cava and a proposal for classifying the anomalies of this vessel. Angiology 2: 85

Hach W (1973) Die Phlebographie beim Beckenvenen- und V. cava-inferior-Verschlußsyndrom. Phlebol Proktol 2: 143

Hach W, Hach-Wunderle V (1994) Die Rezirkulationskreise der primären Varikose. Springer, Berlin Heidelberg Nex York Tokyo

Hach W, Schirmers U, Becker L (1980) Veränderungen der tiefen Leitvenen bei einer Stammvarikose der V. saphena magna. In: Müller-Wiefel H (Hrsg) Mikrozirkulation und Blutrheologie. Witzstrock, Baden-Baden

Kistner RL (1978) Transvenous repair of the incompetent femoral vein valve. In: Bergan JJ, Yao JST (eds) Venous problems. Year Book Medical Publishers Inc, Chicago London

Klippel M, Trénaunay P (1900) Du naevus variqueux osteohypertrophique. Arch Gen Med 3: 641

Lawton RL, Tidrick RT, Brintnall ES (1957) A clinicopathologic study of multiple arterio-venous fistulae of the lower extremities. Angiology 8: 161

Lodin A, Lindvalla N, Gentele H (1961) Congenital absence of valves in the deep veins of the leg. Acta Derm Venorol (Stockholm) 41: 45

Malan E, Puglionisi A (1965) Congenital angiodysplasias of the extremities. J Cardiovasc Surg 6: 255

Martorell F (1949) Haemangiomatosis braquial osteolitica. Angiologia 1: 219

May R, Thurner J (1956) Ein Gefäßsporn in der Vena iliaca communis sinistra als Ursache der überwiegend linksseitigen Beckenvenenthrombose. Z Kreisl Forsch 45: 912

Pratesi F (1972) Classification of angiopathic diseases of the limbs. Folia Angiol 20: 193

Schobinger RA (1977) Periphere Angiodysplasien. Huber, Bern

Servelle M, Trinquecoste P (1948) Des angiomes veineuse. Arch Mal Coeur 41: 436

Sztankay C, Szabo S (1970) Dysplasie iliocave: essai sur la pathogénie des maladies veineuses des membres inférieurs. Rapport du IIIe Congrès International de Phlébologie, Amsterdam 1968. Stenvert u. Zoon, Apeldoorn

Vollmar J (1974) Zur Geschichte und Terminologie der Syndrome nach F.P. Weber und Klippel-Trénaunay. Vasa 3: 231

Vollmar J, Voss E (1979) V. marginalis lateralis persistens – die vergessene Vene der Angiologen. Vasa 8: 192

Weber FP (1907) Angioma formation in connection with hypertrophy of limbs and hemihypertrophy. Brit J Derm 19: 231

Weber J, May R (1990) Funktionelle Phlebographie. Thieme, Stuttgart

Phlebography Following Therapeutic Procedures on the Venous System and Iatrogenic Venous Injury

Phlebography, and in some cases color-coded duplex sonography, can furnish objective evidence of the effectiveness of a therapeutic procedure on the venous system. Modern quantitative instrumented techniques such as phlebodynamometry and Doppler flowmetry provide additional useful information, especially when preoperative data are available as a baseline. Radiography is additionally useful for the detection of iatrogenic venous injury.

Phlebographic Findings After Vena Cava Interruption

Interruptions of the inferior vena cava are intended to prevent recurrent pulmonary embolism in patients with deep venous thrombosis in the pelvis or lower extremity. The lumen of the vena cava can be narrowed by an extraluminal procedure employing special clips or sutures, or a special filtering device can be inserted transvenously to trap potential emboli. The interruption should always be performed distal to the renal veins.

Extravascular Interruptions

Extravascular interruptions of the inferior vena cava are rarely performed today. The operation poses an exorbitant risk to the patient, who often is seriously ill. In the past, complete ligation of the interior vena cava was a popular technique among American surgeons. Cranley (1975) and Kersten and Varco (1978) have published detailed accounts of the problems associated with this type of surgery. Pelvic phlebography demonstrates extensive collateral circulations only a few weeks after the procedure.

Partial vena cava interruption using a grid of sutures (DeWeese and Hunter 1963) or a suture plication technique (Spencer et al. 1965) is very diffi-

cult to detect with radiography or ultrasound. Today these procedures are considered obsolete. Extravascular plastic clips of the kind described by
341 Miles et al. (1984) or Adams and DeWeese (1966)
are demonstrated most clearly by lateral radiographs.

Intravascular Vena Caval Filters

Intraluminal filters and umbrellas have assumed
major importance in the prophylaxis of recurrent
pulmonary embolism. Vena caval filtration is indicated in patients who respond poorly to anticoagulation. The filter device is implanted percu-
ta-neously from the jugular vein using a carrier
system. Since the development of the Mobin-Uddin umbrella (1969), various types of vena caval
342 filter have been designed in recent years. The most
widely used device at present is the Kimray-
Greenfield filter; an advanced autocentering model 343
has recently been developed. A detailed description
of the devices has been published by Günther
and Thelen (1988) and Weber and May (1990). The
recently developed Filcard filter is suitable for temporary treatment during fibrinolysis; it can be removed transcutaneously within 5 days.
The implanted filter is visible on a noncontrast ra- 344
diograph, which will give a general impression of 345

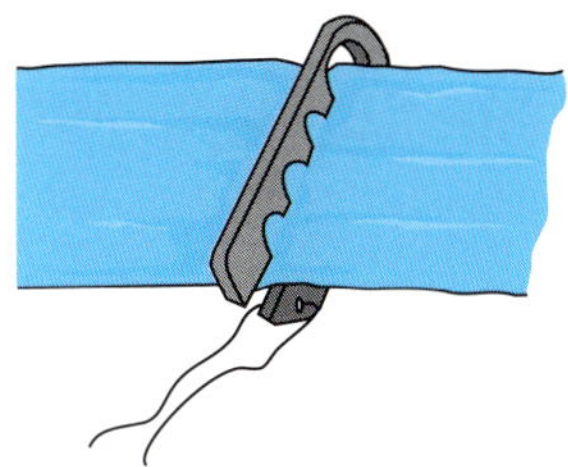

341. Adams-De Weese clip

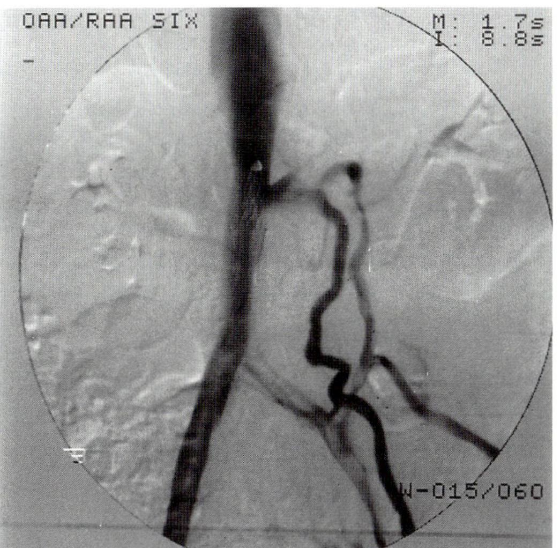

343. Autocentring filter (after Kimray-Greenfield) in the infrarenal position in the inferior vena cava. A 66-year-old woman with post-thrombotic syndrome of the leg and pelvic veins on both sides and recurrent pulmonary emboli despite anticoagulation

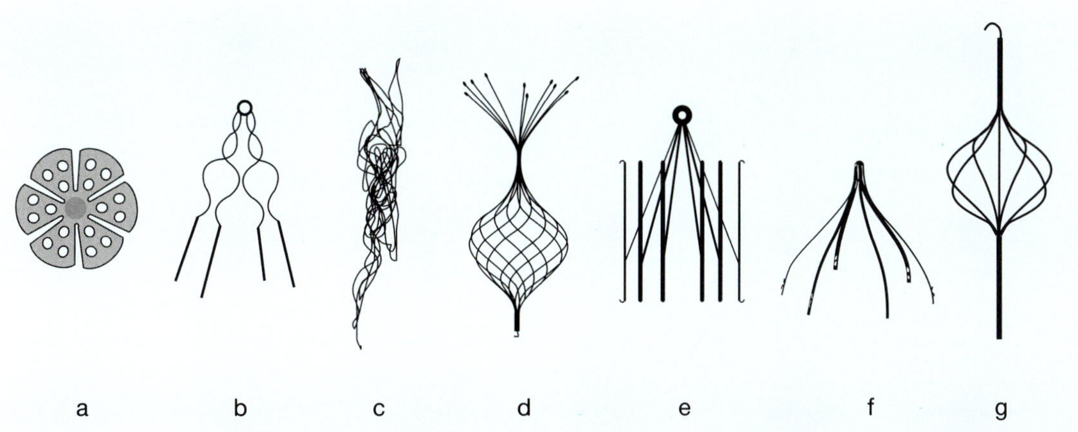

342 a–g. Vena cava filters in clinical use. **a** Mobin-Uddin filter (1969). **b** Kimray-Greenfield filter (1973). **c** Birds nest filter (1984). **d** Günther filter (1985). **e** Autocentring (LEM) filter. **f** Permanent Filcard filter. **g** Temporary Filcard filter

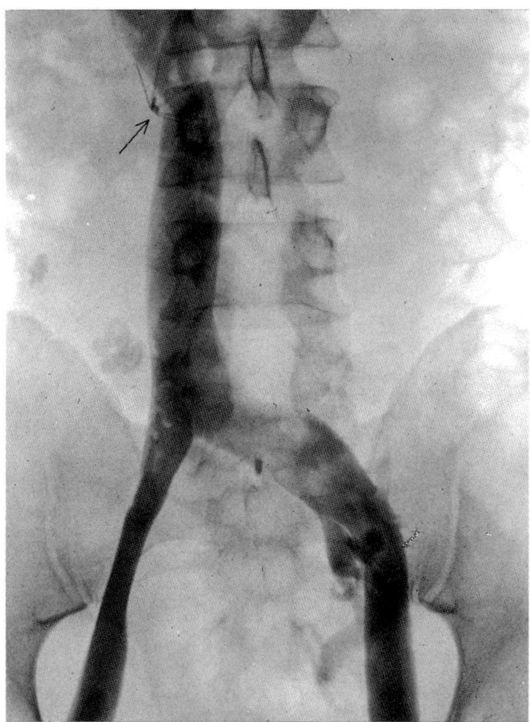

344. Displaced Mobin-Uddin umbrella (→), demonstrated by pelvic phlebography

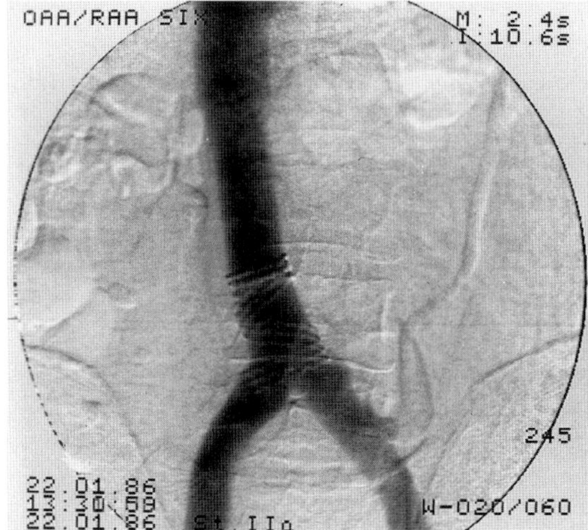

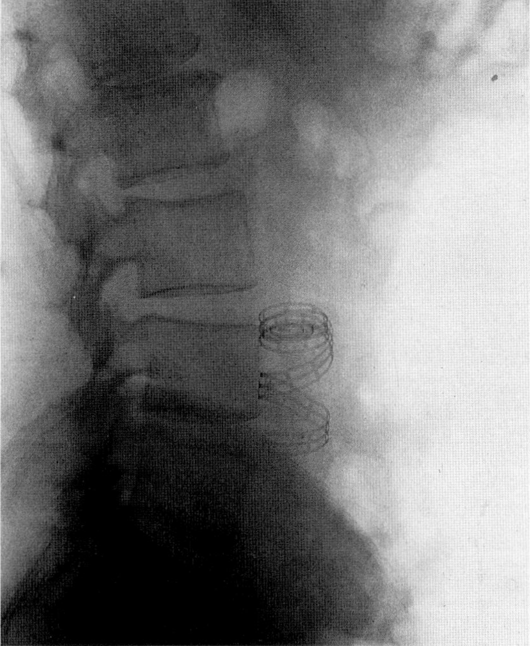

345. Birds nest filter in the vena cava bifurcation in a 64-year-old man with recurrent leg vein thrombi and pulmonary emboli despite anticoagulation. *Top*, digital subtraction angiography. *Bottom*, survey radiogram, lateral view

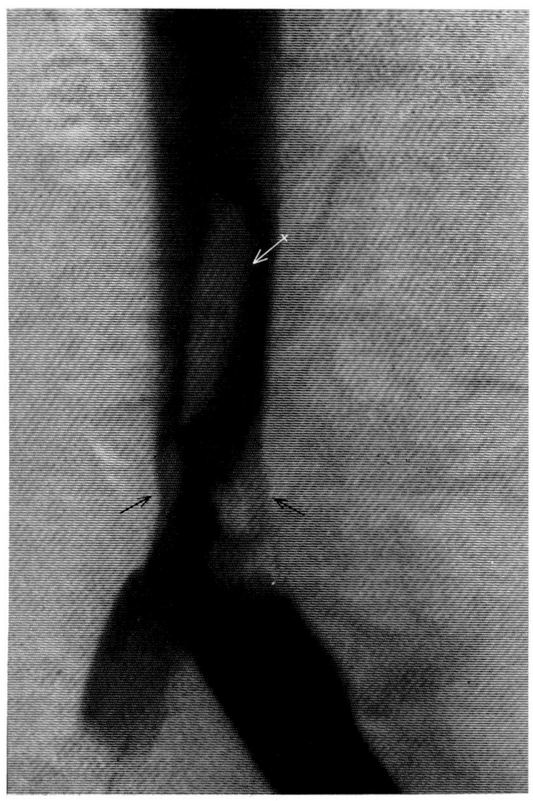

◁

346. Greenfield filter in a 64-year-old man with recurrent pulmonary emboli from the pelvic and leg veins (not shown due to subtraction, indicated by broken line). Trapped emboli in the filter (→), thrombus growing through the grid (↔)

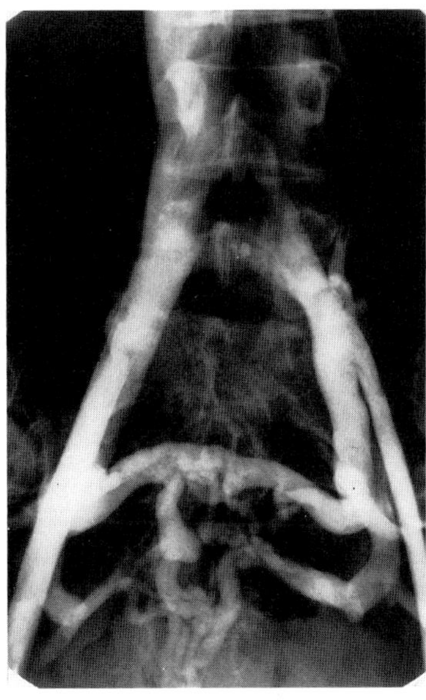
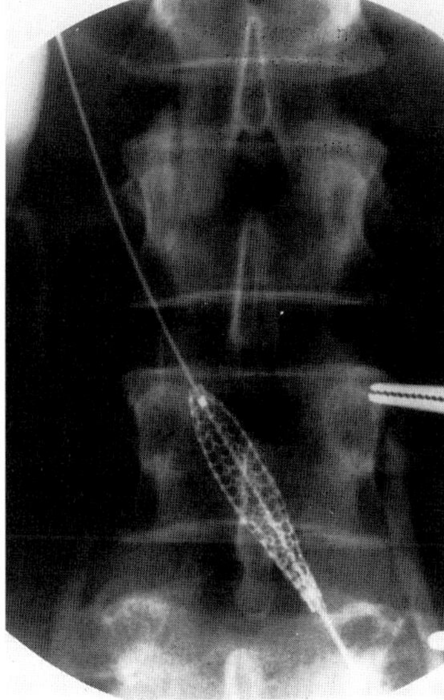
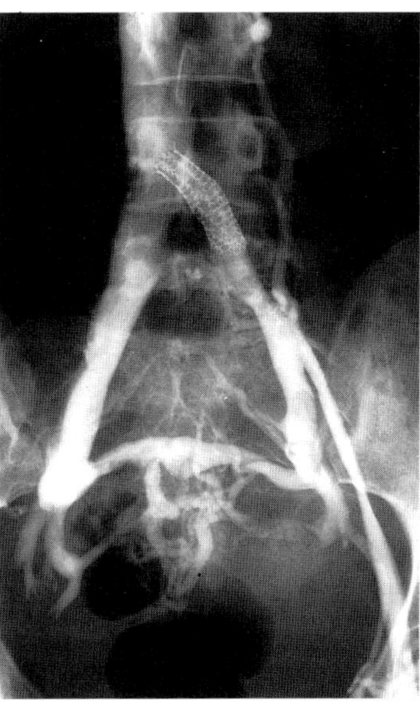

347. Implantation of a Strecker stent in the left common femoral vein in a 41-year-old woman with pelvic vein spur. Symptoms due to insufficiency in the left leg and pathologic pressure increase in the left femoral vein during weight-bearing. *Left,* pelvic vein spur. *Middle,* implantation of the stent following dilatation. *Right,* control phlebography 8 days later; dilated and splinted spur channel. (Operation and radiographic examination by Prof. Dr. Weber, Hamburg)

its status and reveal any proximal migration that
344 may have occurred. A tilted or otherwise abnormal position of the filter is an indication for phlebographic evaluation.

A filter does not provide infallible protection
346 against recurring pulmonary embolism. Small emboli may pass through the mesh. Of particular concern are thrombi that develop above the filter. Real-time sonography and color-coded duplex scanning are also useful for checking filter placement and may occasionally have therapeutic implications.

Percutaneously Implanted Endovascular Prostheses

While percutaneous transluminal dilatation has become a routine treatment for *arterial* stenoses, the procedure is not suited as well for *venous* use because venous stenoses tend to be too elastic to allow for effective dilatation. One approach to this problem has been the development of large-caliber endovascular prostheses, for which initial clinical experience is already available. The indications for endovascular splinting include com-
347 pression syndromes of the inferior vena cava and pelvic veins as well as pelvic venous spurs. Zollikofer (1988) reported on the successful use of the Medinvent prosthesis. The placement of the endovascular splint can be checked by phlebography, but color-coded duplex scanning appears better suited because it also permits an assessment of the vessel wall and perivascular structures. The upper and lower ends of the prosthesis are marked by slight discontinuities in the caliber of the vessel.

Interpositional Grafts

Following the resection of a large-caliber venous segment due to tumor involvement or injury, a ring-reinforced plastic graft can be interposed to
bridge the defect. Usually the upper and lower 348
anastomotic sites can be recognized by a slight incongruity of the vessel lumina. Today, color-coded duplex scanning is generally used to evaluate the function of the graft.

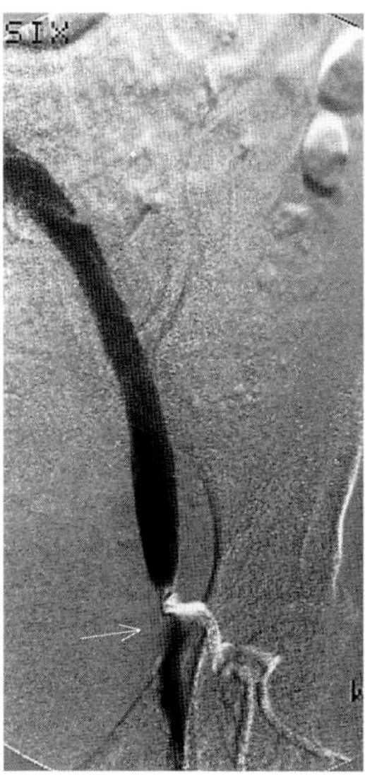
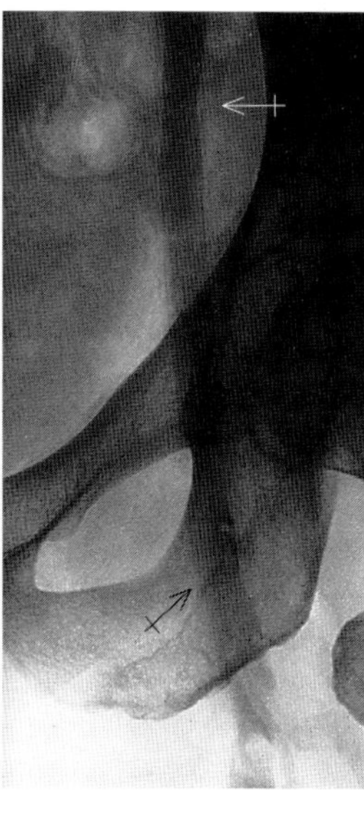

348. Circular stenosis of the left external iliac vein (→) as a result of a longstanding pelvic ring fracture in a 40-year-old woman. Swelling of the leg and hypostatic pain during weight-bearing. Unsuccessful attempt at balloon dilatation. *Left,* digital subtraction angiography before treatment. *Right,* Gore-tex prosthesis strengthened by a ring. Upper and lower anastomoses can no longer be distinguished (↔)

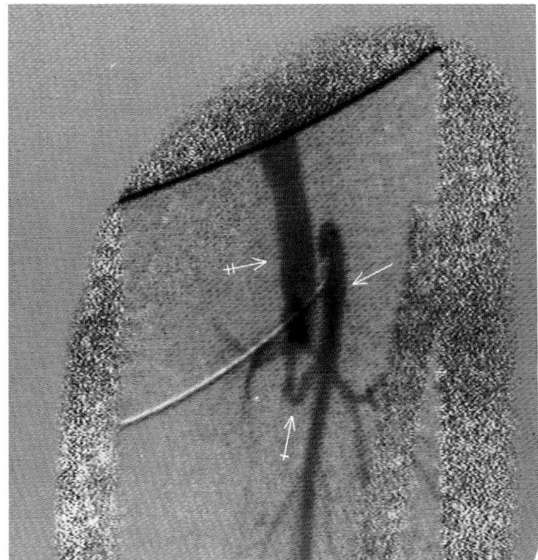

349. Therapeutic arteriovenous fistula in a 19-year-old woman after venous thrombectomy. Demonstrated by digital subtraction angiography with puncture of the common femoral artery (→). Typical bucket-handle appearance of the shunt vein (↔) with a branch of the common femoral vein (⇸)

Phlebographic Findings After Venous Bypass Operations in the Inguinal and Pelvic Region

In patients with an acute or chronic venous outflow obstruction in the femoroiliac system, the circulation can be restored by reconstructive venous surgery. A bypass can be constructed using autogenous great saphenous vein or an alloplastic prosthesis.

For angiography or phlebography following a venous bypass procedure, the contrast medium should always be injected peripheral to the operative site and never close to the anastomoses as this might cause serious complications. *Neither* should the needle be inserted directly into the graft; a transplanted vein can become thrombosed, and puncture of a prosthetic graft can cause detachment, curling, or dissection of the delicate neointima, leading to graft occlusion.

When an alloplastic prosthesis is used, invasive exam- 348
inations are problematic in another respect as well. Implanted plastic materials are exceedingly prone to infection. The bacterial colonization of a prosthesis necessitates its immediate operative removal to avoid sepsis, mycotic aneurysm, and other serious complications. This underscores the importance of maintaining *scrupulous aseptic technique* during contrast radiography.

During the phlebographic evaluation of a bypass, particular attention is given to the outflow conditions at both anastomoses. A transplanted vein can undergo varicose degeneration with passage of time. A vascular prosthesis can develop irregular luminal constrictions caused by mural thrombi, with a strong likelihood of total occlusion within a short time.

Therapeutic and Traumatic Arteriovenous Fistulas

A temporary peripheral arteriovenous fistula may be created in selected cases, or as a matter of routine, to protect a transplant from thrombosis. Permanent use of the shunt for the definitive treatment of post-thrombotic syndrome of the pelvic veins is no longer recommended.

A palpable *thrill* can be detected over a functioning fistula, and stethoscope auscultation reveals a loud bruit that is transmitted proximally in the direction of the vein. The fistula can be demonstrated radiographically by arterial angiography, 349
which may be enhanced by digital subtraction.

A *large-caliber* arteriovenous shunt causes significant compromise of the venous circulation. The

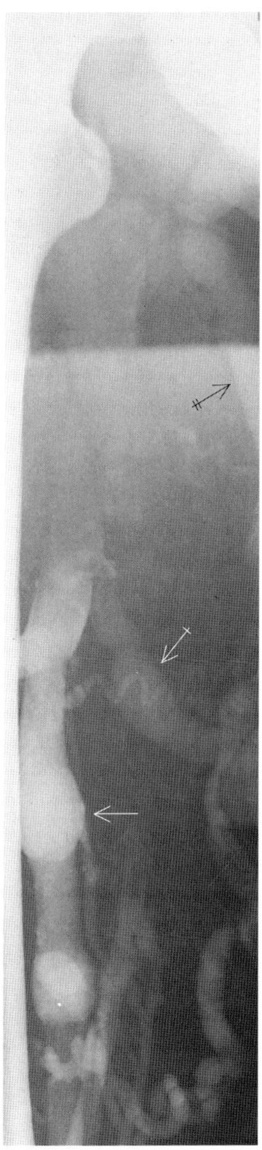

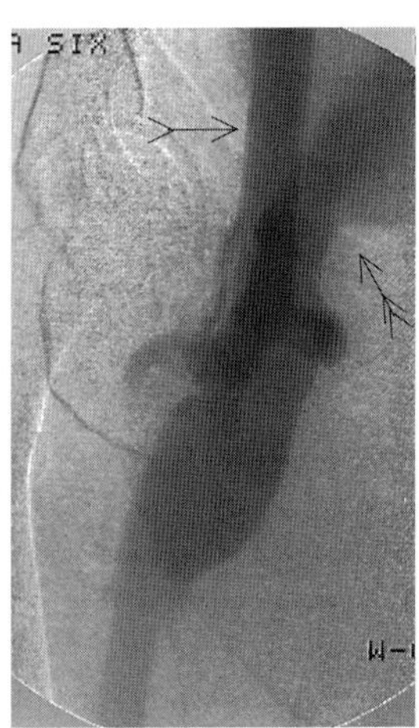

entire leg becomes swollen to the groin, and the
veins are abnormally prominent. The direct entry
of high-pressure arterial blood into the vein prevents peripheral venous return from crossing the
fistula, so the appearance on ascending phlebo- 350
grams is like that of venous occlusion. The contrast
medium flows past the arteriovenous communication through small collaterals, completely sparing
the affected vascular region. This hemodynamic
pattern is easily mistaken for a total occlusion.

An arteriovenous fistula is optimally demonstrated by color-coded duplex scanning, which can also determine the shunt volume and thus the circulatory load. Directional Doppler flowmetry also can detect arterial pulsations in the vein proximal to the shunt, where the direction of the waveform deflection is reversed.

Generally a therapeutic fistula is closed about 6 months after the initial operation. If a suture has already been

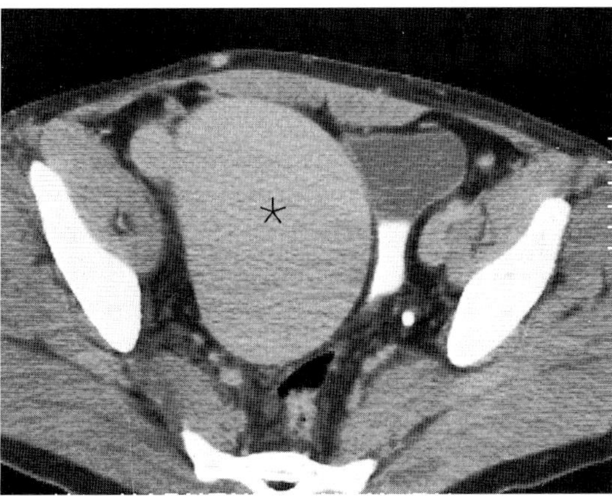

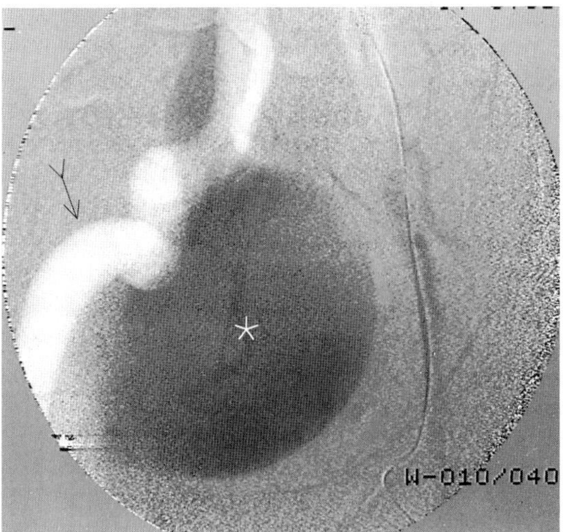

350. Persistent large-luminal therapeutic arteriovenous fistula in the inguinal position after thrombectomy in a 39-year-old man. Function of the fistula over a period of 4 years. *Top left,* ascending pressure phlebography in the middle of the right tigh. Antegrade flow insufficiency; the superficial femoral vein (→) in front of the fistula is not demonstrated. Considerably enlarged stem veins. Extrafascial collateral circulation via Dodds perforating vein (↦) and secondary great saphenous varicosity (⇸). *Top right,* inguinal fistula circuit. External iliac artery (↣) and external iliac vein (⤖). *Bottom left,* huge aneurysm of the external iliac vein (*). Demonstrated by computed tomography. *Right,* aneurysm (*) shown by digital subtraction phlebography

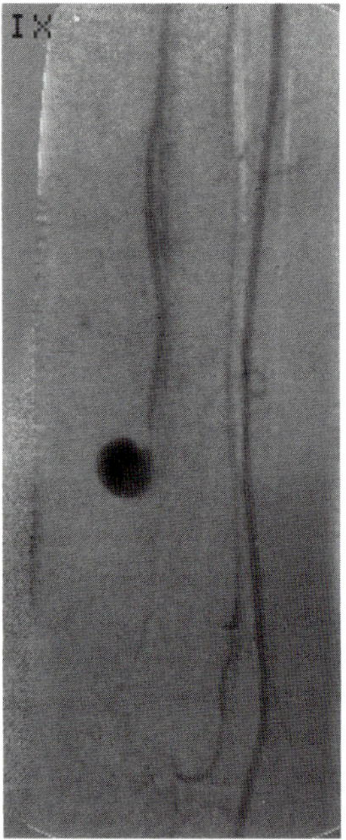

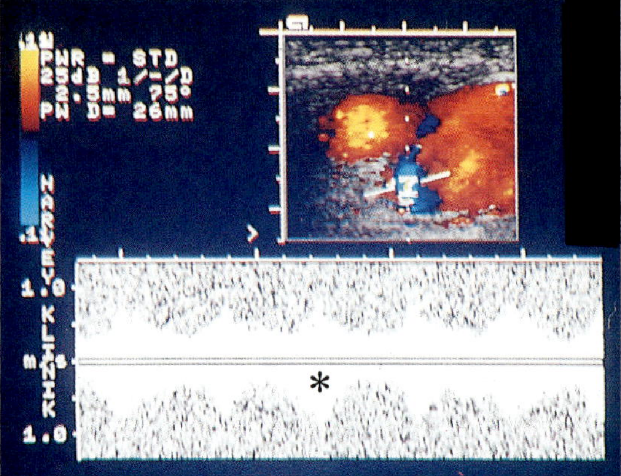

351. Pulsating hematoma with arteriovenous fistula in the distal lower leg after iatrogenic trauma in the posterior tibial artery. *Left,* digital subtraction angiography. *Top right,* color-coded duplex sonogram showing severe flow turbulence. *Bottom right,* arterial pulsations overlayed with loud machine noise (*) in the sample volume

preplaced about the shunt vessel, only a *minor surgical procedure* is needed to reenter and tighten the knot. A large shunt with significant hemodynamic side effects should probably be ligated at an earlier time. If a fistula with a large lumen is not closed within an appropriate
350 period of time, enormous aneurysms and dilatations can form in the vessels.

351 A *traumatic arteriovenous fistula* poses corresponding diagnostic and therapeutic problems. Digital subtraction angiography and color-coded duplex scanning are excellent for localization and hemodynamic assessment of the lesion. The urgency of surgical intervention is decided on an individual basis.

Palma Crossover Venous Bypass

The crossover bypass operation of Palma and Esferon (1960) can ameliorate venous drainage in patients with a unilateral post-thrombotic occlusion of the pelvic veins with deficient collateralization. Patients are *selected* for the procedure based on a synoptic evaluation of clinical and phlebo-

352. Palma crossover venous bypass in a 42-year-old woman with post-thrombotic occlusion of the left pelvic veins. The right great saphenous vein (→) has been anastomosed to the ectatic left great saphenous vein (↔). Demonstrated by digital subtraction phlebography from the left foot

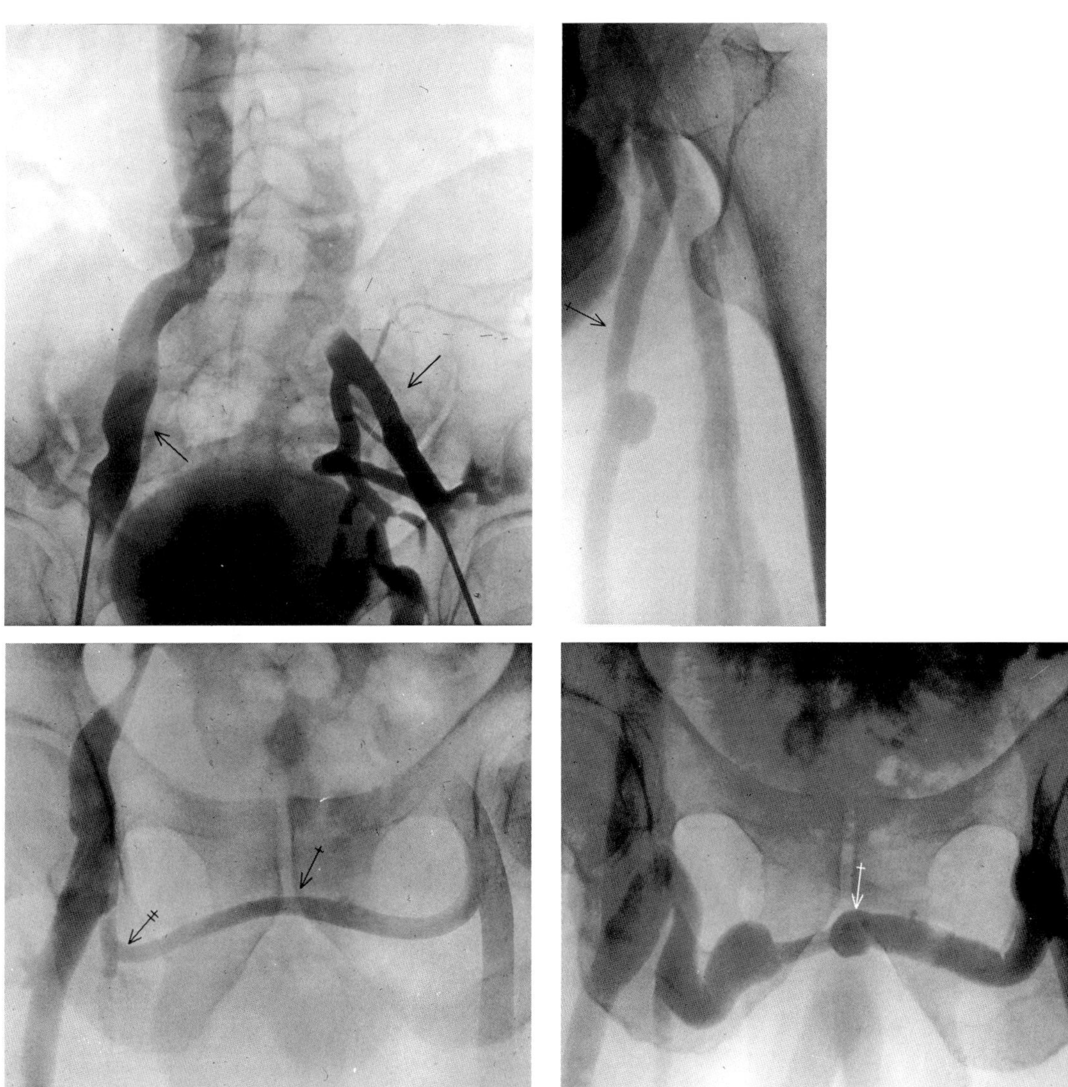

353. Inverse crossover bypass in a 55-year-old man with post-thrombotic syndrome of the left pelvic and leg veins secondary to retroperitoneal fibrosis (Ormond's disease). *Top left,* occlusion of the left common iliac vein. The perivascular fibrosis is evidenced by a paucity of collateralization and the slightly wavy outlines of the pelvic veins (→). Demonstrated by pelvic phlebography. *Top right,* primary varicosity of the left great saphenous vein (→) associated with subtle post-thrombotic changes in the deep leg veins, which show complete recanalization. Demonstrated by ascending pressure phlebography. *Bottom left,* inverse crossover bypass with anastomosis of the varicose left saphenous vein (+→) to the (healthy) right saphenous vein (++→). Hach's variation of the Palma operation. *Bottom right,* further varicose degeneration of the venous bypass at 4 years (+→)

graphic findings and of the femoral venous pressure during exercise. The great saphenous vein of the healthy limb is mobilized to midthigh level, tunneled subcutaneously and suprapubically to the opposite side, and anastomosed to the common femoral vein or the terminal portion of the great saphenous vein on the occluded side.

The function of the transplant is first evaluated
with a Doppler ultrasound probe. *Follow-up phle-* 352
bograms are taken on about the fourth postoperative day, employing unilateral or bilateral ascending phlebography from a foot vein or digital subtraction phlebography. Before concluding the operation, some surgeons pass a fine catheter into a

side branch of the vein to provide a route for continuous anticoagulation of the anastomosis with heparin solution for the first few days. Additionally this catheter allows for postoperative phlebography under sterile conditions, although color-coded duplex scanning is equally useful for postoperative surveillance.

Initially the lumen of the transplanted vein appears small. It is protected from thrombosis, and its caliber expanded, by creating an ateriovenous fistula. Over time the venous conduit will adapt to the increased volume load by physiologic ectasia. The vessel may undergo varicose degeneration af-
353 ter a period of years. As the vessel becomes coiled and kinked, the volume flow through the graft is gradually choked off. In some cases this culminates in a thrombotic occlusion following a trivial precipitating cause. Because of the unfavorable early conditions and late results, more and more surgeons today are abandoning the original Palma operation in favor of a large-caliber alloplastic transplant.

Inverse Palma Crossover Operation

If primary or secondary great saphenous varicosity is present on the side of the post-thrombotic occlusion, the saphenous vein can be utilized as a
353 bypass to the healthy contralateral side (Hach 1980). Because the venous valves are incompetent, blood can flow through the insufficient saphenous vein in retrograde fashion. In this *inverse Palma operation*, then, blood drains from the common femoral vein on the occluded side through the ipsilateral varicose great saphenous vein to the opposite side via the suprapubic route. This procedure is indicated for the dual purpose of improving the collateralization of the occlusion and curing the contralateral saphenous varicosity.

Owing to its large caliber, the transplanted vein has a high transport capacity from the outset, so it may be unnecessary to create an arteriovenous fistula. As the years pass, the bypass is jeopardized in many patients by increasing varicose degeneration and kinking, which can easily lead to occlusion.

Crossover Bypass with a Polytetrafluoroethylene Prosthesis

Today the reinforced polytetrafluoroethylene
(PTFE) prosthesis, routed antepubically, provides 354
a better alternative to the autologous saphenous vein graft for the crossover procedure. It is sometimes necessary to create a temporary arteriovenous fistula on the thrombosed side.

Femoroiliac Crossover Bypass

Anastomoses are always subjected to greater mechanical stresses within the movable portion of the groin. For this reason, and because of its more favorable hemodynamic properties, it is best to perform the bypass with a reinforced PTFE prosthesis, which is routed from the common femoral vein on the occluded side suprapubically to the
contralateral external iliac vein. The procedure is 354
used both for *chonic* venous outflow obstruction
and for *acute occlusion* of the major pelvic veins 355
by a compression syndrome, with or without thrombosis (Hach et al. 1983).

Ilioiliac Crossover Bypass (High Palmer Operation)

Vollmar and Hutschenreiter (1980) have recommended using a reinforced PTFE prosthesis to construct a retroperitoneal bypass between the large axial veins of the pelvis to circumvent an occlusion (usually left-sided) of the common iliac vein.

The bypass can be demonstrated phlebographically by injecting contrast medium from the inguinal fold, provided an anteriovenous fistula has not been created. Care must be taken, however, that the needle tip is not advanced beyond the inguinal ligament, and that aseptic technique is strictly maintained. It is easier to inject the contrast medium through a peripheral route. Digital subtraction angiography is best for evaluating the bypass, but color-coded duplex scanning is also suitable in thin patients.

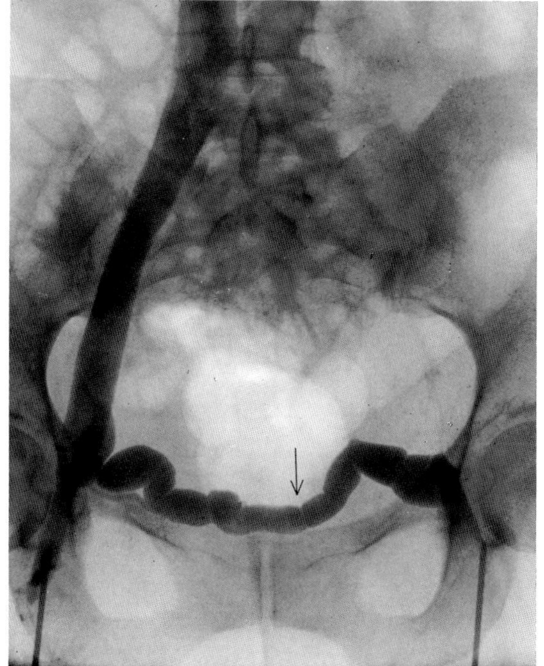

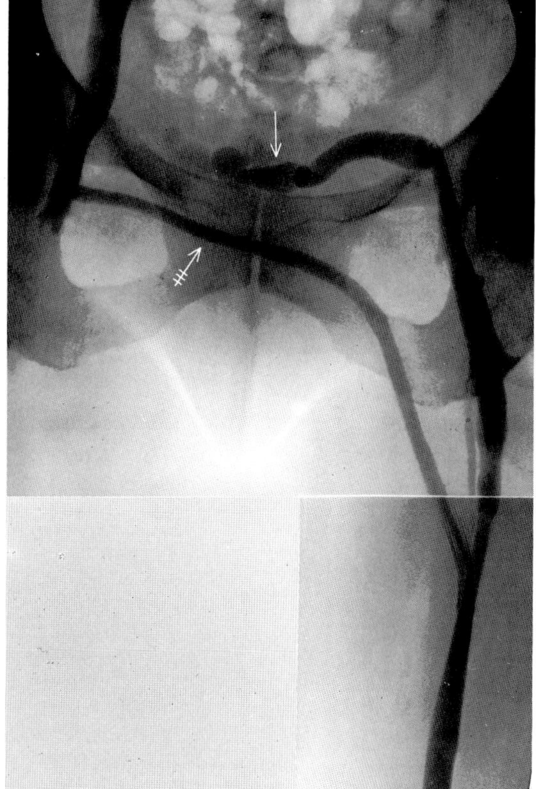

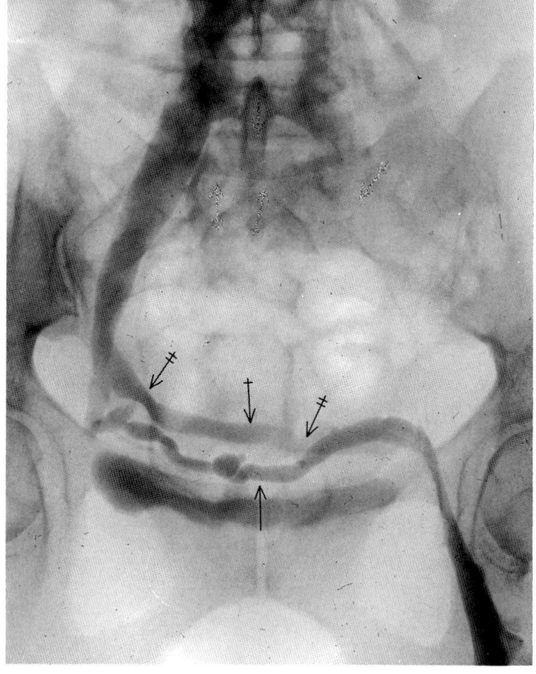

354. Deficient suprapubic collateral in a 47-year-old woman with isolated occlusion of the left pelvic veins and recurrent swelling of the left thigh. *Top left,* visualization of the collateral (→) by pelvic phlebography. *Bottom left,* appearance 3 years after suprapubic femoroiliac bypass (↔) with a polytetrafluoroethylene (PTFE) prosthesis. Luminal narrowing by mural thrombi (⇸), regression of the collateral (→). *Right,* femorofemoral crossover bypass with a PTFE prosthesis (⇻) after spontaneous occlusion of the first bypass. Flow through the suprapubic collateral increased again during the occlusion (→)

Orthotopic Femoroiliac and Femorocaval Bypass

A pelvic venous occlusion can be managed by constructing a bypass between the common femoral vein and the ipsilateral common iliac vein or infe-
356 rior vena cava. Generally this is done in patients with an extravascular compression syndrome or an occluding pelvic venous spur. Hach et al. (1983) also recommend the operation for cases where a severe outflow obstruction has led to a descending type of acute iliofemoral vein thrombosis.

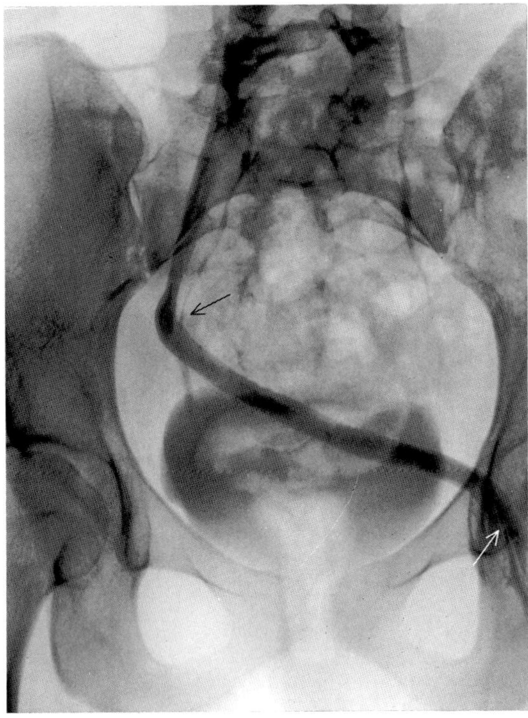

355. Femoroiliac crossover bypass with a ring-reinforced polytetrafluoroethylene (PTFE) prosthesis (→) in a 20-year-old woman. Suspected occluding pelvic venous spur; descending iliofemoral vein thrombosis; lack of outflow at the pelvic level following thrombectomy. Venous hemodynamics returned to normal after the operation

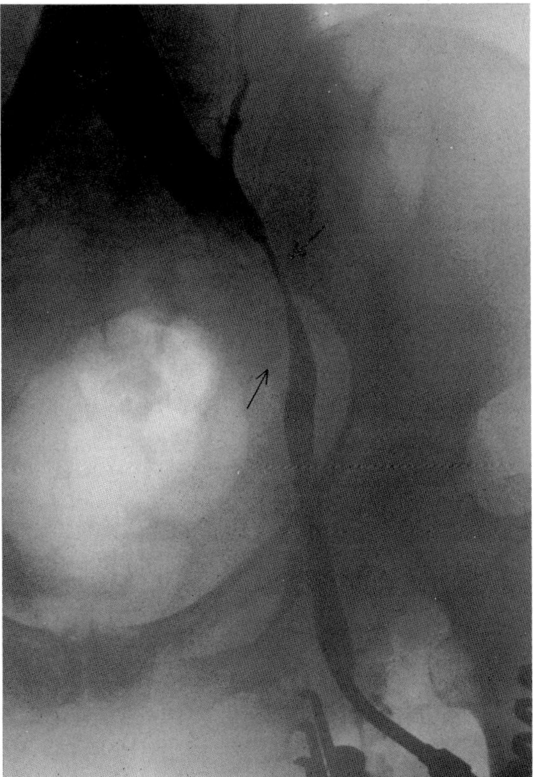

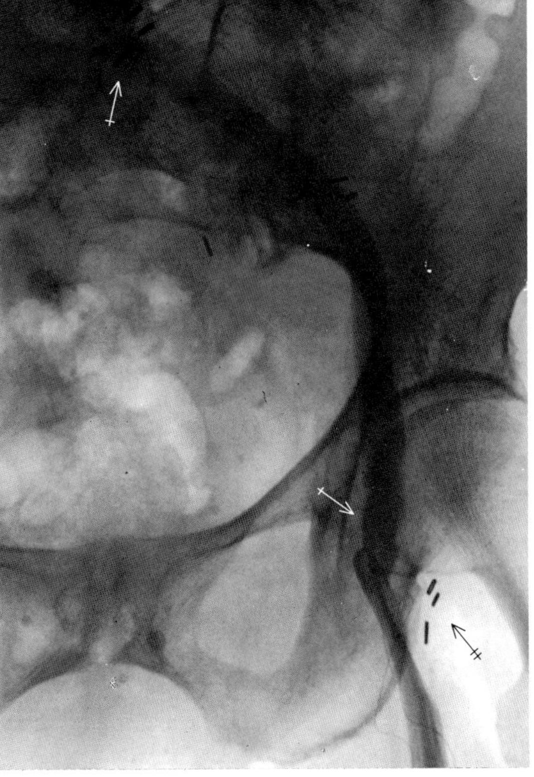

▷

356. Orthotopic femoroiliac bypass with a polytetrafluoroethylene (PTFE) prosthesis in a 65-year-old woman with pelvic venous compression syndrome and descending iliofemoral venous thrombosis. *Top,* extrinsic compression of the external iliac vein (→), demonstrated by intraoperative phlebography from the common femoral vein. Surgical exploration disclosed a matted lymph node mass enveloping the vessels and the ureter. Local reconstruction was not possible. *Bottom,* femoroiliac bypass with a reinforced PTFE prosthesis (↦) and a therapeutic arteriovenous fistula (⇸)

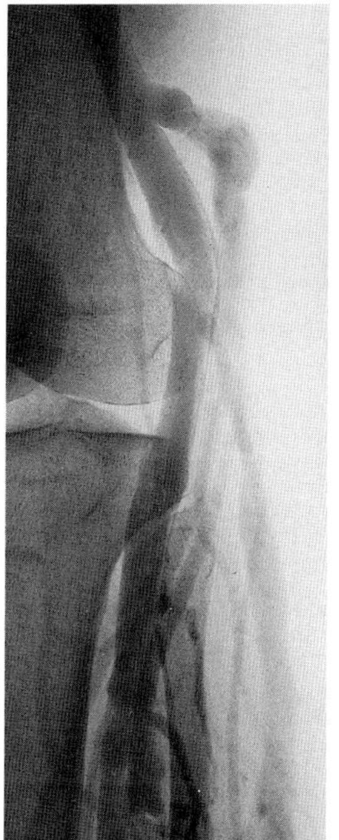
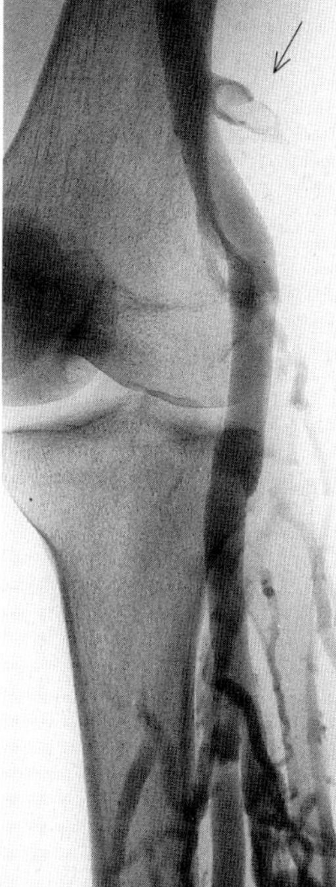

357. Substandard operation for small saphenous varicosity in a 49-year-old woman. *Left,* preoperative phlebogram. *Right,* remaining stump with fresh thrombi. → Pulmonary embolus

Phlebographic Findings After Specific Operations on the Leg Veins

Following a technically sound operation for saphenous varicosity, phlebography should show no pathologic changes other than the sequelae of secondary popliteal and femoral vein insufficiency.
357 The problems associated with recurrent varicosity were discussed earlier (see p. 138). Thrombi may develop in a stump left untreated and cause embolism. Other procedures, many of which are obsolete or seldom practiced today, may leave behind more or less characteristic telltale radiographic signs.

Ligation of the Deep Leg Veins

Ligation of the superficial femoral vein below the entrance of the profunda femoris (Linton and Hardy 1947) and popliteal vein ligation (Bauer 1965) were formerly used in the treatment of post-thrombotic syndrome. They were also utilized in some types of knee surgery. At present, ligation of the common femoral vein is still performed in rare cases for the treatment of septic thrombophlebitis.

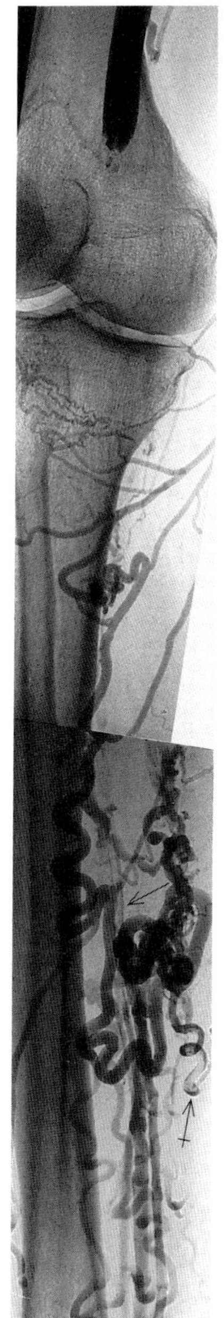

358. Ligation of the popliteal vein during surgery for small saphenous varicosity, with subsequent descending thrombosis in a 58-year-old man. Thrombotic occlusion of the popliteal vein, the proximal veins of the lower leg, and the calf muscle veins. Isolated thrombi in the posterior tibial veins (→) and in residual varices (↔). Demonstrated 2 weeks postoperatively by ascending pressure phlebography, utilizing the overflow effect

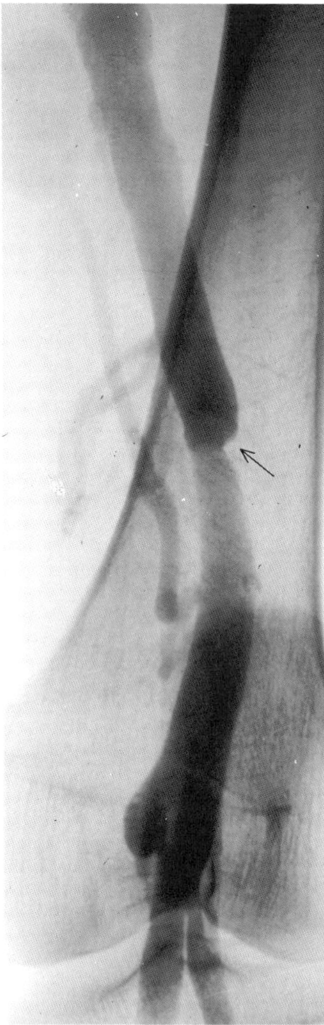
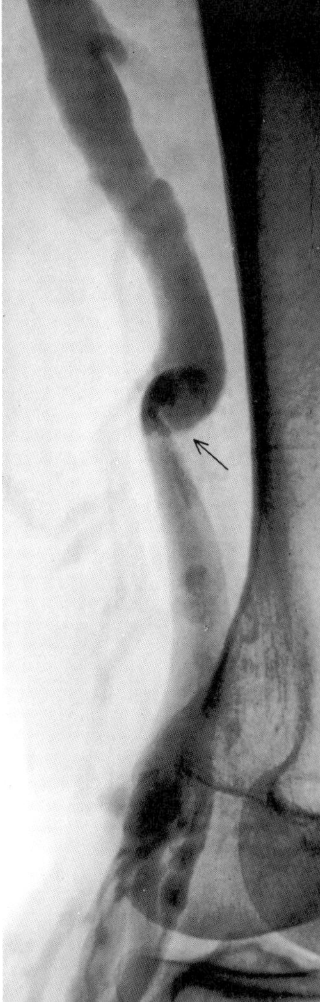
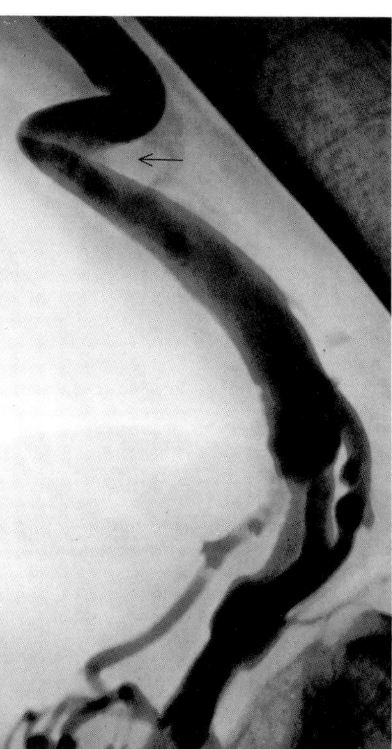

359. Status following a gracilis tendon transfer (Psathakis). *Left, middle,* anteroposterior and lateral projections with the knee extended show compression of the superficial femoral vein by the crossing tendon of the gracilis muscle (→). *Right,* lateral view with the knee flexed shows kinking of the vein by the tendon

The clinical picture and phlebographic findings are characterized by prominent secondary varices in the area surrounding the occlusion. Deep vein ligations also may be necessary during the course
358 of difficult operations, or some may be done inadvertently. The ligation is marked phlebographically by a sharp cutoff of the opaque column, followed later by the appearance of thrombi.

Femoral Venous Bypass of Husni and May

Incomplete recanalization of the superficial femoral vein impairs venous hemodynamics. The Husni-May operation is designed to improve outflow by anastomosing the great saphenous vein to the popliteal vein below the knee (Husni 1970; May 1972). This permits drainage from the deep venous system of the lower leg to the groin via the transplanted saphenous vein.

Long-term follow-ups have shown that the anastomosed great saphenous vein suffers the same fate as in the setting of a spontaneous collateral circulation. The vessel initially adapts to the high volume flow by luminal expansion but then loses its function through secondary varicose degeneration. For this reason the procedure is rarely performed today. Neither has the use of a reinforced PTFE prosthesis proven effective for the bridging of venous occlusions in the lower limb.

We have used the Husni-May bypass to route venous return around an embolizing aneurysm of the superficial femoral vein, but this is an infrequent indication (see p. 204). The function of the transplant can be assessed by phlebography, color-coded duplex scanning, and Doppler flowmetry.

Gracilis Transfer of Psathakis

359 Psathakis (1982) has recommended the construction of an extravascular valve mechanism for the treatment of post-thrombotic syndrome of the popliteal vein and superficial femoral vein with complete recanalization. The valve mechanism is created by transposing the gracilis tendon (or alloplastic tendon) across the proximal segment of the popliteal vein. When the knee joint is flexed, the vessel becomes kinked, creating a barrier to retrograde flow. The indications and the surgical concept itself are controversial.

Ascending phlebography can be used to check the efficacy of the procedure. Several lateral views of the popliteal vein are taken with increasing angles of knee flexion.

Moszkowicz Technique of Low Saphenous Ligation and Intraoperative Sclerotherapy

Low ligation of the great saphenous vein with a retrograde sclerosing injection was described by Moszkowicz in 1927. This procedure is rarely performed today. The sclerosant can easily drain into the deep venous system during the procedure and incite a deep vein thrombosis.

Additionally, it is known that the saphenous veins are resistant to complete sclerosis, especially in younger patients. On ascending pressure phlebography, the sclerosed great saphenous vein will exhibit typical post-thrombotic features with internal webs and luminal irregularities. Often films will also show a great saphenous stump with large branch varices.

Only ascending pressure phlebography is suitable for evaluating recurrent varicosity during the preoperative diagnostic workup. In all cases the entire venous system should be scrutinized, but color-coded duplex scanning is excellent for imaging the great saphenous vein in isolation and may demonstrate post-thrombotic changes.

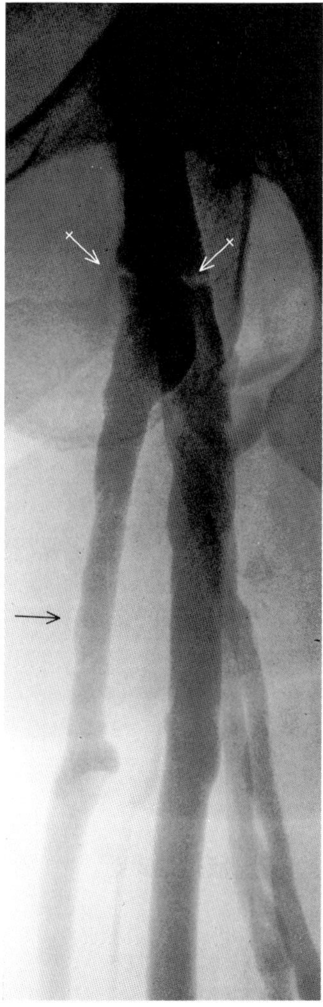

360. Phlebogram following a sclerosing injection into the crosse for saphenous varicosity. Recanalization of the great saphenous vein with internal septations (→). Post-thrombotic wall changes in the common femoral vein (↦)

Sclerotherapy

The injection of a sclerosing solution into a varicose vein causes intimal damage that precipitates the formation of a conglutination thrombus. Today sclerotherapy is a low-risk procedure in the hands of an experienced therapist, but complications are still reported. The main concern for the radiologist is the detection or exclusion of post-thrombotic changes in the deep venous system. Corresponding phlebographic findings tend to be 360
very subtle.

The *efficacy* of sclerotherapy is readily assessed by ascending pressure phlebography. A young patient with severe varicosity of the great or small saphenous vein will not respond to the treatment. The terminal portion of the vein generally remains patent and can be filled by retrograde contrast flow during a Valsalva maneuver. Farther distally, post-thrombotic changes develop in the vessel wall with partial or incomplete recanalization. Older patients are more likely to exhibit a positive response to therapy. Color-coded duplex scanning and ultrasound flowmetry can provide the same quality of information as ascending phlebography within a circumscribed venous segment.

In the *research setting,* phlebography is useful for evaluating and comparing the efficacy of different methods for the treatment of varicose veins. Color-coded duplex scanning is not satisfactory in this regard. Concerning the interpretation of findings in the saphenous veins, it should be noted that post-sclerotherapy recanalization may continue over a period of months, so follow-up examinations should be scheduled for longer intervals.

References

Adams JT, De Weese JA (1966) Partial interruption of the inferior vena cava with a new plastic clip. Surg Gynec Obstet 123: 1087

Bauer G (1965) The long term effect of popliteal ligation in 136 cases of severe bursting lower leg pain and oedema. J Cardiovasc Surg 6: 366

Cranley JJ (1975) Vascular surgery, vol II. Harper und Row, Hagerstown/Maryland

De Weese MS, Hunter DC (1963) Vena cava filter for the prevention of pulmonary embolism. Arch Surg 86: 852

Greenfield LJ, McCurdy JR, Brown PP, Elkins RC (1973) A new intracaval filter permitting continued flow and resolution of emboli. Surgery 73: 599

Günther RW, Thelen M (1988) Interventionelle Radiologie. Thieme, Stuttgart

Hach W (1980) Operative Therapie tiefer okklusiver Venenprozesse. Medica 1: 667

Hach W, Salzmann G, Radovic HW (1983) Die operative Behandlung der deszendierenden Thrombose des akuten Kompressionssyndroms der Ileofemoralvenen durch Bypass mit wandverstärkter PTFE-Prothese. Vasa 12: 249

Husni EA (1970) In situ saphenopopliteal bypass graft for incompetence of the femoral and popliteal veins. Surg Gynec Obstet 130: 279

Kersten T, Varco RL (1978) Vena cava interruption: The why, the how, the uncertainties. In: Najarian JS, Delaney JP (eds) Vascular surgery. Thieme, Stuttgart

Linton RR, Hardy JB (1947) Postthrombotic sequelae of the lower extremity treatment by superficial femoral vein interruption and stripping of saphenous veins. Surg Clin North Am 27: 1171

May R (1972) Venentransplantation beim postthrombotischen Zustandsbild des Beins. Acta Chir 7: 1

Miles RM, Chappell F, Renner OA (1964) Partially occluding vena cava clip for the prevention of pulmonary embolism. Am Surg 30: 40

Mobin-Uddin K, Utley JR, Bryant LR (1975) The inferior vena cava umbrella filter. Prog Cardiovasc Dis 17: 391

Moszkowicz L (1927) Die Behandlung der Krampfadern mit Zuckerinjektionen, kombiniert mit Venenligatur. Zentralbl Chir 28: 1733

Palma EC, Esperon R (1960) Veins transplants and grafts in the surgical treatment of the postphlebitic syndrome. J Cardiovasc Surg 1: 94

Psathakis N (1982) Vereinfachte Technik der Ersatzklappenoperation an der V. poplitea mit der Silikonsehne beim postthrombotischen Syndrom. In: Hach W, Salzmann G (Hrsg) Chirurgie der Venen. Schattauer, Stuttgart

Spencer FC, Jude J, Riemhoff WF, Stonesifer G (1965) Plication of the inferior vena cava for pulmonary embolism: Longterm results in 39 cases. Ann Surg 161: 788

Vollmar JF, Hutschenreiter S (1980) Der quere Beckenvenenbypass (der „hohe Palma"). Vasa 9: 62

Weber J, May R (1990) Funktionelle Phlebologie. Thieme, Stuttgart

Zollikofer CL (1988) Perkutane Implantation endovaskulärer Prothesen. In: Günther RW, Thelen M (Hrsg) Interventionelle Radiologie. Thieme, Stuttgart

Regressive Changes

For the radiologist, the significance of regressive vascular changes relates more to questions of differential diagnosis than to their correlation with clinical symptoms. This is especially true in the diagnosis of post-thrombotic syndrome.

The age-related regressive changes that affect the stem veins include a *decrease in the number of venous valves.* The soleus and gastrocnemius muscle veins already exhibit regressive changes by about
25 years of age. The vessels show fusiform dilata- 361
tion with a marked reduction in valve numbers. In 362
some cases the *dilatation* increases so much over 363
time that the veins assume the aspect of "muscle 364
varices."

Some patients complain of unpleasant congestive complaints and slight swelling on prolonged standing. In most cases, however, calf pain and nocturnal cramps are referable to a static insufficiency, and phlebographic findings are incidental. In other cases the vessels may remain normal to a very old age.

Causes of compression syndromes in the venous system		
Body region	Compressing structure Physiologic	Pathologic
Calf	–	Malignant tumors, tourniquet syndrome, Baker's cyst, muscle hematoma
Knee	Gastrocnemius muscle bellies	Knee effusion, Baker's cyst, popliteal artery aneurysm
Thigh and groin	Peritoneal recess	Malignant and benign tumors, cystic degeneration of adventitia
Pelvis	Crossing arteries	Benign and malignant tumors, pregnancy, perivascular callosities, vertebral osteophytes, arterial elongation and dilatation, arterial aneurysm
Retro-peritoneal space	–	Benign and malignant tumors, aortic aneurysm, hepatic cirrhosis, ascites

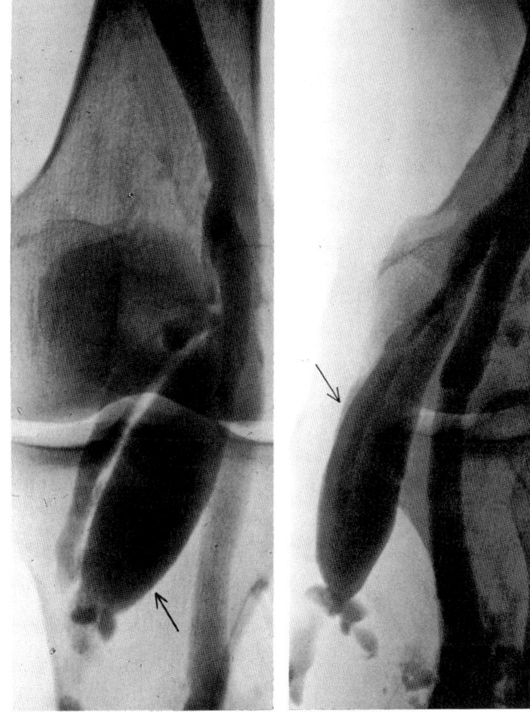

361. Severe regressive changes in the gastrocnemius veins of a 57-year-old woman with stage III great saphenous varicosity. Nonspecific congestive complaints. Fusiform dilatation of the vessels (→) with a reduced number of valves. Demonstrated in the left leg by ascending pressure phlebography, internal rotation (*left*) and lateral view (*right*)

Venous Compression Syndromes

Compression syndromes can be classified etiologically as physiologic or pathologic (Hach 1980). They can affect all venous systems of the lower limb, pelvis, and retroperitoneal space.

The main importance of physiologic compression
365 syndromes lies in their differentiation from pathologic processes. The pathologic syndromes require a complete investigation in all cases, since a mass lesion may represent a malignant tumor, and the outflow impairment caused by the lesion poses an immediate threat of descending thrombosis with all its risks and complications.

Physiologic Causes of Venous Compression

Physiologic compression of the *popliteal vein* occurs during contraction of the two heads of the gastrocnemius muscle. This phenomenon, known as the *popliteal pump* (Hach 1980), can be seen 86
when the patient deliberately or inadvertently contracts the calf muscles during ascending phlebography with a Valsalva maneuver. The posteroanterior film displays the compressed vein as a narrow slit that appears fusiform due to the shape of the muscle belly. On relaxation of the muscles, the vein reexpands at once to its normal caliber.

Differentiation is required from mass lesions in the popliteal fossa, whose compressive effect is usually most apparent in the lateral projection. The compressed segment appears shorter, and its borders are crescent-shaped rather than fusiform. Confusion with thrombosis is unlikely due to absence of the radiographic signs of thrombus.

An impression of the superior femoral vein can be
created by *contraction of the sartorius muscle*, but 87
this is very easy to recognize from its typical appearance.

A compression phenomenon occurs at the junction of the *common femoral vein* and *external iliac*

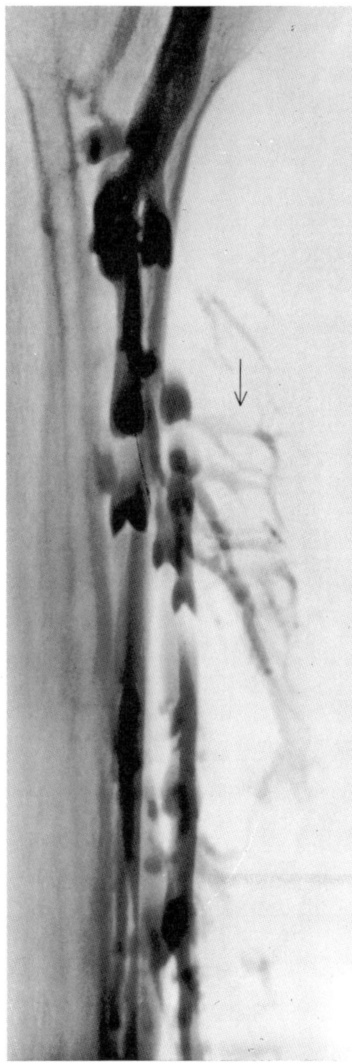

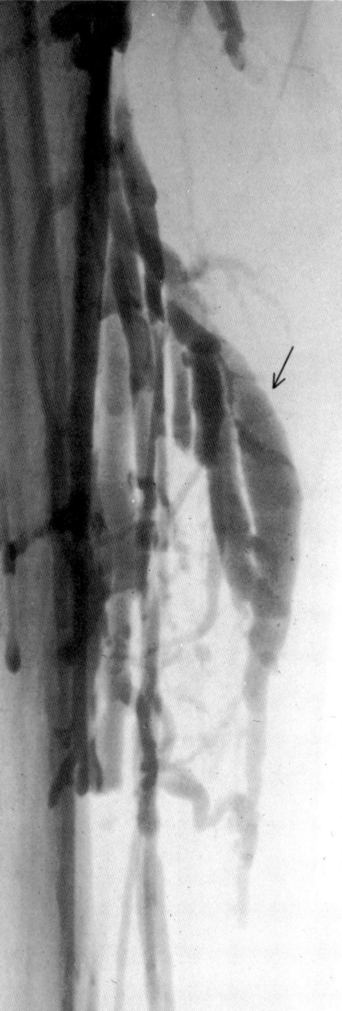

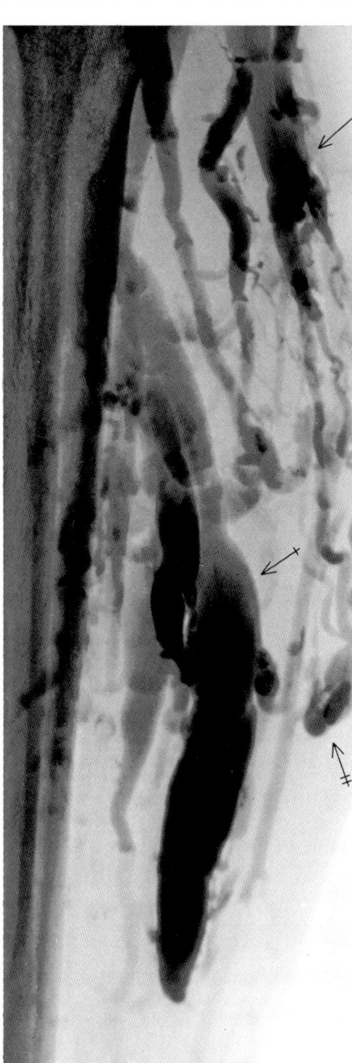

362 *(left)*. Subtle regressive changes in the soleus veins with a reduced number of valves (→). Ascending pressure phlebography in a 27-year-old woman with no subjective complaints

363 *(middle)*. Regressive changes in the soleus veins with a reduced number of valves and fusiform dilatation of the vessels (→). Ascending pressure phlebography in a 33-year-old woman with orthostatic complaints

364 *(right)*. Regressive changes in the gastrocnemius veins (→) and soleus veins (⇸) of a 53-year-old woman with nonspecific congestive complaints in the lower extremities. ⇻ Incompetent May's perforator. Demonstrated by ascending pressure phlebography

366 *vein* due to Gullmo's effect. During straining, the vessel is compressed and narrowed from the medial side but resumes its normal diameter at once when the patient relaxes. *Gullmo's sign* is caused by pressure from the peritoneal sac in the lateral inguinal fossa upon the lacuna vasorum. Some authors (Gullmo 1964; May 1974; Nylander 1961) interpret the sign as indicating a predisposition to femoral hernia. A mass lesion should be considered in the differential diagnosis.

The *pelvic veins* are subject to anatomic compression effects from crossing arteries. These effects are especially common in asthenic patients with increased lordotic curvature of the lumbar spine and in the flat supine position.

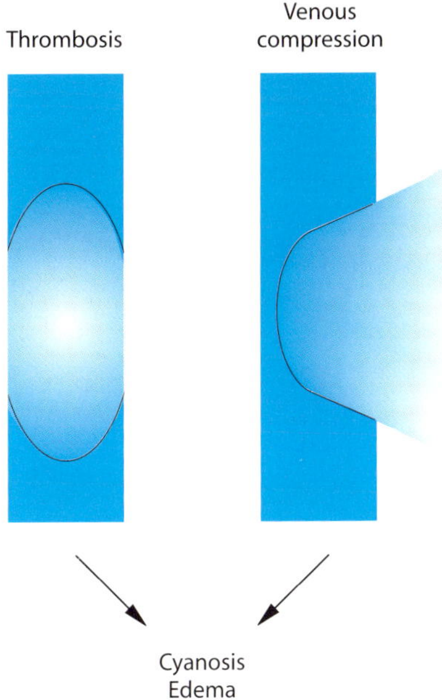

365. Venous occlusion by luminal obturation (thrombosis) and extrinsic compression

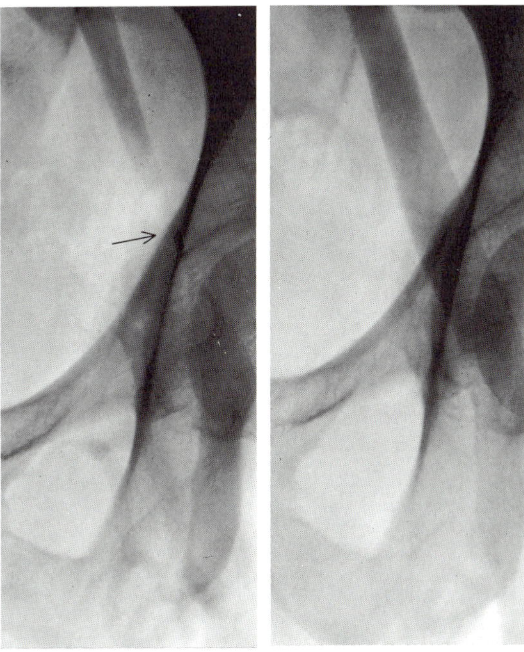

366. Compression of the external iliac artery (→) by the bulging peritoneal sac in the inguinal fovea (Gullmo's sign). Demonstrated by ascending pressure phlebography (*left*) and during normal respiration (*right*)

The *left common iliac vein* is often compressed by
69 the right common iliac artery below the caval bifurcation, the compressed segment appearing as a
filling defect ("invisible zone") on pelvic phlebo-
367 grams (Guilhelm and Baux 1954). The intravascular *pelvic venous spur* of May and Thurner (1956)
is also found at this site. With chronic outflow impairment, the presacral plexuses and ascending lumbar vein can become functional as collaterals.
A less conspicuous physiologic compression effect
is the indentation of the *right external iliac vein* by
the crossing artery a hand's width above the ingui-
70 nal ligament. This finding may be more pronounced in patients with dilatative arteriopathy.
368 The rounded or elongated impression may occasionally require differentiation from a mass lesion.

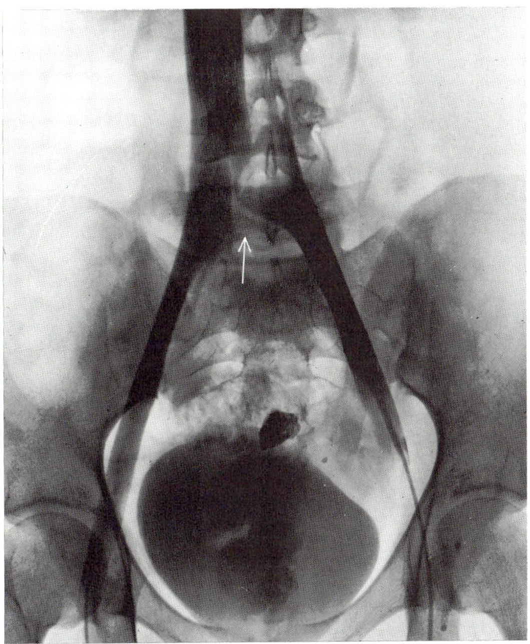

367. Compression of the left common iliac vein ("invisible zone") by the crossing right pelvic artery (→). Demonstrated by pelvic phlebography

Pathologic Compression Syndromes

There are a variety of pathologic conditions that can displace and narrow circumscribed venous segments. Malignant tumors are a relatively frequent cause. Other symptom complexes are rare

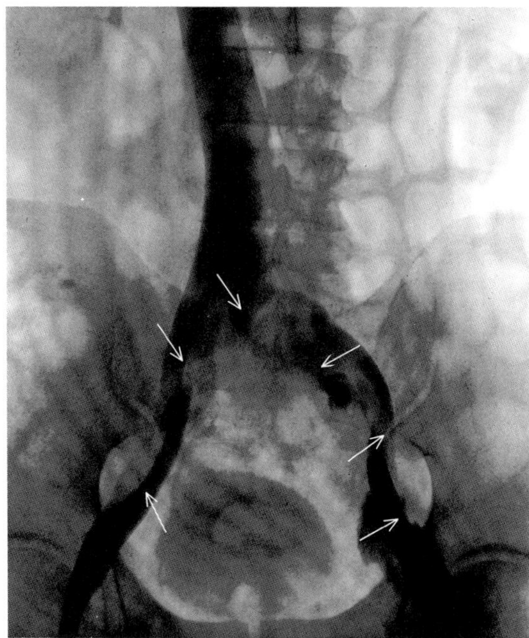

368. Compression of the deep pelvic veins by adjacent arteries (→). Demonstrated by pelvic phlebography in a 59-year-old man with severe dilatative arteriopathy

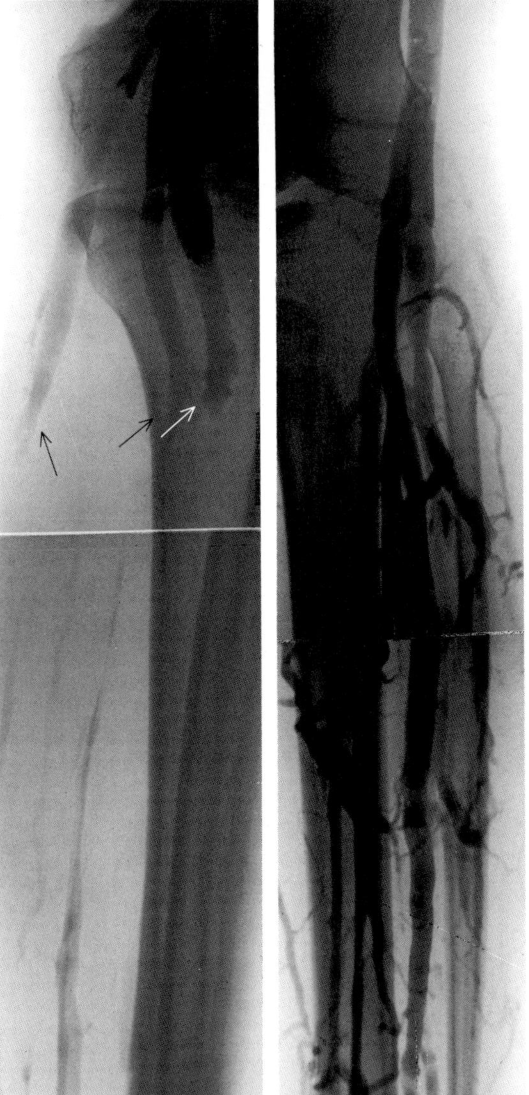

369. Complete compression of the lower leg veins (→) by tourniquet syndrome in a 30-year-old man, caused by excessive compression for control of venous bleeding. Immediate decompression was carried out by fasciotomy, and full recovery ensued. Demonstrated by ascending phlebography before (*left*) and after fasciotomy (*right*) on the left side

and some are even unique, posing problems in the recording and analysis of case data.

A pathologic compression syndrome can develop *insidiously* and then suddenly become manifest by inciting a deep vein thrombosis. Another patient may present with the full-blown symptoms of a severe venous thrombosis, with phlebography revealing a high-grade, hemodynamically significant vascular stenosis justifying a diagnosis of *acute compression syndrome.* Phlebography is the only study that can reliably discriminate these conditions. Due to the potential for confusing thrombosis with an acute compression syndrome, fibrinolysis or thrombectomy should never be undertaken solely on the basis of clinical findings, and phlebographic documentation should be secured *in every case.* In the case of invasive or anticoagulatory treatment, a wrong diagnosis could have fatal consequences.

A pathologic compression syndrome is based either on a disease process in the *vessel wall* itself (cystic intimal degeneration, vessel wall tumor) or a process *extrinsic* to the vessel. B-mode imaging is a useful supplement to phlebography, therefore, and color-coded duplex scanning is particularly useful for bringing out details. Once such a process has become clinically evident, *sonography* is usually the most important investigative technique. Other adjunctive studies of potential benefit are arteriography, computed tomography, and magnetic resonance imaging.

Pathologic compression syndromes are classified according to the vascular region in which they occur. This approach is best for appreciating the specific topographic conditions that prevail in the different regions.

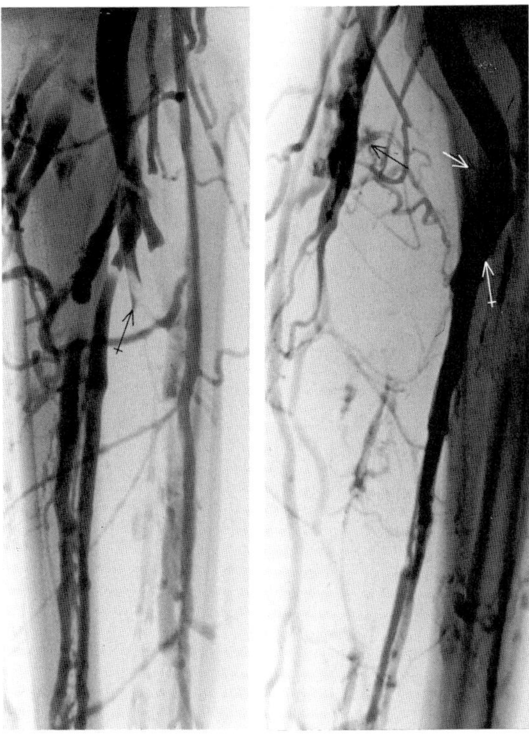

370. Displacement of the deep veins in the left lower leg (→) by muscle swelling 2 months after surgical treatment of tourniquet syndrome following fasciotomy; 64-year-old man who previously underwent reconstruction of the aortic bifurcation with a complicated postoperative course. Films also show thrombotic occlusion of the fibular vein (↔). Demonstrated by ascending pressure phlebography, internal rotation (*left*) and lateral view (*right*)

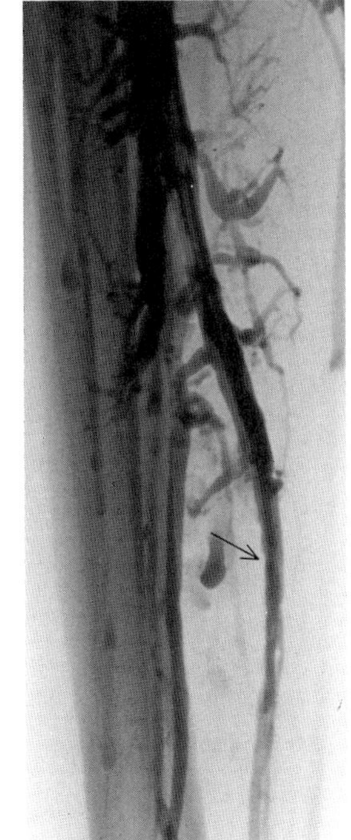

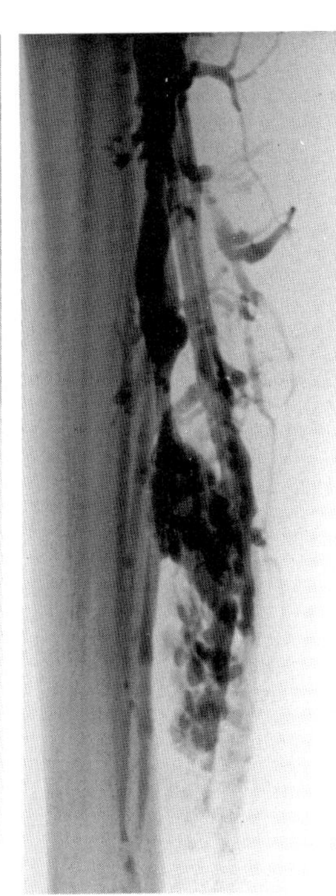

371. Displacement of the posterior tibial veins (→) by cavernous hemangioma in a 22-year-old woman with congestive complaints in the right calf. Demonstrated by ascending pressure phlebography in the early phase of the examination (*left*) and by the overflow effect (*right*)

Compression Syndromes Involving the Crural Veins

Tourniquet syndrome can cause total occlusion of
369 the deep veins below the knee. The disease occurs following the operative revascularization of an ischemic extremity. The interruption of the arterial circulation causes such severe capillary damage that capillary permeability is increased after perfusion is restored. The rapidly progressive intrafascial edema exerts a mass effect on all biologic structures leading to severe circulatory embarrassment, paresis, and tissue necrosis. The diagnosis is based on typical clinical findings, although some cases may require differentiation from deep vein thrombosis. Following the acute stage of the disease, displacement of the deep lower-leg veins by the swollen muscles can persist for
370 months.

The stem veins of the lower leg have a relatively small lumen, so they tend to be displaced more than compressed by mass lesions, most notably
large *hematomas* and *cavernous hemangiomas*. Be- 371
nign *bone tumors* and an expanding callus can also produce mass effects in this region. An extreme case
involved the displacement of both superficial and 372
deep veins by the transfascial growth of a *lipoma*.
Malignant tumors are rare in the lower leg. *Baker's* 373
cysts can sometimes extend well into the calf. 374

Compression Syndromes Involving the Popliteal Vein

Various disorders in the popliteal fossa can be a source of pathologic venous compression. A Baker's cyst or even a large joint effusion in the knee can compromise venous return. A compres-

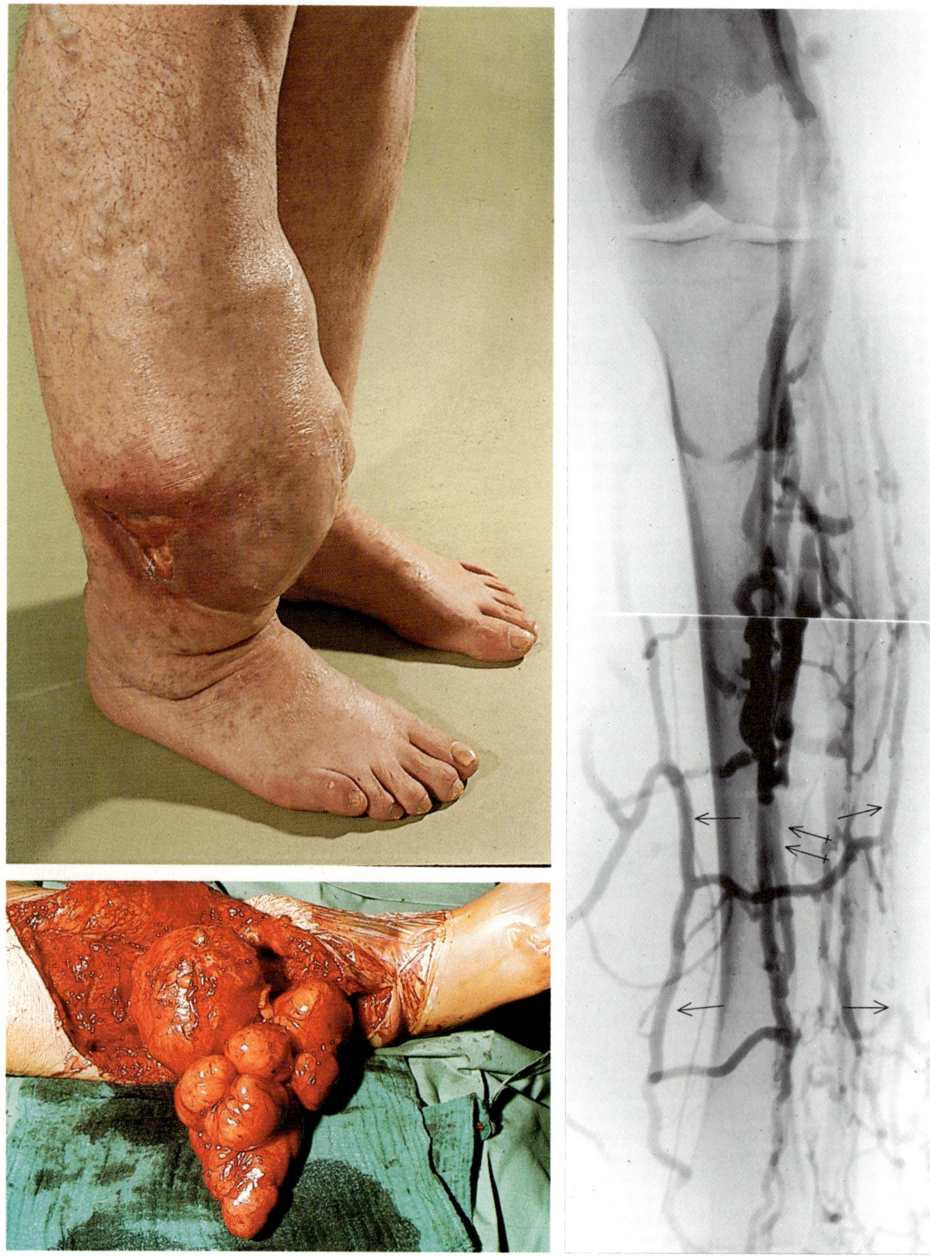

372. Extensive displacement of the superficial vessels (→) and posterior tibial veins (↔) by a large, partly intrafascial lipoma in a 59-year-old woman with chronic ulceration over the tumor. *Top left,* clinical appearance. *Right,* ascending pressure phlebography, internal rotation view. *Bottom left,* appearance at operation

sion syndrome should be suspected clinically in patients presenting with etiologically unclear peripheral edema and joint complaints.

Baker's cyst is a synovial sac protruding through a defect in the posterior fibrous capsule of the knee joint. Emerging between the two heads of the gastrocnemius muscle, the cyst can extend to the midcalf level, where it presents as a tense mass. Usually there is intractable joint effusion caused by chronic irritation from the cyst. Due to the close topographic relationships in the popliteal region, a large Baker's cyst is manifested early by 375
displacement of the popliteal vein and gastrocnemius veins.

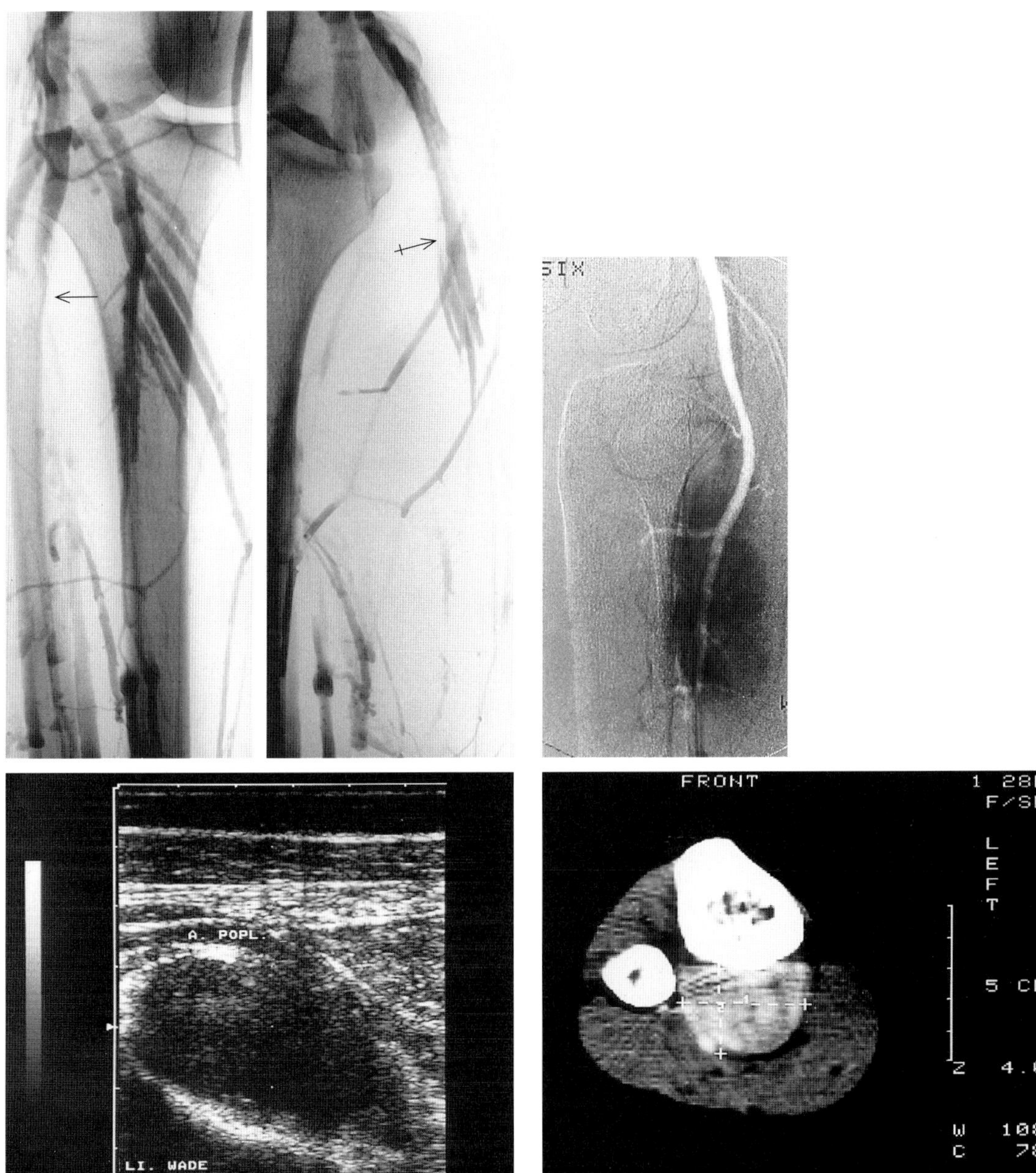

373. Malignant tumor in a 36-year-old woman with discrete tendency toward swelling in the lower leg. *Top left, top middle,* ascending pressure phlebography; fibular vein and gastrocnemius veins not shown. *Bottom left,* tumor demonstrated by sonography. *Top right,* digital subtraction angiography. Well-vascularized tumor with pathologic vessels. *Bottom right,* computed tomography. Histologic diagnosis of carcinoma

The *entrapment syndrome* is usually manifested
by an anomalous course of the popliteal artery
and vein about the medial head of the gastrocnemius muscle, with narrowing of the vessels. Rare-
376 ly, a large *hemorrhagic effusion* in the popliteal
fossa can produce a venous compression effect.
Malignant tumors are uncommon in this region.

A major cause of extrinsic compression of the
popliteal vein is an *aneurysm* of the homonymous 377
artery. Generally the patient seeks medical attention because of the arterial symptoms. The chief
complaint is intermittent claudication due to recurrent small emboli and the slow-growing, pulsating mass in the popliteal fossa.

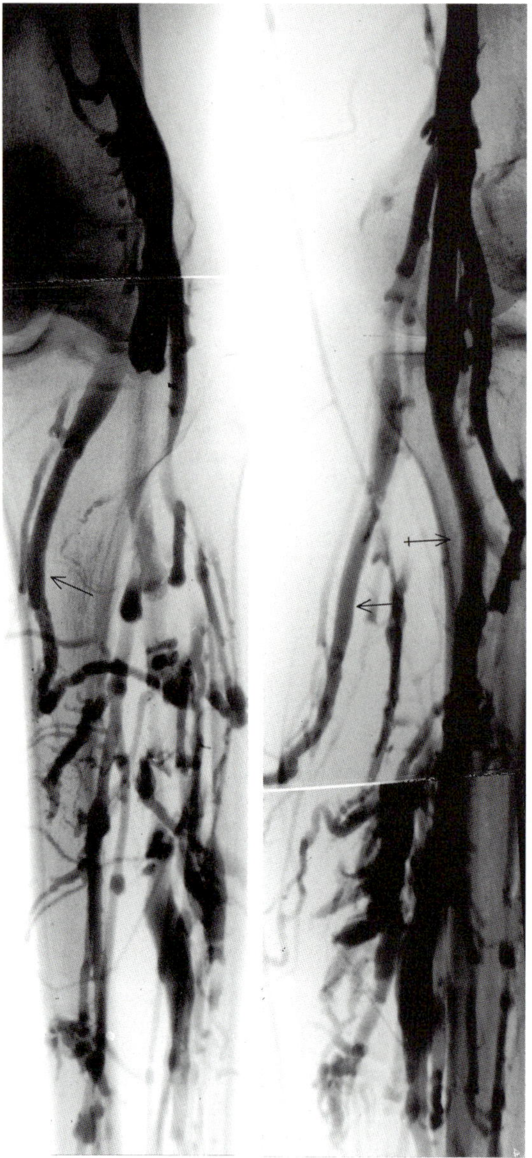

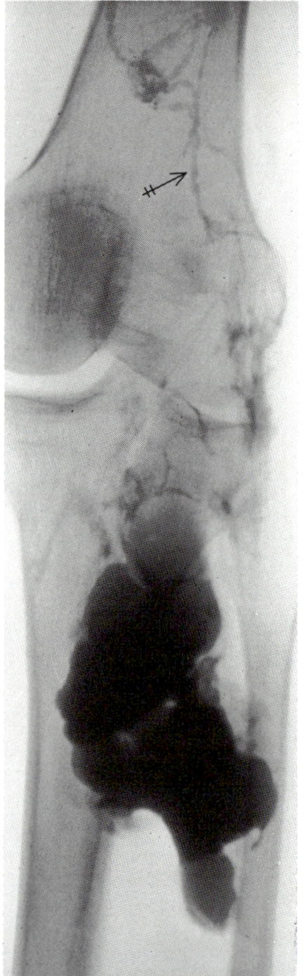

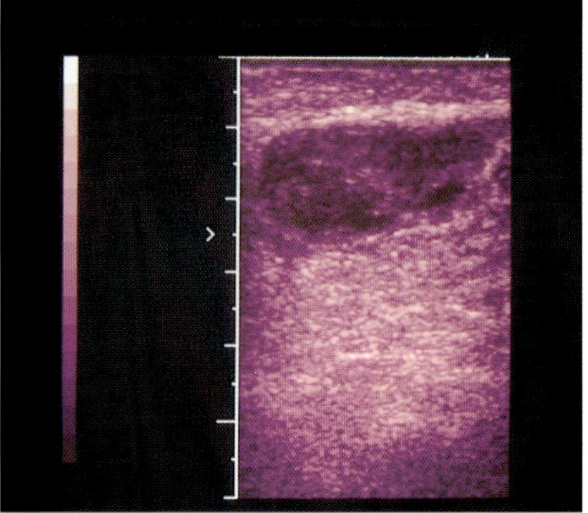

374. Displacement of the tibial gastrocnemius veins (→) and popliteal vein (↔) by a large Baker's cyst in a 47-year-old woman. Initial symptom was swelling of the left leg during a long-distance flight. Demonstrated by ascending pressure phlebography, internal rotation (*left*) and lateral view (*middle*). Opacified cyst (*top right*). Contrast drainage occurs through deep lymphatic channels (⇸). Formation not clearly shown by real-time sonography, color coded (*bottom right*). (Acuson, 7-MHz transducer)

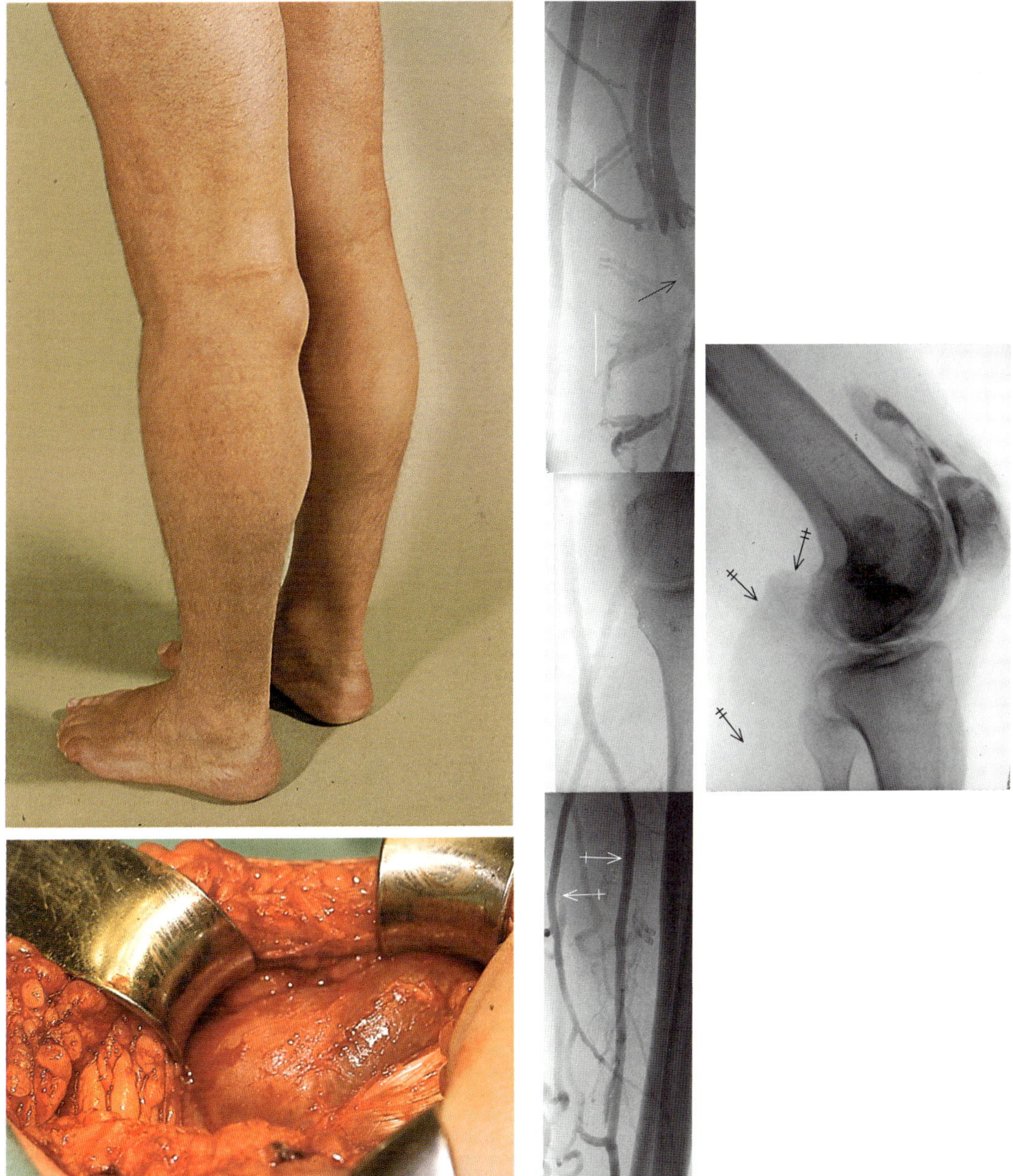

375. Thrombotic occlusion of the popliteal vein (→) associated with a fist-size Baker's cyst in a 58-year-old man with recurrent swelling of the left leg, knee pain, and recurrent knee effusion. *Top left,* clinical appearance. *Middle,* ascending pressure phlebography demonstrates phlebectasia of the reduplicated great saphenous vein (⟷). *Right,* arthrographic appearance of the cyst (⇸). *Bottom left,* appearance at operation

Symptoms are bilateral in almost two thirds of cases. Due to the close anatomic confines of the popliteal fossa, the aneurysm begins to compress the
377 popliteal vein at an early stage and finally occludes the vessel, with regional thrombosis supervening. In some cases thrombosis is the condition that first motivates the patient to consult a physician. Treatment of the popliteal artery aneurysm is surgical. In many patients with spontaneous thrombosis or a severe peripheral embolism, popliteocrural venous reconstruction is no longer possible and amputation may become necessary.

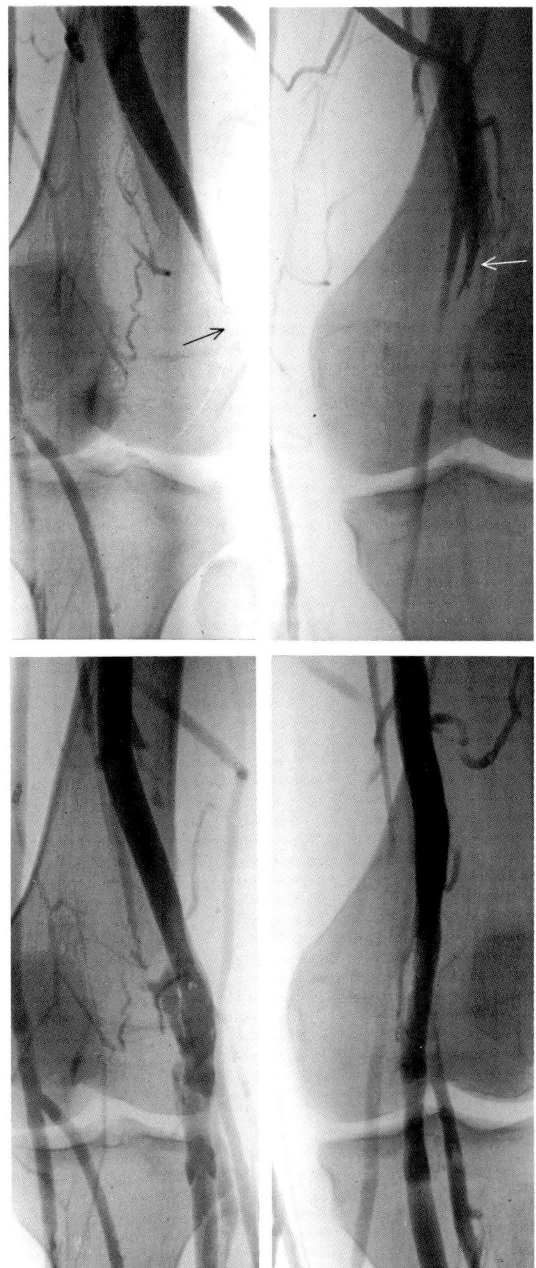

376. Complete compression and displacement of the popliteal vein (→) by traumatic hematoma in an 18-year-old woman who sustained an athletic injury 3 weeks before with subsequent leg swelling. Full recovery ensued after operative treatment. Demonstrated by ascending pressure phlebography, internal rotation and lateral views taken preoperatively (*top*) and 4 days postoperatively (*bottom*)

377. See p. 241

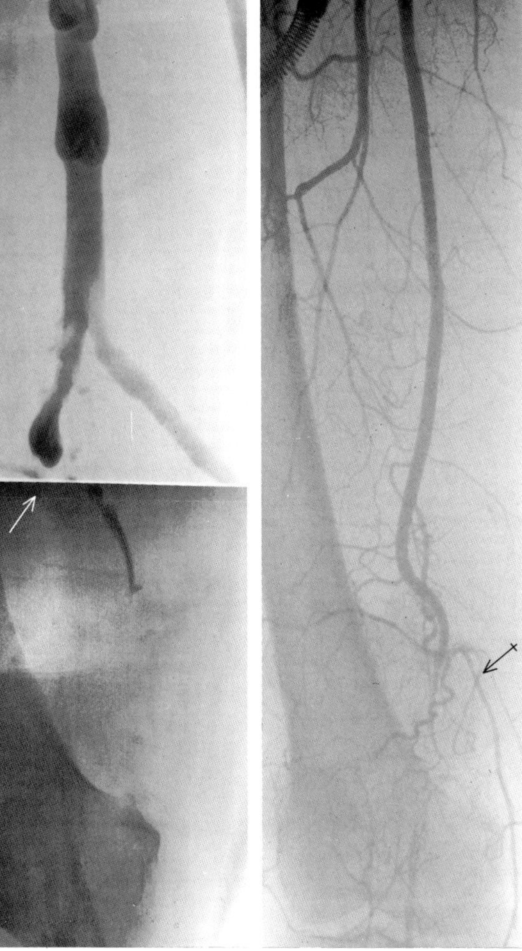

378. Occlusion of the superficial femoral vein by a fist-size tumor metastatic to breast carcinoma in a 62-year-old woman, who presented with the clinical features of acute leg vein thrombosis. *Left,* ascending pressure phlebography shows compressive occlusion of the vein with no evidence of thrombosis (→). *Right,* arteriogram with pathologic vessels (↔)

Compression Syndromes Involving the Superficial Femoral Vein

Pathologic compression effects are less common in the thigh. *Malignant tumors,* especially sarco- 378
mas and metastases, have the greatest causal significance in this region. Occasionally a *luxuriant callus* or *bucket-handle exostosis* leads to venous outflow impairment, and severe *dilatative arteriopathy* is a possible but infrequent cause.

A rare cause of superficial femoral vein compression is *cystic intimal degeneration,* in which the vessel lumen is narrowed by heterotopic pieces of

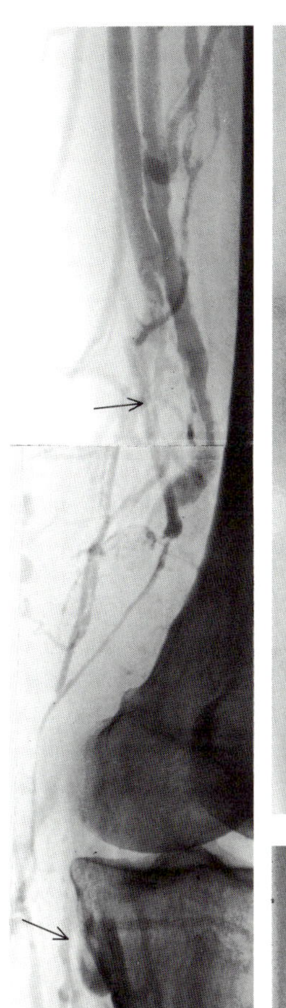

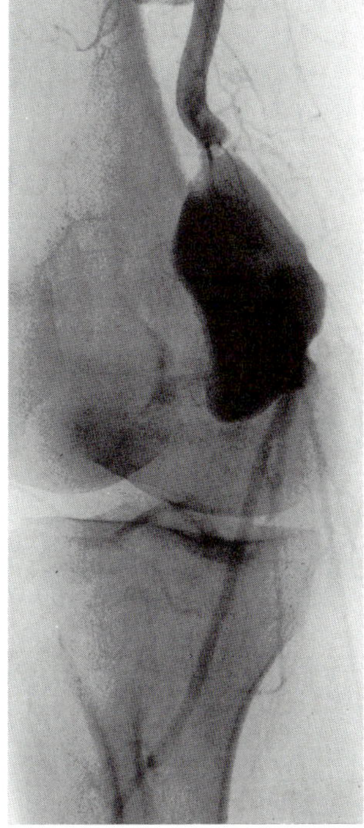

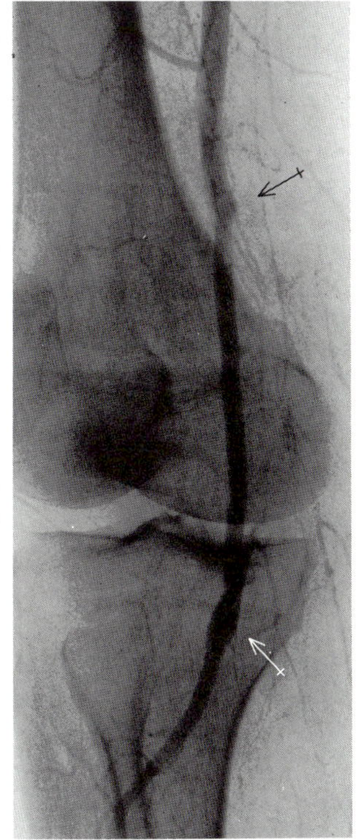

joint capsule within the adventitia that secrete a synovial-like fluid.

Compression Syndromes Involving the Common Femoral Vein

Venous compression in the groin region can result from a malignant or inflammatory *enlargement of the lymph nodes,* which cause a sharply defined, lobulated indentation of the vessel. *Arterial aneurysms* can develop in this region following diagnostic and therapeutic procedures such as cardiac catheterization or angioplasty. Compression by *perivascular callosities* is possible as a sequel to radiation therapy or a protracted inflammatory disorder. 379

Compression Syndromes of the Major Pelvic Veins

Circumscribed narrowing of the pelvic veins should direct suspicion toward a *malignant tumor* 380
such as a pelvic wall sarcoma or lymph node metastasis. The veins also may be displaced by mass lesions of the female genital organs. *Arterial aneu-* 381
rysms are also fairly common in the pelvic region. An important cause of pelvic compression syndrome is perivascular callosities relating to *radia-* 382
tion fibrosis or primary *Ormond's retroperitoneal fibrosis.* This disease should be considered when

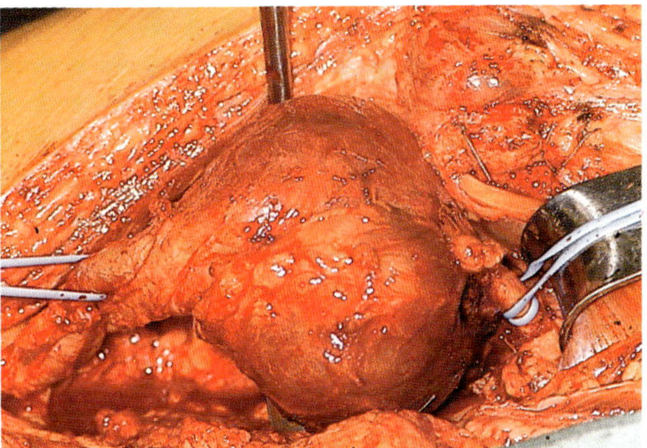

377. Compression and thrombotic occlusion of the popliteal vein by a popliteal artery aneurysm in a 50-year-old man with a long history of chronic venous insufficiency and recurrent ulcerations. The aneurysm was discovered as the source of arterial emboli. *Left,* ascending pressure phlebography shows circumscribed occlusion of the popliteal vein with adjacent post-thrombotic changes (→). *Top middle,* arteriographic appearance of the aneurysm. *Bottom middle,* intraoperative appearance, with tapes passed around the afferent and efferent arterial limbs. *Right,* appearance after aneurysmectomy and interpositional vein grafting (↔)

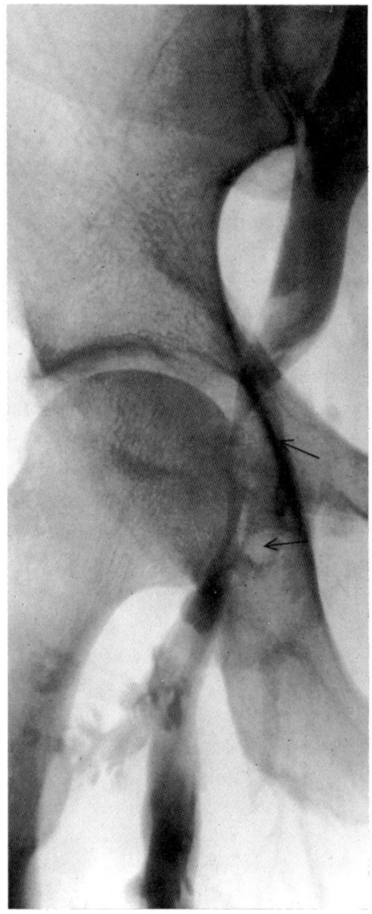

379. Compression of the common femoral vein by Hodgkin's lymphomas (→) in a 42-year-old man

381. Compression of the right external iliac vein (→) and displacement of the internal iliac veins (↔) by a large fibroid uterus. Demonstrated by pelvic phlebography in a 35-year-old woman

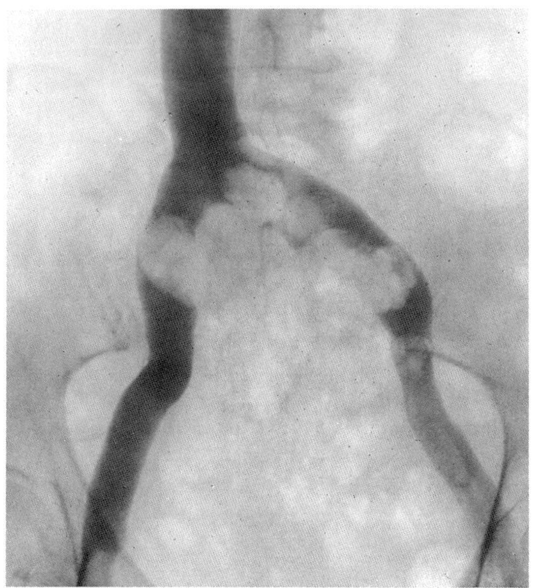

◁

380. The pelvic veins are compressed at multiple sites by metastases from bladder carcinoma in a 71-year-old woman. Demonstrated by pelvic phlebography. (Film courtesy of Dr. K. Seidel, Bielefeld)

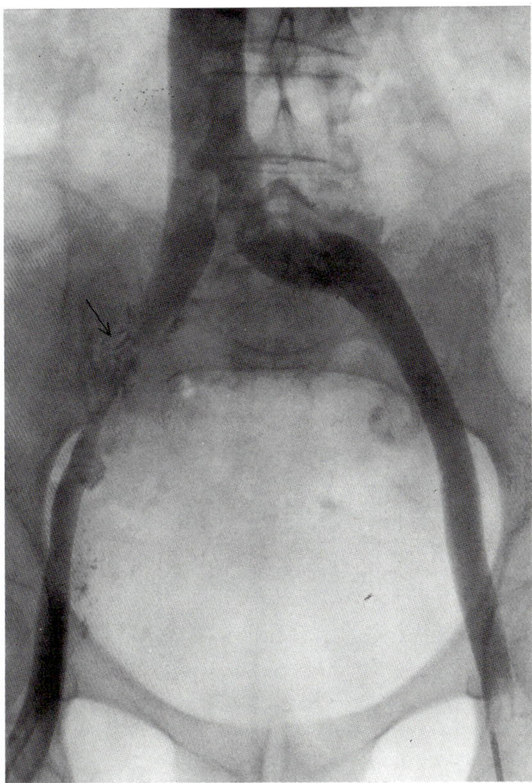

382. Compression of the right pelvic veins (→) by extensive perivascular callosities. Demonstrated by pelvic phlebography in a 46-year-old woman following deep X-irradiation of the lower abdomen

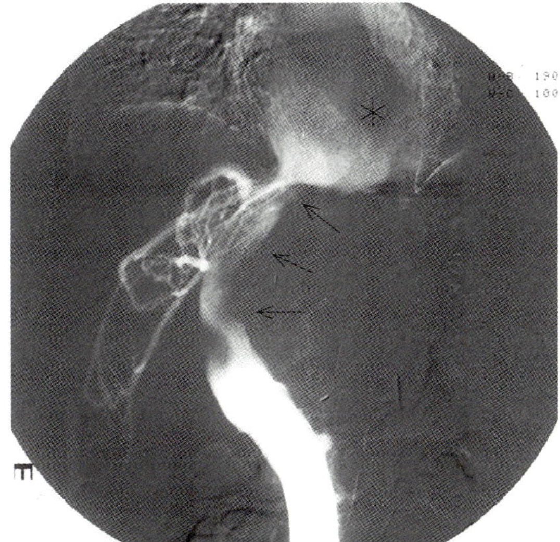

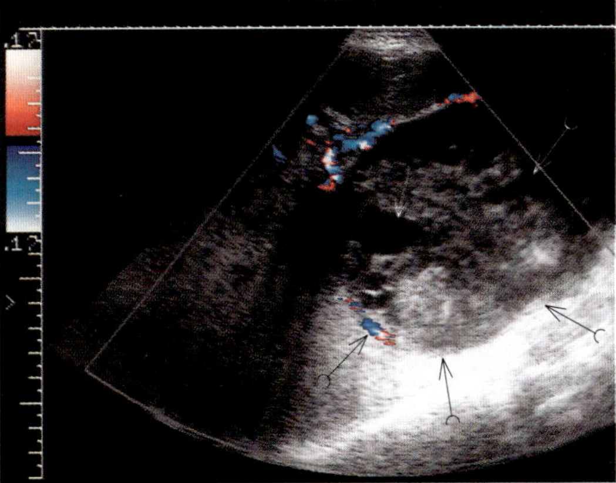

383. Vena cava compression syndrome at the level of the junction with the hepatic veins due to a fist-sized liposarcoma (recurrent tumor) in a 75-year-old woman without major symptoms. *Top*, digital cavogram with impression effect (→). Right atrium (*). *Bottom*, color-coded duplex sonography. → Inferior vena cava (cross-section); ↣ tumor borders

impairment of pelvic arterial and venous circulation coexists with urinary stasis in the kidneys.

Every suspected venous compression syndrome of the pelvic and retroperitoneal region should be evaluated by bilateral pelvic phlebography that includes visualization of the inferior vena cava. This is supplemented as needed by views in the oblique or lateral projection.

Compression Syndromes of the Inferior Vena Cava

Renal malignancies are the principal lesions caus-
383 ing indentation or displacement of the inferior vena cava. Other potential causes are adrenal tumors, soft-tissue sarcomas, neurofibromas, and lymph node metastases. *Hydronephrosis* or a large *aortic aneurysm* can occasionally cause marked displacement of the vein.

As with the pelvic veins, retroperitoneal fibrosis (*Ormond's disease*) can have causal importance, but it is rarely encountered. Finally, ascites and hepatic cirrhosis can exert compression effects on the proximal portion of the vein (Chermet and Bigot 1980).

References

Chermet J, Bigot JM (1980) Venography of the inferior vena cava and its branches. Springer, Berlin Heidelberg New York

Guilhem P, Baux R (1954) La phlébographie pelvienne par voie veneuse, osseuse et utérine. Masson, Paris

Gullmo ALC (1964) Phlebographie der peripheren Venen. In: Diethelm L (Hrsg) Röntgendiagnostik des Herzens und der Gefäße. Springer, Berlin Göttingen Heidelberg New York (Handbuch der medizinischen Radiologie, Bd X/3)

Hach W (1980) Venöse Kompressionssyndrome. Med Welt 31: 502

May R (1974) Chirurgie der Bein- und Beckenvenen. Thieme, Stuttgart

May R, Nissl R (1973) Die Phlebographie der unteren Extremität. Thieme, Stuttgart

May R, Thurner J (1956) Ein Gefäßsporn in der V. iliaca com. als wahrscheinliche Ursache der überwiegend linksseitigen Beckenvenenthrombose. Z Kreislaufforsch 45: 912

Nylander G Hemodynamics of the pelvic veins in incompetence of the femoral vein. Acta Radiol (Stockholm) 56: 369

Pelvic Venous Spur

A "pelvic venous spur" may be found within the left common iliac vein just below the origin of the
74 inferior vena cava. The pathologic anatomy of this lesion was studied in detail by May and Thurner in 1956.

Its *etiology* is presumably based on a chronic irritation of the vein wall by arterial pulsations and by the constriction of the vessel between the artery and the sacral promontory. But the spur has also been detected in newborns, implying a malformative etiology. The lesion consists histologically of loose connective tissue with an endothelial lining. The morphologic type may be classified as lateral,
384 central, or membranous.

A pelvic venous spur is detectable in 11% of the healthy adult population (May 1974). A predilection for females can be explained by the increased pressure on the major pelvic veins that occurs during pregnancy due to uterine enlargement and the increased lordotic curve of the spine. The more frequent occurrence of pelvic vein thrombosis on the left side very likely relates to the venous outflow impairment below the origin of the inferior vena cava.

A spur in the left common iliac vein appears *radiographically* as an oblong filling defect with sharp borders. The vessel is widely indented by ar- 295
terial compression and may be difficult to discern.
The spur projects into this "invisible zone." With 385
chronic outflow impairment, a collateral circulation develops via the presacral pelvic venous plexuses and ascending lumbar vein.

The spur is demonstrated radiographically by pelvic phlebography. Often the lesion is difficult to detect, however, so we recommend taking oblique projections with elevation of the right side. Detailed descriptions of the pelvic venous spur can be found in May (1974) and Weber and May (1990).

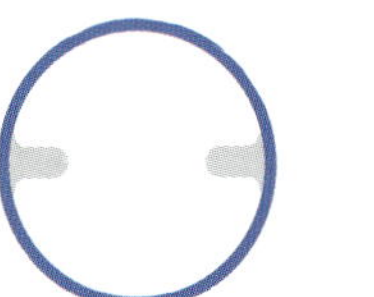
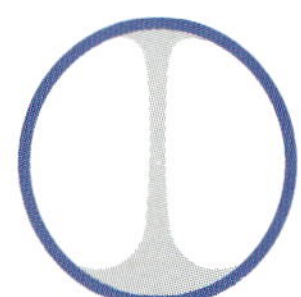
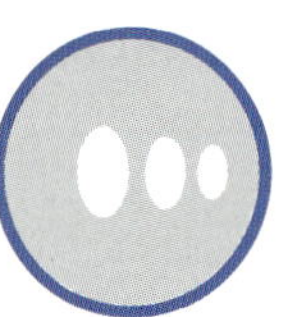

384. Lateral, central, and membranous types of venous spur. (After May and Nissl 1973)

References

May R (1974) Chirurgie der Bein- und Beckenvenen. Thieme, Stuttgart

May R, Nissl R (1973) Die Phlebographie der unteren Extremität. Thieme, Stuttgart

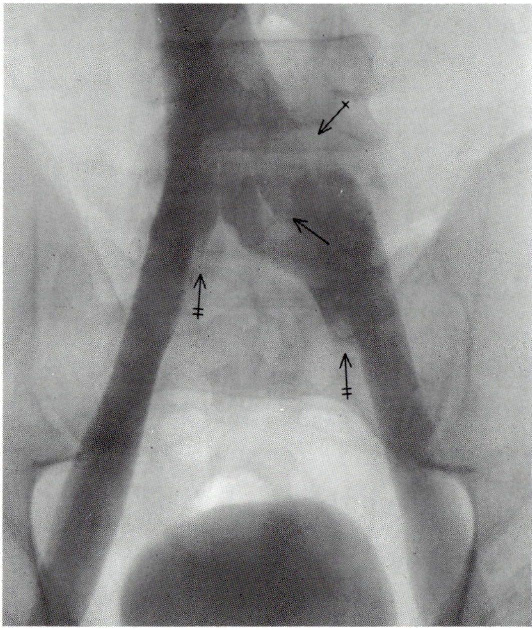

385. The venous spur typically appears on pelvic phlebograms as an oblong lucency (→); ↔ site of crossing of the right common iliac artery; ⇹ inflow effects from the internal iliac veins. Incidental finding in a 38-year-old man

May R, Thurner J (1956) Ein Gefäßsporn in der V. iliaca com. als wahrscheinliche Ursache der überwiegend linksseitigen Beckenvenenthrombose. Z Kreislaufforsch 45: 912

Weber J, May R (1990) Funktionelle Phlebologie. Thieme, Stuttgart

Flow Artifacts and Overlapping Shadows

Flow artifacts and overlapping opacified vessels on phlebograms can sometimes be difficult to distinguish from organic vascular changes. The simplest way to avoid this confusion is to obtain at least two views of each venous segment on different planes or two views separated by a time delay.

Artifacts Caused by Incomplete Mixing of the Contrast Medium

Uneven mixing of blood and contrast medium can cause streaks, stripes, or lines to appear within the vessel lumen. In ascending pressure phle- 386
bography, this artifact is most commonly seen when the contrast medium is directed by manual calf compression from the smaller vessels below

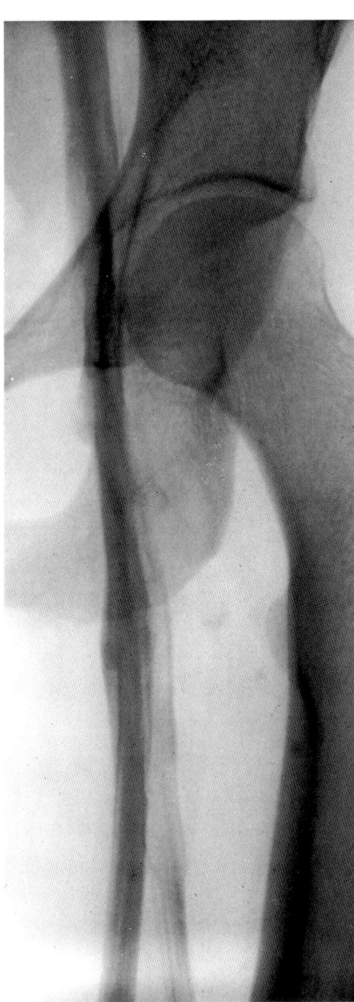

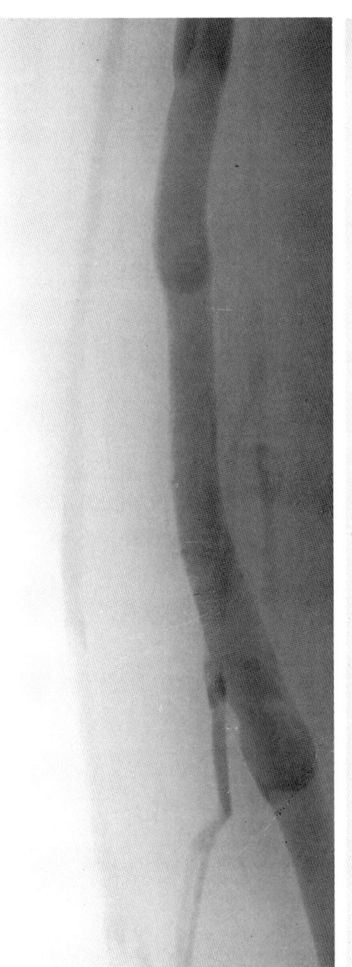

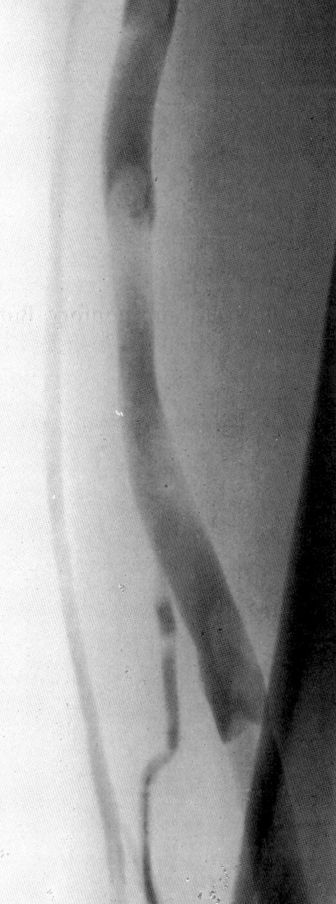

386 *(left).* Intraluminal streaks caused by the nonhomogeneous mixing of blood and contrast medium

387 *(middle, right).* Flow defects associated with the opening of venous valves. *Left,* valves in the closed state, with sedimentation of contrast medium. *Right,* passage of nonopacified blood through the contrast layer simulates a filling defect. Demonstrated by ascending pressure phlebography

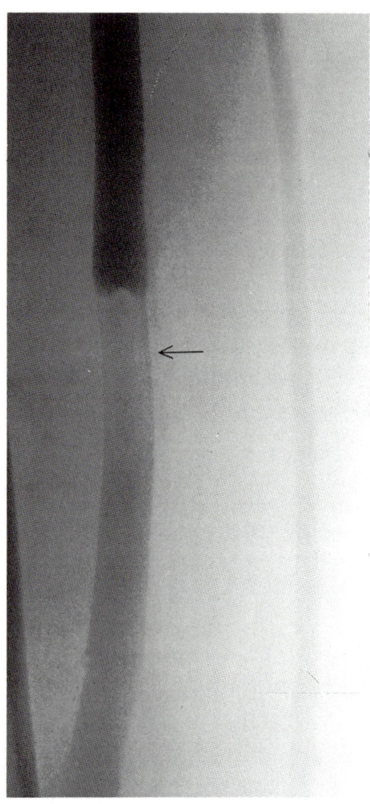

388. Laminar flow effect (→) and contrast sedimentation on the closed venous valve. Superficial femoral vein demonstrated by ascending pressure phlebography

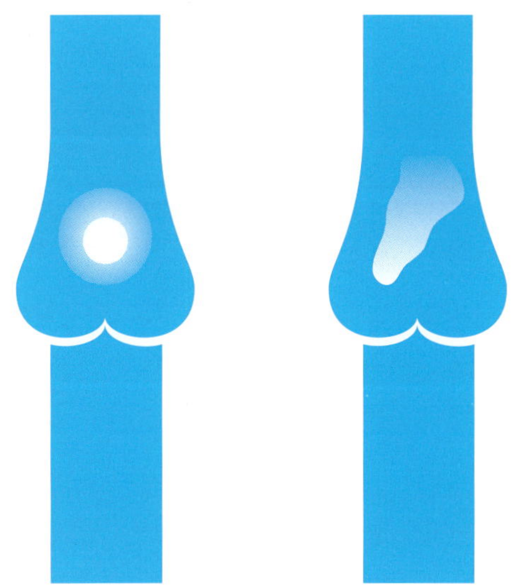

389. Knothole effect (*left*) and chimney effect (*right*)

the knee into the large-caliber superficial femoral vein.

Flow Effects at Venous Valves

Sedimentation of the contrast medium in the venous blood is used as a means of assessing the competency of the venous valves. Owing to its higher specific weight, the contrast medium tends to settle onto the closed valve leaflets when the patient is examined in the semiupright position. 387
When the valves open, the top of the nonopacified blood column flows up through the sedimented contrast layer, giving rise to an artifactual defect that may closely resemble a thrombus. However, these features are very inconstant and vanish at once in the flowing blood stream.

Laminar Flow Effects

The flow velocity is highest at the center of the vein and lower along the vessel walls. As a result, the center of the vein may be cleared of contrast medium while residual dye is still streaming along 388
the vessel walls. Differentiation from the contour sign of a fresh thrombus is easily accomplished by noting the smooth transition from the center stream to the walls. Indeed, the experienced radiologist will use finely controlled manual compression of the calf muscles to elicit this streaming effect as a way to define subtle changes in the vessel wall.

Inflow Effects

Nonopacified blood flowing into an opacified vein can produce various translucent defects on phlebograms. The most familiar is the *knothole effect,* 389
a rounded defect with relatively sharp borders ap- 390
pearing within the opaque column. The observer is looked directly into the lumen of the tributary supplying the nonopacified blood.
Blood entering at a higher flow velocity from an obliquely merging tributary produces the *chimney effect,* a lucent feature that resembles smoke rising from a chimney and dispersing in the wind. Not infrequently, the feature presents a relatively sharp upper border. Inflow effects are seen most commonly in the popliteal vein and thigh vessels.

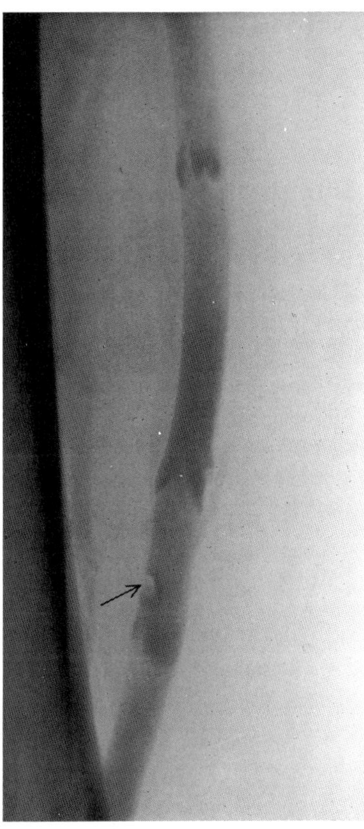

390. Knothole effect in the superficial femoral vein at the entrance of a small tributary (→). Torsion of the venous valves. Demonstrated by ascending pressure phlebography

The flow defect may initially be mistaken for a thrombus, but this question is resolved by taking a second film in a different phase of the examination.

Overlapping Shadows

The overlap or juxtaposition of multiple veins showing different degrees of opacification may create the impression of an elongated filling defect
256 resembling a thrombus. These effects are commonly seen in the vessels of the lower leg. A careful analysis of the roentgenogram will quickly yield a correct interpretation.

Indications and Contraindications for Phlebography

The decision whether to perform an invasive diagnostic procedure is basically a question of its *therapeutic relevance.* Any diagnostic procedure, including phlebography, is appropriate only if it will have significant therapeutic implications or yield information important in making a disability assessment. If effective treatment can be instituted on the basis of clinical findings and noninvasive studies, radiography of the venous system should be withheld. The purpose of phlebograpy, then, is to furnish specific information that will be useful in *planning a specific therapy.* The issue of risk versus benefit must be carefully weighed for each individual case.

Indications

The indications for phlebography have expanded in recent years, because modern methods of treating venous disorders, especially fibrinolysis and the surgical procedures, require a very precise diagnosis. At the same time, major advances have been made in the noninvasive sonographic techniques. *Modern color-coded duplex scanning* can provide impressive documentation of venous disorders; however, it cannot replace contrast phlebography. The sonogram also conveys other types of information that are no less important. Thus, the *combination* of both modalities appears be the optimum approach in many areas for the primary investigation of venous disorders (*Golden Partnership*).

If the patient is to consent to an invasive therapeutic procedure, the therapist must have comprehensive *knowledge of the morphologic situation* that he will encounter. The more precisely the pathoanatomic conditions are known, the more the surgeon can concentrate on the details of the procedure and lower the operative risk. Despite advances in other areas, contrast phlebography still provides *information* on a scope that is unmatched by any other diagnostic procedure. That is why radiography of the veins will continue to be an essential part of the primary diagnostic workup of venous disease. This attitude is reinforced by the very low complication rate of modern phlebographic techniques.

We can distinguish four major areas of applications for phlebography according to the nature of the clinical inquiry. Specific examination techniques are available for each area.

Diagnosis of Diseases of the Extrafascial Venous System

Ascending Pressure Phlebography. The most important disease of the extrafascial venous system is primary varicosity. In principle, varicose veins fall into one of two groups according to the presence or absence of *incompetent transfascial connections* with the deep venous system. The first group includes varicose saphenous veins and varicose perforators as well as certain forms of side-branch varicosity. Causal treatment consists in surgical interruption of the transfascial connection and removal of the varicose venous segments. All other varicose veins are amenable to sclerotherapy.

If the treatment regimen is geared toward sclerotherapy from the outset, for whatever reason, there appears to be no rationale for performing phlebography. Radiographic examination of the veins falls within the diagnostic program of the surgeon. In patients with saphenous varicosity, the first question to be addressed is the *location of*
140 *the points of incompetence.* The proximal point of incompetence defines the site of the transfascial
169 communication, which is virtually constant in the complete forms of varicosity and which defines the incomplete forms. The distal point of incom-
147 petence indicates the limit of the disease process and therefore influences the extent of the surgical procedure.

167 The *preservation of functionally competent veins and venous segments* is a very high priority in modern vascular surgery. In the treatment of saphenous varicosity, this requirement can be met only by early surgical intervention, as long as the reflux circuit associated with the varicosity is still compensated. Clinical symptoms are not very sensitive indicators at this stage, but ultrasound flowmetry provides an effective screening test both for the detection and staging of saphenous varicosity. Today these methods are so advanced that patients can be selected for partial saphenectomy solely on the basis of agreement between clinical and sonographic findings.

Preoperative indications for phlebography in diseases of the superficial venous system
Great and small saphenous varicosity
Transfascial forms of side-branch varicosity
Recurrent varicosity after conservative or operative treatment

The situation is different in patients with a *decompensated reflux circuit.* Even today, secondary popliteal and femoral vein insufficiency is still considered a classic X-ray diagnosis. Certain clini- 157
cal signs point to deep venous damage, such as recurrent ankle swelling, phlebectatic corona, or dermatologic signs of chronic venous statis in the perimalleolar area. There are also typical changes in measurable physical parameters and in duplex scans, which show subtle reflux signals during the calf *de*compression test. But these signs are useful only beyond a certain grade of severity of the antegrade stem-vein insufficiency, whereas phlebography and especially fluoroscopic observation allow for early detection. They enable the surgeon to plan the operation for a decompensated reflux circuit from the outset as a complete ablative procedure on the extrafascial venous system. Leaving a single incompetent connection between the venous systems will spoil any chance for restoration of normal deep venous outflow while enabling the progression of secondary popliteal and femoral vein insufficiency and recurrent varicosity. There is no question that modern, painless phlebographic technique causes far less risk and inconvenience to the patient than would be caused by a second operation or a lifetime of conservative aftercare.

The patient who seeks medical help desires to have his *disease cured* and his subjective complaints eliminated. But he is also curious about his prognosis, for it is likely that talks with other doctors and with fellow sufferers have exposed him to highly diverse opinions. In particular, there is still widespread ignorance regarding the significance of the decompensation of venous reflux circuits. Only roentgenograms can provide a comprehensive assessment of the patient's condition, especially as regards the prospect for a cure by prompt surgical intervention or any complaints that may persist following the operation.

On the one hand, the venous surgeon must meet his obligation to remove diseased vascular segments to the extent that an adequate resection demands. But at the same time, even laypeople are becoming increasingly aware of the need *to limit a surgical procedure to the extent required.* The modern science of reflux circuits defines the surgery that is appropriate and does not permit a "minimum" or "maximum" operation. Phlebography lays the diagnostic groundwork for making this assessment, and the phlebogram provides *unique documentary* evidence that can answer any questions that may arise later on.

The formulation of a differentiated operating plan seems especially useful for younger surgeons who are just entering the field, and even an experienced phlebologist can quickly adjust to "operating from the X-ray." He will surely appreciate the benefits of fast and reliable orientation and receiving an advance look at the morphology and anomalies that he will encounter at operation. This particularly applies to severe recurrent varicose veins following surgical treatment or sclerotherapy.

In the various forms of incomplete saphenous varicosity as well, contrast phlebography is essential for making a complete and precise diagnosis. This cannot be accomplished with color-coded duplex scanning or Doppler flowmetry. Phlebography provides the basis for an individually formulated plan of operation. The more specific the information requested of the radiologist by the clinician, the more precisely the radiologist will be able to answer the clinician's questions through selective delineation of the vascular regions of interest.

Diagnosis of Perforator Incompetence

Ascending Pressure Phlebography. Primary incompetence of one of the many perforating veins in the leg can occur as an isolated entity or in conjunction with other venous outflow disturbances. *Precise localization* of the incompetent perforator is a necessary prelude to selective op-
205 erative treatment. For this task, ascending phlebography with the Valsalva maneuver is superior to other modalities in its ability to furnish comprehensive information on the morphologic status of all pelvic and lower limb veins, and to document those findings.

Known clinical and instrumental methods for the diagnosis of incompetent Cockett's perforators offer a *sensitivity* of 70% or less. The accuracy of ascending phlebography with a Valsalva maneuver is no better, so phlebography cannot serve as the gold standard for this type of investigation. The cause lies in the complicated flow conditions in Cockett's perforators. Diagnostic confidence is increased by the simultaneous application of multiple techniques. *Varicography* can be used in selected cases as part of a specific preoperative investigation, but ascending phlebography with a Valsalva maneuver, when combined with clinical data, is generally sufficient to formulate a treatment plan even if individual perforating veins are not depicted.

Color-coded duplex scanning also can detect incompetent Cockett's perforators, but the procedure appears to have no value as a screening test.

Diagnosis of Deep Venous Disorders

Ascending Phlebograph and Ascending Pressure Phlebography. A classic indication for phlebography is for the early diagnosis of *deep venous thrombosis* in the pelvis and lower limb. *Color-* 253
coded duplex scanning is a valuable adjunct, as it can provide detailed information on the condition of the thrombus, vessel wall, and perivascular tissues. All other studies, including real-time sonography, are useful only for screening.

Without proper treatment, deep vein thrombosis can give rise to a fatal pulmonary embolism. The belated initiation of appropriate treatment will yield unsatisfactory results and lead to post-thrombotic syndrome. Thus, any suspicion of deep vein thrombosis, whether from clinical symptoms or physical measurements, warrants an immediate radiographic examination. The *optimum mode of treatment* cannot be decided upon until the phlebograms have been seen. The decision for anticoagulation, fibrinolysis, or surgery is guided by the differentiated hemodynamic conditions as portrayed on the X-ray films. The phlebo- 262
grams are also used in deciding whether the patient should be ambulatory with a compression
bandage, or whether he should be immobilized 263
due to pelvic vein involvement. In every case, however, the clinician is free to select his treatment method only during the first 8 days or perhaps less; after that time the prospects for a complete cure quickly decline.

Color-coded duplex scanning is not an effective alternative to phlebography in the primary investigation of deep vein thrombosis. Both modalities are equivalent in their ability to detect a clinically relevant thrombosis, but otherwise they are dissimilar. *Phlebograms* can clearly depict a non-occluding thrombus or tiny clots within the valve pockets – details that are very easily missed on sonograms. Individual venous valves are not routinely portrayed by ultrasound, and collateral circulations are not detected at all with color-coded duplex scanning. On the other hand, the *ultrasound examination* conveys a vivid impression of the status of the vein wall and perivascular structures. A reasonable estimate can be made as to the *age of the thrombus* and its composition. These aspects of primary diagnosis have led to the current concept of applying *both methods simultaneously*. It is advantageous to obtain the phlebograms first to avoid prolonged searches with the ultrasound probe.

Fibrinolysis and operative thrombectomy must be *monitored* and documented to determine their efficacy. In the past, this could be accomplished only by phlebography. But the therapist knows the specific vascular region of interest in a given case, and color-coded duplex scanning appears perfectly suited for secondary regional evaluations. *Repeated phlebograms* during the course of fibrinolytic therapy have become obsolete.

In cases where anticoagulation, thrombolysis, and surgery are contraindicated due to the patient's age, poor health, or other causes, a rationale for phlebography does not exist. Color-coded duplex scanning may provide adequate evaluation of these cases. On the other hand, the radiographic
264 exclusion of an *acute venous compression syndrome is an essential step before an invasive therapeutic procedure* is carried out.

Phlebography has an important role in the investigation of unexplained chronic swelling of the lower extremity. Many of these cases involve a *post-thrombotic syndrome*. Ascending phlebography provides detailed information on the conditions of venous drainage. It informs the attending physician on the extent of post-thrombotic changes,
279 the degree of recanalization, and the function of the collateral circulations. A comprehensive work-up that includes clinical signs and symptoms, radiographic findings, and the results of functional physical measurements of venous hemodynamics is essential for formulating a differentiated plan of conservative or operative treatment. In less favorable cases, patients will require compression stockings of a higher pressure grade than in cases with optimum recanalization. For patients in the stage of late post-thrombotic syndrome, operative treatment should be considered as an option. Phlebography is particularly useful in these cases for differentiating *secondary great saphenous vari-* 286
cosity from compensatory phlebectasia and for locating incompetent perforators.

Cavernous hemangiomas frequently communicate 334
with the deep venous system. Since the feasibility of operative treatment depends on the caliber, number, and location of the feeding and draining vessels, ascending phlebography is an indispensable part of the preoperative workup. If a needle can be directed into a tumor vessel, direct opacification is recommended. In patients with combined angiodysplasias, *arteriography* should be 339
added to identify arteriovenous shunts that may be accessible to selective ligation. The use of the digital subtraction technique is advantageous in these cases.

Regressive vascular changes are sometimes recognized as the cause of localized leg swelling in older patients. *Primary femoral vein insufficiency* is very uncommon in younger patients. Tumors of the vessel wall are another unusual diagnosis. When a diagnosis has been confirmed by real-time or duplex sonography, further evaluation becomes necessary.

In *disability assessment practice,* a common inquiry is whether exposure to a harmful influence has left residual objective changes in the deep venous system. Phlebography is an invaluable tool in this type of investigation. But since there is no *curative* indication, the patient must be thoroughly counseled regarding possible complications, with a witness present. It is also recommended

Indications for phlebography in diseases of the deep venous system
Investigation of deep vein thrombosis in the leg
Monitoring response to fibrinolytic therapy
Differential diagnosis of venous compression syndromes
Differential diagnosis of localized edema
Diagnosis of secondary popliteal and femoral vein insufficiency (with a decompensated primary reflux circuit)
Specific conservative and surgical treatment of post-thrombotic syndrome
Diagnosis of primary femoral valve incompetence
Preoperative investigation of vascular tumors
Questions relating to disability assessment

that written consent be secured since phlebography, as an invasive method, is not a procedure to which the patient is obliged to submit as part of the disability assessment process.

Diagnosis of Diseases of the Pelvic Veins and Inferior Vena Cava

Digital Subtraction Phlebography, Ascending Phlebography, Occlusion Phlebography. The same indications and principles apply to the radiographic evaluation of suspected *pelvic vein thrombosis* as for deep vein thrombosis in the leg. Early diagnosis is essential so that fibrinolysis or thrombectomy, if needed, can be instituted without delay.

In patients with extensive pelvic and leg vein thrombosis, it is no longer possible to demonstrate all the pelvic vessels by performing ascending phlebography through a foot vein. But the surgeon needs to identify the proximal tail of the thrombus to ensure that a temporary or perma-
343 nent venous interruption is placed safely above the tip of the thrombus. Digital subtraction phlebography has proven very advantageous for this purpose. The multiinjection technique may yield more information and narrow down the problem in selected cases. The contralateral pelvic veins should also be examined in every patient, first to exclude a thrombosis and then to ensure good visualization of the inferior vena cava.

264 It is important to recognize the *descending form* of pelvic vein thrombosis, which is frequently caused by a mechanical outflow obstruction that may be accessible to surgical treatment. The definition of the descending form is based solely on the phlebographic diagnosis.

Phlebography is also used in *post-thrombotic syndromes* of the pelvic veins to identify patients that
354 could benefit from a vascular surgical procedure. With a unilateral occlusion that is poorly collateralized and associated with chronic stasis edema, the Palma crossover operation or other reconstructive procedure may be appropriate. Besides X-ray findings, venous pressure measurements are also considered in selecting patients for reconstructive venous surgery.

Indications for phlebography in diseases of the pelvic veins and inferior vena cava
Investigation of acute pelvic vein thrombosis
Monitoring response to fibrinolytic therapy
Differential diagnosis of venous compression syndromes
Specific treatment of post-thrombotic syndrome
Diagnosis of intrapelvic and retroperitoneal tumors, and identification of the organ(s) involved
Trauma
Questions relating to disability assessment

Contraindications to phlebography
Contrast medium intolerance
No relevance to treatment or disability assessment
Severe systemic illness
Advanced age
Pregnancy
Phlegmasia cerulea dolens
Severe peripheral arterial circulatory disturbance
Severe inflammatory processes
Severe lymphedema

Contraindications

An absolute contraindication to phlebography exists in patients whose prior history includes a *severe allergic reaction* to the contrast medium. Even with appropriate prophylaxis of an anaphylactic response, a second examination should not be performed.

Care is taken to elicit an *accurate history* of allergic complications. It is not uncommon for a patient to misinterpret a vagovasal reaction experienced in a previous contrast examination. Consideration should also be given to the *product previously* used. The nonionic contrast media, with their very low rate of side effects, were not available prior to 1985.

The phlebographic findings should aid the attending physician in making a sound therapeutic decision. There is no justification for performing any invasive diagnostic procedure unless there is good reason to believe that it will contribute to therapeutic planning. Such a rationale is often lacking in patients with *severe systemic diseases, elderly patients,* and during *pregnancy*.

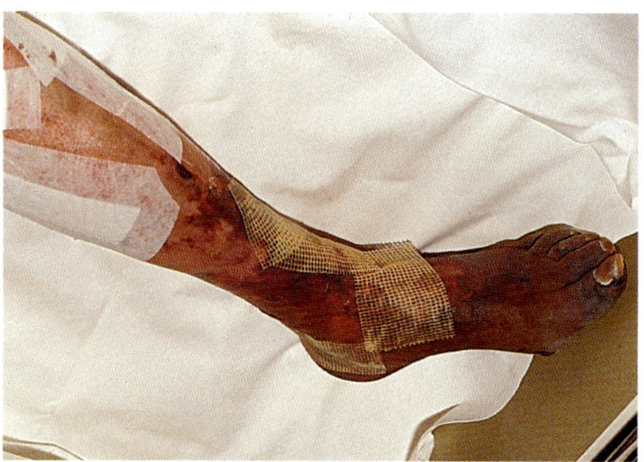

391. Phlegmasia cerulea dolens progressing to venous gangrane in a 67-year-old woman with metastatic rectal carcinoma, 2 weeks before her death. Adhesive bandages were applied following unsuccessful surgical intervention

Severe regional disorders in the lower extremity can lead to significant local complications due to the mechanical trauma of the venepuncture and contrast injection. In particular, an advanced stage of *arterial circulatory impairment* would seem to contraindicate phlebography.

391 *Phlegmasia cerulea dolens* results from the thrombotic occlusion of all main stem veins and leads to the collapse of the venous circulation. A drainage route no longer exists for an injected contrast bolus, which would cause endothelial damage with a high risk of local complications. Phlebography is also contraindicated in any patient with a *severe inflammatory process* involving the lower extremity.

The puncture wound caused by the injection needle can seriously exacerbate an existing *lymphedema* and lead to protracted problems of fistula formation. Therefore, it must be very carefully examined whether phlebography is indicated, in particular with regard to the therapeutic consequences.

Complications of Phlebography and Their Management

When modern nonionic contrast media are used and attention is given to essential technical principles, serious complications of phlebography are very rare (also see p. 53). Nevertheless, the examining physician must be prepared for them at all times and be ready to institute immediate, appropriate treatment should the need arise.

All severe adverse reactions represent an anaphylactic response to the *contrast medium*. Other side effects bear a direct or indirect causal relationship to the *examination* itself. They include orthostatic collapse, vasovagal syncope, deep vein thrombosis, and superficial thrombophlebitis. Local extravasation of the contrast medium can lead to blistering and skin necrosis under unfavorable conditions. In practice it is useful to classify the complications of phlebography into the two broad categories of systemic and local reactions.

Systemic Reactions

The systemic complications of phlebography include anaphylactic reactions to the contrast medium and the various forms of hypotensive circulatory disturbance.

Various types of *allergic drug reactions* are recognized (Kerp and Kasemir 1982). The side effects of

Complications of phlebography
Systemic reactions
Anaphylaxis
Anaphylactic shock
Urticaria
Quincke's edema
Bronchial asthma
Hypotensive circulatory disturbances
Sympathicotonic form
Asympathicotonic form
Vagovasal syncope
Thyrotoxic reaction
Local reactions
Phlebothrombosis
Thrombophlebitis
Tissue inflammation by extravascular contrast medium

Behavior of blood pressure and pulse in general systemic reactions

Circulatory disturbance	Blood pressure	Pulse
Anaphylactic shock	↓	↑
Sympathicotonic form	↘	↘
Asympathicotonic form	↓	→
Vagovasal syncope	↓	↓

contrast media are representative of the anaphylactic type (type I), which may be manifested clinically as anaphylacic shock, urticaria, Quincke's edema, or bronchial asthma.

Anaphylactic Shock

Any intravascular injection of contrast material can evoke a potentially life-threatening anaphylactic response. Thus, the radiologist must know the characteristic features of anaphylactic shock and be prepared to intervene at once with appropriate therapy.
The mortality rate associated with the intravenous use of *ionic* contrast media, according to the collective statistics of Hach, Helmig, May and Schmitt (Hach 1985), is less than 1:86000 (see p. 261). Anaphylactic shock was observed and successfully treated in two cases from this series. Benness and Fischer (1989) and Katayama et al. (1990) report that the complication rate is decreased by a factor of 5 when *nonionic* contrast media are used.

Prospective studies comparing the effects of ionic and nonionic contrast media are proscribed by ethical considerations. It may be that precise statistical data on the mortality risk of nonionic contrast media cannot be obtained. According to Schmiedel (1987), the statistical determination of differences between a 1:75000 and 1:150000 risk would require study populations numbering 2–3 million, clearly an impractical goal.
Based on the data of the Pharmaceutical Commission of the Association of German Physicians, Reiser (1988) estimates that the incidence of fatal complications related to intravascular contrast media is 1:500000 (11:5.6 million). Data relating specifically to contrast phlebography are not available.

Pathogenesis of Anaphylactic Shock. Anaphylaxis is based upon an *immediate hypersentivity* (type I) reaction. Previous exposure of the patient to the allergen has led to the formation of antibodies bound to receptors on mast cells, basophils, and platelets. The contrast medium combines with the antibodies to form an antigen-antibody complex, which in turn causes cell damage with release of chemical mediators that incite the dramatic clinical manifestations. Kerp and Kasemir (1982) list four important *mediators* of immediate hypersensitivity in humans: histamine, slow-reacting substance of anaphylaxis (SRS-A), eosinophil chemotactic factor of anaphylaxis (ECF-A), and platelet-activating factor (PAF).

Allergic drug reactions (modified from Kerp and Kasemir 1982)

Type of allergic reaction	Example of reaction	Example of causative drug
Immediate type		
Anaphylactic type (type I)	Anaphylactic shock	Contrast medium
	Urticarial exanthema	
	Quincke's edema	
	Bronchial asthma	
Cytotoxic type (type II)	Hemolytic anemia	Quinine
Immune complex type (type III)	Serum sickness	Xenogenic sera
Delayed type (type IV)	Contact dermatitis	Chromiun, nickel

Histamine plays a leading role in the pathogenesis of anaphylactic shock. It is stored in the granules of mast cells and basophils. Its pharmacologic action consists in a generalized vasodilation and increased capillary permeability. This results in plasma loss from the circulating blood with hemoconcentration, a rise in blood viscosity, and a drop in blood pressure. Histamine also causes bronchospasms by stimulating smooth muscle contractions.

Histamine produces its effects by binding to specific *H receptors* present in nearly all organs and tissues. The H1 receptors activate the inositol phosphate/Ca2+ messenger system (Beaven et al. 1987). In the effects mediated by H2 receptors, cyclic adenosine monophosphate (cAMP) functions as a "second messenger" for cellular signal transduction (Hegstrand et al. 1976). So far no details are known about the H3 receptors (Arrang et al. 1987).
Besides the immune response, there is evidence that contrast media can also produce side effects by *other mechanisms* such as activation of the complement system, changes in the permeability of cell membranes, disturbances of the electrolyte balance by calcium binding, or direct effects on the central nervous system.

Clinical Manifestations of Anaphylactic Shock. Anaphylactic shock develops within minutes after injection of the contrast medium. Its onset is heralded by *nonspecific prodromal symptoms* that include itching of the head, palms, and soles of the feet, a furry sensation about the lips, and a heavy tongue (stage I). This is followed by apprehension, an ascending flush, and progressive dyspnea with an inspiratory stridor. *Urticaria* develops rapidly (stage II). The sudden dilatation of the peripheral arteries and the fall in cardiac output lead to a precipitous *drop in blood pressure*. The circulatory collapse is accelerated by hypovolemia and hemoconcentration and by constriction of the pulmonary vessels. The patient looks ashen and is covered with cold sweat. Central reactions are slowed. Finally there is *loss of consciousness* with convulsions and passage of stool (stage III) and frank *organ failure* (stage IV). Untreated, the condition can terminate fatally due to central respiratory arrest.

The diagnosis must be made quickly on the basis of clinical signs. An important early sign is a *weak, rapid pulse* with rates up to 200/min. Tachycardia may not develop, however, in patients with coronary artery disease.

The anaphylactic response to a contrast medium also may commence with *acute respiratory distress*. The expiratory stridor of an asthamatic episode distinguishes that condition from laryngeal edema, which is marked by an inspiratory stridor. In rare cases the edematous swelling may spread to involve the bronchi, causing pulmonary diffusion defects and making the clinical picture more dramatic.

In the rare *cerebral form* of anaphylactic shock, acute brain edema or direct chemotoxic effects lead to severe vomiting and headache, followed shortly by loss of consciousness and generalized convulsions. Intestinal cramping and vomiting are typical in cases where abdominal symptoms predominate.

Treatment of Anaphylactic Shock. The primary measure in the treatment of anaphylactic shock is the immediate establishment of a *secure peripheral intravenous line* through a plastic indwelling catheter. If the peripheral veins are already collapsed, the line may be inserted into the external or internal jugular vein or the common femoral vein, preferably with the immediate placement of a central venous catheter. Finally, the subclavian vein can also be used.

Initially the phlebographic needle is left in the foot to provide a route for administering medications should the need arise. Once the vein has collapsed due to shock, however, there is a danger that the sharp needle point will perforate the vessel wall. Moreover, the lumen of standard phlebographic needles is too small for effective emergency therapy. Another potential danger is the persistence of injected medications in the peripheral vessels, producing a very delayed effect or no effect until the recovery of circulatory function, when overdosing occurs.

Volume therapy begins by elevating the lower extremities on the footboard of the X-ray table to produce an autotransfusion effect. In order to remedy the hypovolemic deficiency, the rapid infusion of 500–1000 ml crystalloid solution followed by plasma substitutes (polypeptide solutions) can be administered, but plasma expanders (hydroxyl starch solution) are more effective for anaphylactic shock.

Patients with hemodynamic cardiac arrest will require immediate *cardiopulmonary resuscitation,* beginning with a precordial punch. For closed-chest cardiac massage, 15 sternal compressions are applied to every two lung inflations in the one-man technique, or five compressions to one lung inflation in the two-man technique. Ventilation is performed mouth-to-nose or with an Ambo bag and mask connected to an emergency oxygen cylinder. The most favorable conditions, of course,

Treatment of anaphylactic shock following contrast injection
Bring patient to supine position; establish intravenous line with large-bore indwelling cannula.
Epinephrine; administer 1/2–1 ml of 1:10 dilution by intravenous injection; if necessary, repeat in 2–10 min.
Ringer solution; administer 500–1000 ml by rapid infusion.
Plasma expander; administer 500 ml or more by rapid infusion.
Methylprednisolone; administer contents of one ampule, dissolved in 10 ml distilled water, by intravenous injection.
Dopamine; administer one ampule, diluted 50 mg/10 ml in a 250-ml infusion solution, by continuous intravenous drip at rate of 20–40 drops/min or more, maintaining the systolic blood pressure at 80 mmHg.
Cardiopulmonary resuscitation; may take precedence over other measures.

are established by intubation. Today buffer therapy for acidosis following circulatory arrest is administered only in a hospital setting where blood gas analysis is available.

The primary treatment of shock includes the administration of *epinephrine* to improve circulatory status. We dilute one ampule of epinephrine 1:10 with physiologic saline and administer $^1/_2$–1 ml of the solution by intravenous injection. An injectable ampule with this solution also may be used. The injections can be repeated at intervals of 2–3 min. The patient's blood pressure and heart activity are closely monitored during this time, with arrhythmia signifying overdose. Epinephrine is considered the agent of choice for anaphylactic shock and is life-saving in many patients. It also exerts a significant bronchodilating action.

After the blood pressure has risen to measurable levels and volume replacement is completed, Gersmeyer and Yasaegil (1978) recommend continuation of treatment for shock with *dopamine*, a biologic precursor of epinephrine. It is best administered with an automated perfusor or infusor. Continuous drip infusion is acceptable in emergencies. This may be done by dissolving 50 mg of dopamine in 250 ml isotonic saline and adjusting the drip rate to the blood pressure. A rate of 20 drops/min provides an average dose of 200 μg/min; if necessary this dose can be doubled or tripled, or increased even more in extreme situations. An alternative to high dosing is to *combine* dopamine with norepinephrine. For this we add 1 ml of norepinephrine (one ampule) along with 10 ml dopamine to 250 ml of physiologic saline in an intravenous bottle and match the drip rate to the blood pressure.

Intravenous *corticosteroids* have proven beneficial for antiallergic treatment in anaphylactic shock. The recommended dose is 1000 mg methylprednisolone or 1000 mg prednisolone. Corticosteroids take about 15 min to act, so epinephrine, which acts immediately, should be administered first.

Antihistamines have an even slower onset of action than corticosteroids, so they do not have a role in the emergency treatment of anaphylactic shock, but should instead be used at a later stage of treatment.

Cerebral symptoms in a severe anaphylactic reaction result from a direct chemotoxic action of the contrast medium on the central nervous system or from cerebral edema. *Diuretic therapy* should be instituted as rapidly as possible. We administer 20–40 mg of *furosemide* intravenously. Pulmonary edema and laryngeal edema also require the prompt administration of diuretics in high doses.

Diazepam is beneficial in patients with severe apprehension or cerebral convulsions. A dose of 5–10–20 mg, depending on response, is given by intravenous injection while respiration is monitored.

Sequence of Therapeutic Measures in Anaphylactic Shock. To successfully manage the dramatic situation of anaphylactic shock, the attending physician and staff must *work calmly* and delibrately. A professional atmosphere is essential so that assistants can respond briskly to the physician's orders and avoid mistakes. Even without personal experience in intensive care medicine, the proposed treatment measures should be carried out in a systematic, straightforward manner.

If the patient reports any suspicious general reactions during or after phlebography, the examination should be halted at once and the X-ray table brought to a horizontal position. *A small pulse* with a rate *higher than 120/min* signifies impending danger. The phlebographic needle and its infusion line are left in place on the foot. Immediately the physician places a tourniquet on the arm and establishes a secure intravenous line with a large-bore cannula. If the *blood pressure* falls significantly, $^1/_2$–1 ml of a 1:10 dilution of epinephrine 1 mg is injected right away. Then a plasma expander is rapidly infused through the indwelling plastic cannula. The epinephrine injections are repeated at 3-min intervals until the blood pressure rises to about 80 mmHg, while the heart is monitored for dysrhythmias.

Meanwhile a second assistant has opened the patient's collar and removed any oral dentures. The legs have been elevated onto the footboard of the X-ray table. The assistant summons an *ambulance* for transfer to the hospital.

Emergency treatment is continued during the infusion therapy. The patient is given one ampule of *methylprednisolone* 1000 mg, and O_2 is administered from an emergency cylinder. If convulsions are present, 10 mg diazepan is now given intravenously, and furosemide is administered as required.

Cardiopulmonary resuscitation can be instituted while the patient is still on the X-ray table. The physician applies five cardiac compressions for each lung inflation by an assistant.

The physician should *intubate* a nonbreathing patient only if he has fully mastered the technique. Endotracheal tube insertion is particularly difficult in emergency situations. The apnea can be bridged by mask-and-bag or mouth-to-nose ventilation.

Anaphylactic shock can recur within hours after the initial episode, so the patient should be placed in the *intensive care unit* and observed for at least 24 h. The physician accompanies the patient to the hospital with the necessary medications. Dopamine started by slow intravenous drip in the radiology unit should be continued during the transfer.

Prevention of Anaphylactic Shock. The first step in the prevention of anaphylaxis is to take a careful medical history, giving specific attention to an allergic diathesis and previous adverse reactions to contrast injections. In patients at risk, an *indwelling cannula* is introduced into the brachial vein on the radial side of the forearm. Fifteen minutes before the examination, 1000 mg methylprednisolone is administered by intravenous injection. Premedication with an H1 anatagonist and an H2 antagonist is also recommended; one, two, or three ampules of each are given by slow intravenous injection (for at least 2 min) according to body weight (<45 kg, 45–90 kg, >90 kg). The line is kept patent with heparinized saline solution (5000 units *heparin* in 100 ml physiologic saline). After a *trial injection* of 2 ml contrast medium into the brachial vein, the physician observes the patient for 2–3 min, which is sufficient for a positive reaction. It should be noted, however, that an *allergic response does not depend on dose,* and that contrast outflow can be greatly delayed by the underlying venous disorder when the phlebographic needle has been used for the trial injection.

The examining physician must be prepared for the possibility of anaphylactic shock. The necessary equipment and medications are stored in an easily accessible drawer and are regularly checked and replaced as needed. Also, an outline of treatment measures should be clearly posted in the examination room.

It is advisable to prepare the medical personnel for emergencies and instruct them in the use of the equipment. Efficiency is improved by *occasional practice* in a simulated emergency.

Emergency equipment required for severe adverse contrast reaction
Stethoscope and sphygmomanometer
Rubber tourniquet
Guedel tube, Safran airway
Rubens bag and ventilation masks
Intubation set and ventilation equipment
Indwelling cannulas and infusion set
Intravenous poles and tourniquet

Recommended stock of pharmacologic agents for anaphylactic shock
Plasma expanders Two 500-ml bottles and two infusion sets
Circulatory agents Epinephrine; one pack of ten 1-ml ampules *Dopamine;* 10-ml ampules, 50 mg
Corticosteroids Methylprednisolone; two bottles with ampules of distilled water, 10 ml
H1 Antagonists Dimethindene 4 mg; one pack of five 4-ml ampules
H2 Antagonists Cimetidine 200 mg; one pack of ten 2-ml ampules
Bronchodilators Theophylline 240 mg; one pack of five 10-ml ampules
Diuretics Furosemide 40 mg; one pack of five 4-ml ampules
Sedatives Diazepam 10 mg; one pack of five 2-ml ampules

Urticaria

Urticaria occurs in approximately 1% of patients who receive contrast injections and most commonly affects the upper half of the body. The eruptions coalesce to larger plaques and cause severe pruritus. Mild nausea is reported by some patients.

Burning, itching, runny nose, sneezing, and coughing signify involvement of the mucous membranes. There is associated watering of the eyes and conjunctivitis.

Treatment by the injection of 10–20 ml of 10% calcium gluconate is sufficient for most mild allergic cutaneous and mucosal contrast reactions. Calcium is contraindicated in patients taking digitalis.

The agent of choice is an H1 antagonist such as dimethindene, administered in a dose of one to three ampules, depending on body weight, by slow intravenous injection. This may be combined with an H2 antagonist (e.g., cimetidine) in a corresponding dose.

In severe cases, treatment with a corticosteroid is indicated. A dose of 40–120 mg methylprednisolone or 60–180 mg 16-methylene prednisolone should be adequate. Onset of action takes about 15 min.

The severe pruritus and conjunctivitis associated with a urticarial reaction can be relieved by applying cold compresses soaked in ice water.

A sensation of warmth in the face, hands, tongue, genitalia, or other body regions is rarely reported when nonionic contrast media are used. It is based on a pharmacologic vasodilating action of the medium and should not be confused with an allergic response.

Treatment of urticarial cutaneous and mucosal reactions
Calcium 10–20 ml of 10% solution intravenously (contraindicated by digitalis use)
Dimethindene 4–8–12 mg (one to three ampules) by slow intravenous injection
Cimetidine 200–400–600 mg (one to three ampules) by slow intravenous injection
Methylprednisolone 40–120 mg (one to three ampules) intravenously
Cold compresses

Treatment of Quincke's edema and laryngeal edema following contrast injection
Methylprednisolone 1000 mg (one ampule) intravenously
Dimethindene 4–8–12 mg (one to three ampules) by slow intravenous injection
Cimetidine 200–400–600 mg (one to three ampules) by slow intravenous injection
Calcium 10–20 ml of 10% solution intravenously (contraindicated by digitalis use)
Furosemide 20–40 mg (one to two ampules) by slow intravenous injection; may be repeated
Diazepam 5–10 mg (half to one ampule) by slow intravenous injection
Oxygen insufflation
Hospitalization

Quincke's Edema

Circumscribed Quincke's edema can occur in any part of the body. Laryngeal involvement is a life-threatening condition marked by increasing dyspnea with an inspiratory stridor, and energetic therapy is required. High doses of corticosteroids are administered at once, e.g., methylprednisolone (one ampule 1000 mg) or prednisolone (100 mg) and either one or two ampules of 10% calcium gluconate. The patient also receives one to three ampules of dimethindene and cimetidine. Additionally, a potent diuretic is administered; we prefer 20–40 mg of furosemide injected intravenously at a rate no faster than 4 mg/min.

Intravenous diazepam, 5–10 mg, can effect good sedation in highly apprehensive patients.

A patient with laryngeal edema is transfered by ambulance to a hospital where he can be moni-

Treatment of asthma attack following contrast injection
Bring patient to upright sitting position
Calcium 10–20 ml of 10% solution by slow intravenous injection (contraindicated by digitalis use)
Theophylline 240 mg (one 10-ml ampule) intravenously; for se vere attack, give up to six ampules by intravenously drip in 250 ml physiologic NaCl
Methylprednisolone 40 mg (one ampule) intravenously
Oxygen inhalation

tored in an intensive care setting. Recurrence is possible after a favorable initial therapeutic response.

Bronchial Asthma

The contrast injection as well as psychological influences can precipitate an asthma attack in predisposed individuals. This condition is easily diagnosed. The bronchospasm caused sudden, severe dyspnea with an expiratory stridor and the secretion of a viscous, glassy mucus.

Before specific treatment is instituted, the patient should be brought to an *upright sitting position,* supported by his arms, to improve ventilation. Constricting articles of clothing are removed. Initial drug treatment consists of 10 ml calcium gluconate 10% and theophylline (one 10-ml ampule, 0.24 g) administered by slow intravenous injection. Usually a severe attack is quickly arrested by a higher dose of theophylline, e.g., six 10-ml ampules 0.24 infused by intravenous drip in 250 ml of solution. The injection of corticosteroids, such as 40 mg of methylprednisolone, produces an effect in 10–15 min. A half to one ampulle of terbutaline sulfate should also be administered subcutaneously. A rapid effect is also achieved with fenoterol administered by metered-dose inhaler.

Recommended stock of pharmacologic agents for mild adverse reactions during phlebography
Crystalloid solution *Ringer* (two 500-ml bottles) and infusion sets
Plasma expanders *Hydroxyl starch solution* (two 500-ml bottles) and infusion sets
Carrier solution for medications *Isotonic saline solution, 0.9%* (two 250-ml bottles)
Circulatory agents *Etilefrin* 10 mg; one pack of six 1-ml ampules
Antihistamines Dimethindene 4 mg, one pack of five 4-ml ampules Cimetidine 200 mg, one pack of ten 2-ml ampules Calcium gluconate 10%; one pack of five 10-ml ampules
Corticosteroids *Methylprednisolone* 40 mg; one pack with three ampules and diluent
Bronchodilators *Theophylline* 240 mg; one pack of 10-ml ampules *Fenoterol* in metered-dose inhaler 0.2 mg

Functional Hypotensive Circulatory Disturbances

Disturbances of circulatory regulation occur in 0.5%–1% of patients undergoing phlebography. They are generally a result of vasovagal syncope. Unlike intra-arterial injections, which cause pronounced vasodilatation, the injection of contrast medium into a vein does not cause a fall in blood pressure. Often the patient will lose consciousness even before the contrast medium is administered, in which case a causal relationship can be confidently excluded.

Three forms of hypotensive circulatory disturbance – the sympathicotonic form, asympathicotonic form, and vasovagal syncope – are distinguished according to the response of the pulse and blood pressure. The radiologist must know these forms so that he can differentiate them from anaphylactic shock and treat them accordingly.

Sympathicotonic Form. These patients already show a *history* of proneness to hypotensive circulatory disorders. They may complain of general weakness, fatigue, or hypersentivity to weather changes. Dizziness or even loss of consciousness can result from exposure to particular physical, psychological, or climatic stresses.

Orthostasis has a particularly detrimental effect in patients with severe varicose veins. During standing, up to 2 l blood can pool in the dilated vessels of the lower extremity, so this volume is removed from the active circulation. This decreases the cardiac stroke volume by 40%; the heart rate rises, while the blood pressure and blood-pressure amplitude fall slowly and steadily to levels that are difficult to measure (Siegenthaler and Veragut 1970). Finally the patient *collapses*. He appears ashen, is covered with cold sweat, and is unresponsive to verbal cues.

When the patient *lies flat*, his circulatory status quickly returns to normal. A cup of black coffee will hasten the recovery. Very few patients require volume replacement with plasma expanders such or treatment with circulatory agents. In patients considered to be at risk, the phlebographic examination can be initiated with the patient in a more recumbent position.

Asympathicotonic Form. The asympathicotonic or hypodynamic form of hypotensive circulatory disturbance is very rare. Its primary form is known as *Shy-Drager syndrome*, of which about 100 cases have been described to date in the world literature (Gersmeyer and Yarsagil 1978). As a secondary complication, it occurs mainly in *severe neurologic disorders* with a failure of sympathetic centers in the setting of polyneuritis, polyradiculitis, tabes dorsalis, or other diseases. During standing, the blood pressure falls while the pulse rate remains unchanged or rises slightly.

Vasovagal Syncope. Vasovagal syncope, known colloquially as *fainting*, is of major practical importance. It can have various precipitating causes such as fear or fright; prolonged standing; confrontation with medical instruments, syringes, or blood; or just the thought of undergoing a diagnostic or surgical procedure. It can also be triggered by a violent peritoneal stimulus, a blow to the solar plexus, or acute pain.

During an episode of vasovagal syncope, the patient becomes deathly pale, and his skin is cold and clammy. He may remark that he is about to faint, then ceases to respond to external stimuli and collapses. The correct diagnosis is based on the combination of a *slow pulse rate with hypotension*.

Once recumbent, the patient recovers rapidly from the syncopal attack. But his circulatory status remains labile for 1 h or more, so he should lie flat in a quiet, well-ventilated room at the institute. During this time he should be watched by an assistant, who periodically checks his pulse and blood pressure.

Though it is most prevelant in young patients, vasovagal syncope can affect virtually anyone. It is prudent, therefore, to organize the *preparations for phlebography* in a way that will lower the risk. Prolonged standing in a hot, crowded waiting area should particularly be avoided. The physician can have an assistant explain to the patient what will happen during the examination. This should be done in a calm, unhurried manner. A trusting atmosphere will do much to alleviate the patient's fears and help him assimilate what he is told in an objective fashion.

The *circumstances surrounding the examination* can be important in preventing a vasovagal reaction. The examination room should be large, brightly lit, and well ventilated. The patient does not need to see instruments, catheters, and equipment that are not part of the procedure. Order in the examination room also conveys a sense of concern for the individual.

While the foot bath is being administered in the changing room, the patient should not feel unduly cramped or confined. If it is necessary for the patient to stay in the small room for a prolonged period, verbalizing this to the patient will make the experience easier to tolerate. Hot or constricting articles of clothing should be removed. On the other hand, there is no reason to institute exaggerated precautions against syncope. If the examination routine gives the patient the sense that he is being attended to by an experienced staff trying to conduct the procedure in a purposeful, efficient manner, he will feel safe in the atmosphere of a conscientious routine.

It can happen to any physician that the puncture of a vein in the foot is not successful even after two or three attempts. In such a case, it is better to arrange a new appointment. The phlebographic investigation should be carried out rapidly and purposefully. It can usually be completely within 2–3 min. If further images are necessary, we recommend that the patient lies down for a short while before the examination is continued.

Differential Diagnosis of Systemic Hypotensive Circulatory Disturbances During Phlebography. In the *sympathicotonic form* of hypotensive circulatory disturbance, it takes 5–10 min or even longer for collapse to occur under an orthostatic stress. This situation is unlikely to arise in the position used for phlebography, where the patient is semiupright with the lower extremities relaxed. In *anaphylactic shock,* severe circulatory disturbances are usually accompanied by other allergic symptoms such as urticaria, facial edema, or dyspnea with stridor.

In cases of *secondary asympathicotonic hypotension,* it may be assumed that the radiologist has been apprised of the severe underlying neurologic disease. In case of collapse, the pulse rate remains normal or is only slightly elevated.

Thus, a reasonable axiom is that every severe circulatory disturbance associated with a small, rapid pulse noted shortly after contrast injection should be interpreted as an anaphylactic reaction and treated accordingly. This complication is very rare compared with *vasovagal syncope.* The two symptom complexes are readily distinguished from each other by the difference in the pulse.

In the almost 50 000 phlebographic examinations that we have conducted to date, we have seen only two cases of a severe anaphylactic circulatory reaction (0.0001 %), as opposed to about 200 episodes of vasovagal syncope (0.4 %). We have additionally noted a marked correlation between the frequency of complications and the personal experience of the examining physician. We have seen no instances of a sympathicotonic or asympathicotonic response.

Local Reactions

The principal local complication of contrast phlebography is iatrogenic thrombosis, which must be classified by its location as intrafascial (deep) or extrafascial (superficial). Another significant local complication is tissue inflammation or skin necrosis caused by extravascular injection of the contrast medium.

Deep Vein Thrombosis After Phlebography

Phlebothrombosis of the deep leg and pelvic veins is a serious condition that generally leads to postthrombotic syndrome and frequently to pulmonary embolism. In recent years several authors, using the 125I fibrinogen uptake test, have demonstrated higher rates of thrombosis associated mainly with the use of ionic contrast media and, to a lesser degree, with nonionic media. Reiser et al. (1983) report that the incidence ranges from 1 %–52.7 % in the first group to 0 %–7.4 % in the second group. Albrechsson and Olsson (1979) used phlebography to objectively document the presence of single or multiple small thrombi in cases of this kind.

While the above-cited radionuclide studies usually covered small groups of only about 50 patients, clinical experience is available for much larger populations. Helmig (1983, personal communication), for example, reported one incidence of deep vein thrombosis of the lower leg in a series of more than 30 000 phlebographic examinations. May (1979, 1983, personal communication) observed no complications in over 20 000 examinations. Schmitt (1979, 1983) documented one case of small thrombi in the calf muscle in 60 000 roentgen examinations of the veins. We have personally observed two cases of postphlebographic deep vein thrombosis in almost 20 000 extremities. Ac-

Osmolality and iodine content of comparable contrast media

Chemical or generic name	Brand name	Osmolality at 37 °C (mosm/ kg H2O)	Iodine content (mg/ml)
Ionic media			
Iothalamate	Conray 60	1540	282
Diatrizoate	Angiografin	1530	306
Ioxithalamate	Telebrix 300	1600	300
Amidotrizoate	Peritrast	1500	300
Ioxaglate	Hexabrix	490	320
Nonionic media			
Metrizamide	Amipaque	470	300
Iohexol	Omnipaque	720	300
Iopromide	Ultravist	610	300
Iopamidol	Sulutrast 300	616	300
Iomeprol	Imeron 300	521	300
Comparison			
Blood	–	300	–

cordingly, the incidence of clinically apparent thrombosis following the use of *ionic contrast media* is 4:86 000. In almost 40 000 examinations with *nonionic media,* we have found no instances of thrombosis detectable by clinical evaluation.

Based on the experience of European examiners reporting the largest case numbers, it appears that the small thrombi detected by the radiofibrinogen test and documented to a degree by phlebography have no clinical relevance as long as certain precautions are taken. Foremost among these prophylactic measures are a *brief contact time* of a 60 % contrast medium with the vein wall and the use of more heavily diluted contrast solutions. *Physical thromboprophylaxis* involves clearing the contrast medium from the veins at the end of the examination by massage, active leg movements against a resistance, and especially by early ambulation with a properly applied compression bandage.

Tiny thrombi in the deep and superficial veins that produce no clinical symptoms are often discovered incidentally during routine phlebography. In a series of 100 consecutive examinations, we found them in 18 % of cases.

The radionuclide studies on the frequency of iatrogenic thrombosis offer statistical proof of the superiority of nonionic contrast media over the high-osmolality media. Thus, phlebography can be made a very low-risk procedure through optimal technique and conscientious thromboprophylaxis.

Superficial Thrombophlebitis

In contrast to clinically relevant deep vein thrombosis, inflammatory changes more commonly affect the pedal vein used for injection of the contrast medium. The incidence in our series was 1.54 %. May (1979) and Salzmann et al. (1980) reported superficial thrombophlebitic complications in 5 %–20 % of cases where ionic media were used. The series examined by radionuclide studies noted in the previous section also exhibited a relatively high incidence of superficial vein thrombosis.

Local thrombophlebitis has various *causes.* Because the contrast medium is most concentrated at the injection site, it causes the greatest osmotic damage to endothelial cells at that location. The medium is injected under a high manual or mechanical pressure which greatly distends the vessel wall and imposes a severe mechanical stress upon the intima. Additionally, the sharply beveled needle can directly damage the delicate endothelial layer at many sites.

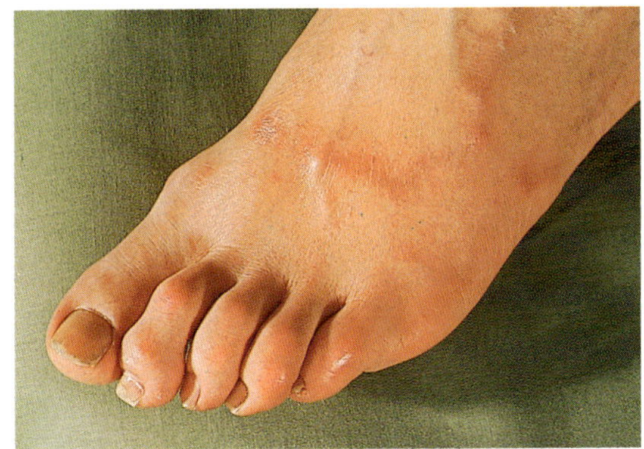

392. Thrombophlebitis of the injected vein 4 days after phlebography

Patients with a *post-thrombotic syndrome* show a relatively high incidence of thrombophlebitic reactions. There are several reasons for this. When deep venous channels are blocked by occlusions, it is almost inevitable that contrast medium will drain through the delicate superficial collaterals in relatively high concentration. The outflow obstruction also leads to prolonged contact between the contrast agent and vein wall, especially in secondary varices. Moreover, the preexisting damage to the venous system in itself leads to an aggravated general risk of thrombosis.

Postinjection thrombophlebitis is always an *innocent complication.* Nevertheless, it can be upsetting to anxious patients. About a 2- to 5-cm segment of the vessel appears hardened and is tender to pressure. The thrombus is solidly fused to the vein wall and cannot be expressed through a stab incision. The recommended *treatment* consists of cold compresses, the local application of heparin ointments or etofenamate, and use of a padded compression bandage until the tenderness and mild perivascular infiltration have resolved.

The risk of injection-site thrombophlebitis can be reduced by *prophylactic measures.* These include the appropriate selection of a vessel for the venipuncture. The veins on the dorsum of the foot are much more delicate than the dorsal vein of the great toe. Contrast medium injected into a varix may remain there for several minutes, even in the foot. Thus, varicography is more likely to incite a

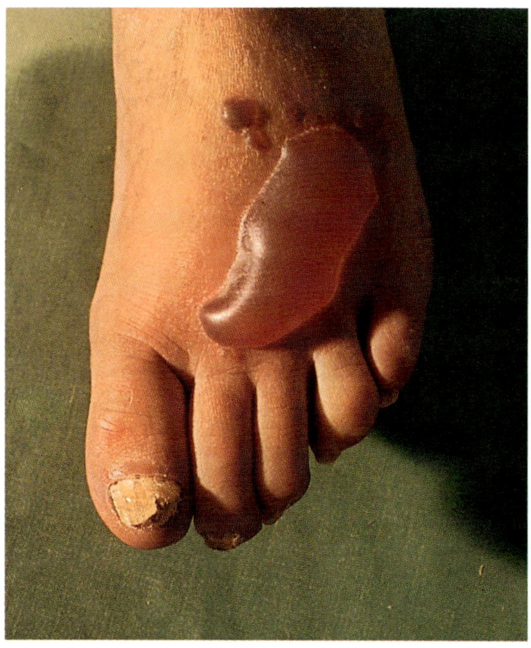

393. Blistering caused by extravascular contrast injection

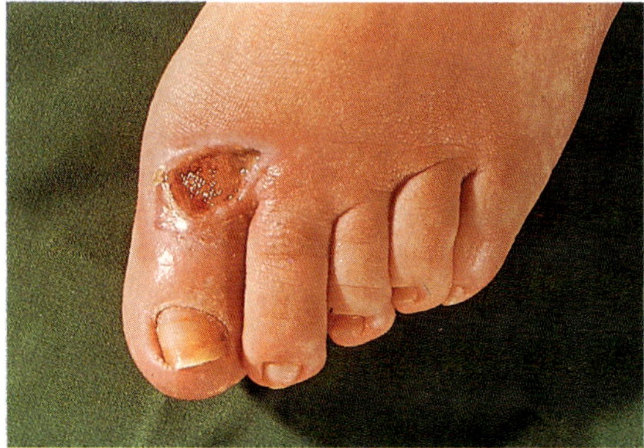

394. Refractory ulcer caused by extravascular contrast injection

phlebitis than other techniques, and special attention must be given to effective medical and mechanical thromboprophylaxis. The best way to protect a delicate vein from overdistention is to apply fingertip pressure during the injection. With some experience, the examiner can use this technique to match the pressure of the contrast injection to individual circumstances.

Even a competent *great saphenous vein* can react sensitively to contact with a high dose of contrast medium and become thrombosed. Direct injection into the vessel should be avoided if at all possible, especially as it does not convey significant diagnostic information.

Extravascular Injection and Skin Necrosis

The extravenous injection of contrast medium is easily detected. If the examiner places the tip of his index finger lightly over the tip of the injection needle, he can easily detect the slightest extravasation.

An extravenous injection must be terminated at once. The paravascular fluid can be disbursed in the tissue by gentle digital massage. Cold compresses and heparin ointments provide effective local anti-inflammatory therapy.

Any concentrated solution such as contrast medi- 393
um will incite an inflammatory response in tissue,
which in unfavorable cases leads to *blistering*. Lat- 394
er the lesion may progress to circumscribed *skin necrosis* with a poor healing potential. The condition may persist for weeks or months. Initially there is considerable pain and associated disability. If the skin defect does not respond to granulation-promoting treatment in a reasonable amount of time, skin grafting is recommended.

Apparently, *skin necrosis* after contrast extravasation is very uncommon. In the few cases published to date, Reinhardt (1979) estimated that the volume of extravasate was 10–15 ml. The affected patients had significant peripheral edema, which greatly delayed clearing of the medium. There has been no instance of skin necrosis in the 50 000 examinations performed by the authors.

In patients with *autoimmune disorders*, necrosis may occur in the area of the injected vein. This complication is rare and cannot be predicted. It is thought to be due to a hypersensitive angiitis with an abnormal reactivity of the vessel wall to the instilled solution. We personally have observed two such cases in patients with lupus erythematosus and cryoglobulinemia. Two cases of peripheral gangrene after phlebography were published by Lea Thomas (1970), one in a girl with aplasia of the deep veins and another in a young woman with complete thrombosis of the leg veins in the postpartum period.

References

Albrechtsson U, Olsson CG (1979) Thrombosis after phlebography. A comparison of two contrast media. Cardiovasc Radiol 2: 9

Arrang JM, Garbarg M, Lancelot JC, Lecomte JM, Pollard H, Robba M, Schunack W, Schartz JC (1987) Highly potent and selective ligands for histamine H_3-rezeptors. Nature (London) 327: 117

Beaven MA, Maeyama K, Wolde Mussie E, Lo TN, Ali H, Cunha-Melo JR (1987) Mechanism of signal transduction in mast cells and basophils: studies with RBL-$_2$ H_3-cells. Agent actions 20: 137

Benness GT, Fischer HW (1989) Reactions to ionic and non-ionic contrast media. Radiology 170: 282

Gersmeyer EF, Yasargil EC (1978) Schock und hypotone Kreislaufstörungen. Thieme, Stuttgart

Hegstrand LR, Kanof PD, Greengard P (1976) Histamine-sensitive adenylate cyclase in mammalian brain. Nature (London) 260: 163

Katayama H et al. (1990) Adverse reactions to ionic and nonionic contrast media. Radiology 175: 621

Kerp L, Kasemir HD (1982) Allergie und allergische Reaktionen. In: Kühn HA, Schirmeister J (Hrsg) Innere Medizin. Springer, Berlin Heidelberg New York

Lea Thomas M (1970) Gangrene following peripheral phlebography of the legs. Br J Radiol 42: 528

May R (1979) Thrombosis, a sequel to phlebography. Comment 1. Cardiovasc Radiol 2: 15

Reinhardt K (1979) Blasenbildung mit anschließender Hautnekrose nach paravenöser Kontrastmittel-Injektion am Fußrücken bei einer Patientin mit Ödem und tiefer Phlebothrombose. Röntgenblätter 32: 277

Reiser W (1988) Kontrastmittelnebenwirkungen: Allergoide Reaktionen. Vortrag anläßlich des 3. Frankfurter Gesprächs über digitale Radiographie (Bad Nauheim, 5. bis 8. Oktober 1988)

Reiser M, Buttermann G, Gulotta U, Reimann JH, Feuerbach S (1983) Zur Frage der Thromboseentstehung durch Phlebographie. Röntgenberichte 12: 1

Ring J, Messmer K (1977) Incidence and severity of anaphylactoid reactions to colloid volume substitutes. Lancet I: 466

Salzmann P, Windorf B, Ehresmann U, Wolf V (1980) Kontrastmittelschäden bei der Phlebographie. In: Loose KE, Loose DA (Hrsg) Gefäß, Patient, Therapie. Witzstrock, Baden-Baden

Schmiedel E (1981) Sicherheitspharmakologische Untersuchungen von Röntgen-Kontrastmitteln. Kolloquium mit Krankenhaus-Apothekern. Konstanz, 23. 10. 1981

Schmiedel E (1987) Pharmakodynamik und Verträglichkeit von Kontrastmitteln. Röntgenblätter 40: 1

Schmitt HE (1979) Thrombosis, a sequel to phlebography, Comment 3. Cardiovasc Radiol 2: 17

Siegenthaler W, Veragut U (1970) Blutdruck. In Siegenthaler W: Klinische Pathophysiologie. Thieme, Stuttgart

Subject Index

Springer and the environment

At Springer we firmly believe that an international science publisher has a special obligation to the environment, and our corporate policies consistently reflect this conviction.

We also expect our business partners – paper mills, printers, packaging manufacturers, etc. – to commit themselves to using materials and production processes that do not harm the environment. The paper in this book is made from low- or no-chlorine pulp and is acid free, in conformance with international standards for paper permanency.

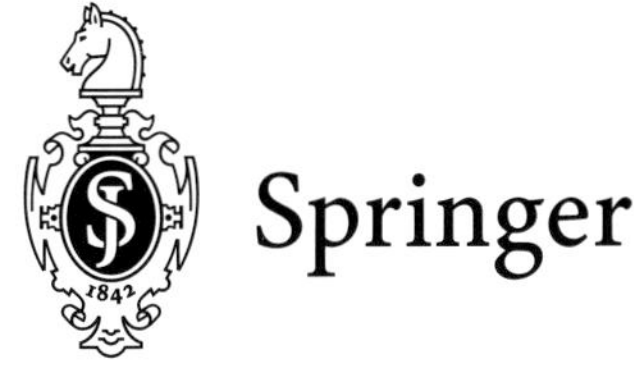